# Advanced Renal Care

Edited by

## Nicola Thomas

*RN, BSc (Hons), PG Dip (Education), MA*
*Research Lead Nurse, SW Thames Renal and*
*Transplantation Unit, St. Helier Hospital, Carshalton,*
*Surrey, and Senior Lecturer, City University, London*

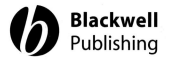

**Blackwell**
Publishing

Editorial offices:
Blackwell Publishing Ltd, 9600 Garsington Road, Oxford OX4 2DQ, UK
    Tel: +44 (0)1865 776868
Blackwell Publishing Inc., 350 Main Street, Malden, MA 02148-5020, USA
    Tel: +1 781 388 8250
Blackwell Publishing Asia Pty Ltd, 550 Swanston Street, Carlton, Victoria 3053,
Australia
    Tel: +61 (0)3 8359 1011

First published 2004 by Blackwell Publishing Ltd

Library of Congress Cataloging-in-Publication Data
Advanced renal care/edited by Nicola Thomas.
    p. ; cm.
Includes bibliographical references and index.
ISBN 1-4051-0933-5 (pbk. : alk. paper)
1. Chronic renal failure–Treatment.
[DNLM: 1. Kidney Failure–therapy. 2. Renal Replacement Therapy. WJ
342 A244 2003] I. Thomas, Nicola.

RC918.R4A34925 2003
616.6′1406–dc22
2003023483

ISBN 1-4051-0933-5

A catalogue record for this title is available from the British Library

Set in 10/12.5 pt Palatino
by Graphicraft Limited, Hong Kong
Printed and bound in India
by Replika Press Pvt Ltd

The publisher's policy is to use permanent paper from mills that operate
a sustainable forestry policy, and which has been manufactured from pulp
processed using acid-free and elementary chlorine-free practices. Furthermore,
the publisher ensures that the text paper and cover board used have met
acceptable environmental accreditation standards.

For further information on Blackwell Publishing, visit our website:
www.blackwellpublishing.com

# Contents

# Preface

This book is aimed at experienced members of the multiprofessional team working in nephrology, dialysis and transplantation. Each chapter is written by an expert who is passionate about their speciality. The topics covered have developed from the structure of an advanced renal care module that I have managed and taught for 5 years. There appeared to be a need for a book aimed at experienced renal practitioners, one that critically reviewed contemporary practice and evaluated current issues in renal care.

The book is relevant for all members of the multiprofessional team, whether they be dieticians, nurses, physicians, social workers or technicians. There are an ever increasing number of specialised practitioners working in renal care, such as clinical psychologists and renal pharmacists, and this book is aimed at them too. Everyone involved should be aiming for the highest standards of quality care. Understanding the whole person and all the physical, social and psychological effects of established renal failure is a fundamental prerequisite to achieving best practice.

Health care has altered almost beyond recognition in the 20-odd years since I began my career in renal nursing and exciting initiatives continue to develop, such as user/carer involvement that seeks to ensure the patient and family is placed firmly at the centre of care. The publication of the Renal National Service Framework (Part One) puts nephrology, dialysis and transplantation back in the spotlight. Renal practitioners are sometimes accused of being rather blinkered in their outlook. Hopefully this book will help broaden practitioners' minds into thinking about the benefits of working in partnership with other specialities, as well as recognising the importance of the individual roles. The aim is the same – to give those who have renal failure the best possible quantity and quality of life, and to care with sensitivity and understanding.

New terminology is gradually being adopted in renal care. An example is the use of the phrase 'established renal failure' (ERF) instead of 'end-stage renal failure' (ESRF), the latter implying a rather pessimistic outcome. I have therefore used ERF throughout the book together with other terms that more accurately relate to current practice, such as 'allowance' instead of 'restriction'. I have tried not to use derogatory labels such as 'the renal diabetic' and 'the elderly'. The book has instead been written in a style that I hope promotes the renal speciality for what it is – dynamic and involving, wide-ranging and rewarding.

It has been a privilege to work with the expert contributors to this book to whom I am extremely grateful. Among the many others who have helped, I am particularly appreciative to my colleagues at City University for their ever constructive criticism, and to my husband Paul for his continuing encouragement and support.

*Nicola Thomas*

# Contributors

**Nicola Thomas** RN, BSc (Hons), PG Dip (Education), MA, Research Lead Nurse, SW Thames Renal and Transplantation Unit, St. Helier Hospital, Carshalton, Surrey, Senior Lecturer, City University, London, and Past President EDTNA/ERCA and EDTNA/ERCA Education Board Chair

**Cordelia Ashwanden** RN, Cert Ed, BSc (Hons), MSc, PhD, Consultant Lecturer and Former Haemodialyis Unit Manager, and EDTNA/ERCA Scientific Programme Co-ordinator

**Jane Bentley** RN, RHV, BA (Hons), MSc, Research Fellow, Adult Nursing–Care for Older People, City University, London

**Peter Bentley** RN, BSc (Hons), PGCEA, MSc, Lecturer, Applied Biological Sciences, City University, London

**Celia Eggeling** DPsych, CQSW, Counselling Psychotherapist and Social Worker, Renal Unit, St. Helier Hospital, Carshalton, Surrey

**Cathal Gallagher** BD, FPC, Programme Co-ordinator Living Well Programme, Whipps Cross University Hospital NHS Trust, London

**Sandra Y. Gann** BA, CQSW (accred.), Dip PST, Medical Social Worker and Psychosexual Therapist, Department of Urology, Barts and the London NHS Trust, London

**Judith A. Hurst** RN, BSc (Hons), PGDip (Education), MSc, Senior Lecturer, Adult Nursing Specialising in Renal Care, City University, London, and EDTNA/ERCA Education Board Member

**Karen J. Jenkins** RN, Dip HE Professional Practice, Nurse Consultant Renal Medicine, East Kent Hospitals NHS Trust, Canterbury, Kent, and President of ANSA (Anaemia Nurse Specialist Association) 2003–2005

**Mike Kelly** FPC, Renal Counsellor, Barts and the London NHS Trust, London

**Anne M. Keogh** RN, BA (Hons), DipN, Nursing and Health Care Consultant, Clinical Solutions Ltd, and Past President EDTNA/ERCA

**Althea Mahon** RN, BSc, Nurse Consultant Peritoneal Dialysis, Barts and the London NHS Trust, London, President Elect, EDTNA/ERCA

**Catherine Morgan** RN, BSc (Hons), MSc, Nurse Consultant, Renal Services, Mid-Essex Hospital Services NHS Trust

**Gurch Randhawa** BSc (Hons), MSc, Principal Research Fellow, Institute for Health Services Research, University of Luton

**Martin Steggall** RN, Dip N, BSc (Hons), MSc, Lecturer, Applied Biology and Urology, City University, London, and Honorary Specialist Urology Nurse (Erectile Dysfunction), Barts and the London NHS Trust, London

**André Stragier** Former Chief Renal Technician, Catholic University of Louvain, UCL St. Luc, Brussels, Belgium, and EDTNA/ERCA Communication and Public Relations Officer

**Debbie Sutton** BSc (Hons) SRD, Renal Research Dietician, Wessex Renal and Transplant Unit, Queen Alexandra Hospital, Portsmouth, and Renal Nutrition Group Chair 2000–2003

**Raymond Trevitt** RN, BSc, Dip HSM, Transplant Nurse Specialist, Barts and the London NHS Trust, London, and EDTNA/ERCA Transplant Special Interest Group Chair

**Sara Youngman** RN, MSc, Clinical Nurse Manager, Renal Unit, St. Helier Hospital, Carshalton, Surrey

# Chapter 1
# Current Trends in Renal Care

*Nicola Thomas*

## Introduction

The care of those with established renal failure (ERF) has improved at a fast pace in recent years. For those working in renal care, the changes are immense and it is becoming increasingly challenging to keep up-to-date with new technology and at the same time achieve the standards of care proposed by national and international guidelines.

This chapter aims to provide an overview of the trends in renal care. The overall acceptance rate of patients for renal replacement therapy (RRT) will be put in an international context, whilst current debates on inter-professional working and workforce planning will be presented. The chapter concludes with a review of renal care associations and a list of useful websites.

## Historical perspective to renal replacement therapies

Haemodialysis (HD) as a routine treatment for renal failure was initiated in the 1960s, and failure to provide sufficient hospital-based services stimulated the development of home haemodialysis, followed by continuous ambulatory peritoneal dialysis (CAPD) in the late 1970s.

The first successful renal transplant, between identical twins, was reported in 1951. Subsequent development of immuno-suppressive drugs enabled transplantation from cadaveric unrelated donors, and today renal transplantation is also carried out between living related and unrelated donors and recipients.

In the 1980s, acceptance rates onto renal replacement therapy, particularly for older people, remained low (EDTA, 1985), and for many years there has continued a mismatch between the amount of renal care provision and demand. The National Renal Review conducted in 1992 highlighted regional variations in acceptance rates for dialysis and transplantation resulting in the issue of national renal purchasing guidelines in 1994. Today, the annual acceptance rate for patients onto RRT remains static (UK Renal Registry, 2002).

Home haemodialysis numbers have declined in recent years, but the number of satellite haemodialysis units doubled between 1993 and 1998. The proportion of patients on hospital and satellite haemodialysis has continued to rise, whilst peritoneal dialysis (PD) is falling slightly. In 2002, 56% of all new patients (on day 90 of dialysis) were receiving haemodialysis (UK Renal Registry, 2002).

## Acceptance rates on renal replacement therapy

In 2001, the Kidney Alliance (an umbrella body representing all organisations involved in renal services) suggested that acceptance rates for RRT were rising, but there remained geographical inequalities (Kidney Alliance, 2001). There were some areas in the UK that did not have autonomous renal services or satellite dialysis units; therefore both hospital and community-based services need to be expanded to enable patients to have a choice of treatment.

Inequalities remain today. The annual acceptance of new patients in the UK in 2002 has been the same for the previous 4 years. At 93.2 per million population (pmp) for adults and 1.7 pmp for children it was lower than in most other Western European countries (UK Renal Registry, 2002).

## UK Renal Registry

The UK Renal Registry was established by the Renal Association with support from the Department of Health, the British Association of Paediatric Nephrologists and the British Transplant Society as a resource for the development of patient care in renal disease (Table 1.1).

The Registry provides a focus for the collection and analysis of standardised data relating to the incidence, clinical management and outcome of renal disease. It thus acts as a source of comparative data, for audit/benchmarking, planning, clinical governance and research. The UK Renal Registry monitors indicators of the quality as well as quantity of care, with the aim of improving the standard of care. There is currently a concentration on data concerning renal replacement therapy, including transplantation. At a later date there will be an extension to other forms of treatment of renal disease.

**Table 1.1**  Functions of the UK Renal Registry.

| |
|---|
| • To collect demographic and descriptive data for comparison and planning. |
| • To facilitate comparative audit by means of a carefully defined data set. |
| • To collect data on indicators of quality of care to facilitate: |
|    — audit against recommended national standards |
|    — improved care |
|    — identification of good practice. |
| • To produce national and local outcome data. |

The most recent UK Renal Registry report at the time of writing was the 2002 report. This report referred to activity in 2001 and covered 72% of the UK adult population. The 2003 report will cover up to 80% of the UK.

## Summary of the UK Renal Registry 2002 Report

The acceptance rate in England for RRT estimated from the 1998 Renal Survey [92 per million population (pmp)] is lower than that of other developed countries; in 2000, for example, rates in Spain and Germany were 132 and 175 pmp respectively. Both Wales (128 pmp) and Scotland (107 pmp) had a higher acceptance rate than England despite having smaller ethnic minority populations.

Diabetic nephropathy as a cause of renal failure, seen in 18% of new patients, is not increasing and remains lower than in the USA and much of Europe.

The annual growth in the number of those receiving RRT in the UK is 7%, largely occurring for haemodialysis (HD). Of prevalent patients, 46.6% are transplanted, 37.1% are on HD and 16.3% receive peritoneal dialysis (PD). PD is more common in the young, especially in those with diabetes. The number on RRT is predicted to rise for the next 20 years until a steady state position is reached, with a future prevalence approaching 60 000 patients. Figure 1.1 shows patients accepted for RRT in the UK from 1980–2001.

The 1-year survival of established patients in England and Wales is 84% for dialysis and 97% for those who have been transplanted. For dialysis patients, 1-year survival is 90% for those under 65 and 77% for older patients. For those with diabetes on dialysis, the figures are 82 and 72%, respectively.

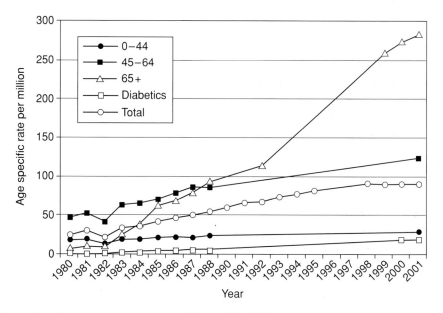

**Figure 1.1**  Patients accepted in the UK for RRT. (With permission from the UK Renal Registry, Bristol.)

# Rationing of renal replacement therapy

There are many possible reasons why the UK lags behind other European countries in the number of patients that are offered dialysis. One possibility is that age plays a factor, with family doctors not being fully aware of the options for older people with renal disease. However, as Lamping et al. (2000) suggest, age alone should not be used as a barrier to referral and treatment and the benefits of dialysis in elderly people should always be considered. Indicators of the ability to benefit from treatment, rather than chronological age, should be used to develop policies that ensure equal access to care for all (see Chapter 7).

Stanton (1999) has suggested a sociological approach to understanding why there still appears to be 'covert' rationing of dialysis in the UK, and proposes that comparisons with other countries are most influential in breaking the hold of this covert rationing. In other words, policy making by embarrassment can be successful.

It is important to put the UK situation in an international context and the ongoing DOPPS study compares dialysis practices in 12 countries, including the UK.

# Dialysis Outcomes and Practice Patterns Study (DOPPS)

DOPPS is an on-going observational study of haemodialysis patients that is seeking to identify dialysis practices that contribute to improved mortality and hospitalisation rates, health-related quality of life and vascular access outcomes.

There have been many research papers published that have reported on DOPPS outcomes. Pisoni et al. (2002) reported on a DOPPS study that has used the same data collection protocol for more than 6400 HD patients to compare vascular access use at 145 American dialysis units and 101 units in five European countries (France, Germany, Italy, Spain, and the UK).There were some startling findings:

- In Europe, 84% of new HD patients had seen a nephrologist for more than 30 days compared with 74% in the USA.
- Twenty five percent of European and 46% of American patients did not have a permanent access placed prior to starting HD.
- Large differences in vascular access use exist between Europe and the USA.

However, it is important to put these findings into a national rather than European context, as the UK may well fall behind other European countries in terms of vascular access formation prior to dialysis.

# Prediction and prevention

The predicted number of people on RRT will continue to rise for the next 20 years until a steady state position has been reached, with a future prevalence approaching 60 000 patients. By 2010, the current prevalence will have increased from about 30 000 to between 42 000 and 51 000, depending on assumptions about acceptance rate and patient survival. Much of the rise in demand will occur even if there is no increase in the current acceptance rate. This growth will occur disproportionately in the older people treated by HD. The most realistic figures are over 45 000 patients (900 pmp), or a 4.5% average annual increase over the next decade (Roderick et al., 2002).

In an attempt to reduce the increasing prevalence of ERF, the National Kidney Research Fund (NKRF) was successful in obtaining funding from the Department of Health to initiate a 3-year awareness and community education campaign entitled 'ABLE – A Better Life'. The aim of the ABLE programme is to highlight the incidence of kidney disease in ethnic groups, to reduce the incidence of ERF amongst such groups and, where it cannot be avoided, to ensure early referral, optimal treatment and equality of access to dialysis and transplantation.

Lightstone and Woolnough (2002) have suggested that the impetus generated by this initiative will improve the prognosis and reduce the increasing rates of ERF. More importantly, successful health awareness projects within ethnic communities will pave the way for more effective implementation of preventative and therapeutic strategies in the wider community.

# Challenges for the renal team

There are many challenges facing the renal team and it is possible that the time is now right to focus on prevention of renal failure, as well as on care in the immediate pre-dialysis phase. It is well documented that early diagnosis and prompt treatment of renal disease processes may prevent progression to ERF and the need for RRT. Co-morbidities are reduced and the prognosis and quality of life on RRT are improved (Vora et al., 2000).

Late referral is also a challenge, but the evidence for timely referral is sound. Jungers et al. (2000) found that the prevalence of cardiovascular disease (CVD) was nearly twice as high in patients referred less than 6 months before starting RRT than those who had benefited from effective nephrological care for more than 3 years in the pre-dialysis period. Considering that CVD is the major cause of death in ERF patients, this is a significant finding.

Sesso and Belasco (1996) also found health benefits for those who had an early referral. Indeed, mortality rates were higher (the hazard ratio of mortality was 2.77 times that of the early diagnosis group) in patients who were referred to a nephrologist within the 6 months before commencing than those who had

**Table 1.2**  Challenges facing renal care professionals.

- Providing true 'patient-centred' renal care.
- Increased numbers of patients requiring RRT.
- Increased numbers of patients with co-morbidities.
- Increased numbers of older patients.
- Decreased numbers of health care professionals with appropriate knowledge and skills.

had an earlier referral. Most of these deaths were of cardiac origin that could have been prevented with dialysis care. There are many papers written on the importance of good pre-dialysis care, and an in-depth review is beyond the scope of this book. Readers are referred to Hurst (2002) for a more detailed analysis.

In summary, the challenges are the rapid and sustained rise in the number of adult patients treated with RRT over the past two decades and the acceptance rates that are low in the UK compared to other European countries. An increasing proportion of patients have associated co-morbidities, particularly diabetes and vascular disease. Population projections show that growth in numbers of patients with ERF will continue until at least 2030.

Renal care should be patient-centred, and patients and their families should have an increasing role in developing and directing renal replacement therapies. It is likely that patients who play a central role in the management of their illness do well on dialysis.

In many parts of the country the availability of staff with the required knowledge and skills to care for those with renal disease is inadequate and there are implications for future planning of the workforce. Table 1.2 summarises the main challenges facing renal care professionals today.

# Multi-professional working

Patients with renal disease require the management and support of many different health care professionals and good multi-professional team working is essential for high quality patient-centred care. It is not only integrated working between the renal health care professionals that is paramount, but also close working relationships with primary care providers such as family doctors and practice nurses.

## Workforce planning

The British Renal Society (BRS) established a multi-professional National Renal Workforce Planning Group in January 2001 to prepare recommendations for establishments and staffing levels across each professional group involved in renal health care. Professional staffing recommendations have now been made

**Table 1.3** Summary of adult renal workforce requirements for the UK (total number of practitioners). [From 'The Renal Team: A Multi-Professional Renal Workforce Plan for Adults and Children with Renal Disease', 7 pp., with permission from the British Renal Society (2002).]

| | 2001 establishment | Current requirements | 2010 requirements |
|---|---|---|---|
| Renal physicians | 290 | 512 | 803 |
| Renal transplant surgeons | 81 | 130 | 130 |
| Renal transplant donor coordinators | 87 | 87 | 144 |
| **Renal histocompatibility scientists** | | | |
| Consultant scientists | 14 | 48 | 75 |
| Health care scientists | 252 | 468 | 734 |
| Renal dietitians | 180 | 464 | 738 |
| Renal social workers | 73 | 356 | 555 |
| Renal clinical psychologists | 7 | 106 | 168 |
| Renal clinical technologists | 225 | 272 | 583 |
| Renal pharmacists | 97 | 425 | 669 |
| Renal administrators and managers | 65 | 165 | 312 |
| **Nurses** | | | |
| Haemodialysis | 2330 | 2127 | 4223 |
| Peritoneal dialysis | 250 | 312 | 524 |
| Ward based (renal and transplant) | 1834 | 2958 | 4760 |
| **Health care assistants** | | | |
| Haemodialysis | 876 | 1441 | 2860 |
| Peritoneal dialysis | 51 | 65 | 109 |
| Ward based (renal and transplant) | 746 | 1228 | 1978 |

for the UK and they are intended to complement the Renal National Service Framework (NSF).

The report is intended to provide advice and guidance on the workforce requirements to care for adults and children with renal disease. Table 1.3 summarises the specialist renal workforce requirements for the UK to 2010 for adult practitioners in absolute numbers.

The plan highlights the need for an increase in specialist renal practitioners and the changing pattern of skills and competencies required. There are also some current gaps in service provision, for example renal pharmacists. The BRS recommends that a national recruitment and retention plan for renal health care practitioners is developed in collaboration with the Workforce Development Confederations and as part of the renal NSF implementation strategy.

## National Service Framework (NSF)

As outlined in the Department of Health (1997) paper 'The New NHS', the Government will work with the professions and representatives of users and carers to establish clearer, evidence-based NSFs for major care areas and disease groups. That way, patients will get greater consistency in the availability and quality of services, right across the NHS. The Government will use them as a way of being clearer with patients about what they can expect from the Health Service.

So the NSFs will:

- Set national standards and define service models.
- Put in place programmes to support implementation.
- Establish performance measures against which progress within an agreed timescale will be measured.

The Renal NSF aims to raise standards, reduce variations in services and improve the health care of renal patients. The development process started in 2002 and two parts will be produced and published at intervals comprising standards in:

(1) Dialysis and transplantation (published January 2004)
(2) Prevention, primary care, acute renal failure and end of life care

## Renal care associations

There are a number of multi-professional renal care associations in the UK and across the world. Although three of these associations are described in detail here, website addresses for other associations are given at the end of the chapter.

### British Renal Society

The British Renal Society (BRS) is a multi-professional group created to improve standards of care for renal patients and their families. The BRS provides a forum for the discussion and dissemination of knowledge in the area of renal care. The BRS is a charity registered with the Charity Commission for England and Wales and has a primary mission as follows:

- To promote clinical research and education in the subject areas of renal disease and RRT, which includes dialysis and transplantation in the UK.
- To provide funding and facilities for research projects.
- To provide a forum for discussion of renal care.
- To facilitate multi-professional working, to monitor, maintain and improve standards of patient care and comfort.

The BRS holds an annual conference for renal professionals, with oral and poster presentations, debates and speciality meetings, and various social activities.

The BRS wishes to promote clinical research in the subject areas of renal disease and RRT in the UK. The Society has received substantial charitable donations to support research in these areas. A research committee reflecting the multi-professional nature of renal health care has been established to independently award grants on the basis of scientific merit and clinical relevance.

## The European Dialysis and Transplant Nurses Association/ European Renal Care Association (EDTNA/ERCA)

EDTNA/ERCA is an association of individual members. The members of the Association are professionals working in the field of renal care and are drawn from a number of European states and other countries worldwide. At the end of 2002 the Association had more than 5000 members from more than 75 countries.

EDTNA/ERCA is a multi-disciplinary association, and full membership is open to members of the paramedical staff (nurses, teachers, dieticians, technicians, social workers and others) from Europe. International members and other interested colleagues have a status as associate members.

The Association has an annual international conference, a scientific journal, a newsletter and educational publications such as monographs, books and standards/guidelines. The conference and most publications are translated into seven European languages. Educational events on a national or local level are also organised.

The Association has a Research Board (RB) and the main work of the RB is the running of the Collaborative Research Programme (CRP). Over the past years the CRP has investigated vascular access care, nutrition, water treatment, hepatitis C and other topics. Results have been published (Lindley et al., 2000; Nevett et al., 2000; Van Waeleghem et al., 2000) and guidelines written (see www.edtna-erca.org).

The Education Board (EB) of the Association provides opportunities for continuing professional development. Both a core curriculum for basic (Fuchs et al., 2002) and post-basic (Küntzle and Thomas, 1995) nephrology nursing courses has been developed. The Association has also published clinical standards for fundamental aspects of care such as psychological support for patients, plus standards for specific treatment modalities, such as HD and PD (Van Waeleghem and Edwards, 1995).

The Association has recently started accrediting post-basic renal nursing courses that are running across Europe. The aim is to demonstrate that certain schools are running good-quality courses and it encourages free movement of nurses across differing countries in Europe.

Within the Association, inter-professional working is promoted and there are special interest groups (SIGs) for dieticians, technicians, social workers and those working in paediatrics and transplantation. There is also a *Journal Club* offering a worldwide on-line educational forum (see www.edtna-erca.org).

## *Association of Renal Technicians (ART)*

The Association of Renal Technologists was founded as the Association of Renal Technicians in 1975 following a number of seminars organised under the direction of the Department of Health, the first of which took place in 1973 at the Falfield Hospital Engineering Centre.

The original mission was much the same as now – to promote the field of work shared by technicians and engineers working within the sphere of renal medicine. Principally aimed at National Health Service staff, the Association also has among its numbers employees of various medical companies with interests in renal medicine as well as a few with less obvious links.

Current projects include the development of a training programme using the City University in London, a joint voluntary register of clinical technologists in conjunction with the Institute of Physics and Engineering in Medicine (IPEM), and an affiliation agreement with IPEM to allow for a wider sharing of information and ideas.

## Summary

The challenges today are looking after increased number of patients and those with special needs – older people, those with diabetes and other chronic conditions. In order to give good-quality care, professionals need to have access to continuing professional development and should be members of one of the increasing number of renal care associations. Practice should be based on evidence and health-care professionals should work in partnership with patients and their families.

## Useful renal websites

Anaemia Nurse Association: www.anaemianurse.org.
Association of Renal Technicians: www.artery.org.uk.
British Renal Society: www.britishrenal.org.
DOPPS: www.dopps.org.
EDTNA/ERCA: www.edtna-erca.org.
Hypertension Dialysis and Clinical Nephrology: www.hdcn.com.
International Society of Nephrology: www.isn-online.org.
Kidney Alliance: www.kidneyalliance.org.uk.
National Kidney Federation: www.kidney.org.uk.
National Kidney Research Fund: www.nkrf.org.uk.
Renal Association: www.renal.org.
Renal Registry: www.renalreg.com.
UK Transplant: www.uktransplant.org.uk.
UK Transplant Co-ordinators: www.uktca.co.uk.

# References

British Renal Society (2002) *The Renal Team: A Multi-Professional Renal Workforce Plan for Adults and Children with Renal Disease.* www.britishrenal.org/workfpg.

Department of Health (1997) *The New NHS.* HMSO, London.

Department of Health (2004) *The National Service Framework for Renal Services. Part One: Dialysis and Transplantation.* www.doh.gov.uk/nsf/renal.

European Dialysis and Transplant Association (EDTA) (1985) Combined report on regular dialysis and transplantation in Europe. *Nephrology Dialysis and Transplantation* **16**.

Fuchs, S., Küntzle, W. and Thomas, N. (eds) (2002) *European Core Curriculum for a Basic Course in Nephrology Nursing.* European Dialysis and Transplant Nurses Association/European Renal Care Association, www.edtna-erca.org.

Hurst, J. (2002) Pre-dialysis care. In: *Renal Nursing,* 2nd edn (Thomas, N., ed.). Baillière Tindall, Edinburgh.

Jungers, P., Chokroun, G. and Robino, C. (2000) Epidemiology of end-stage renal disease in the Ile-de-France area: a prospective study in 1998. *Nephrology Dialysis and Transplantation* **12**, 2000–2006.

Kidney Alliance (2001) *End-Stage Renal Failure – A Framework for Planning and Service Delivery.* www.kidneyalliance.org.uk.

Küntzle, W. and Thomas, N. (eds) (1995) *European Core Curriculum for a Post-Basic Course in Nephrology Nursing.* European Dialysis and Transplant Nurses Association/European Renal Care Association, Gent, Belgium.

Lamping, D.L., Constantinovici, N., Roderick, P., Normand, C., Henderson, L., Harris, S., Brown, E., Gruen, R. and Victor, C. (2000) Clinical outcomes, quality of life, and costs in the North Thames dialysis study of elderly people on dialysis: a prospective cohort study. *Lancet* **356** (9241), 1543–50.

Lightstone, E. and Woolnough, L. (2002) *Preventing Kidney Disease: The Ethnic Challenge in Brent.* National Kidney Research Fund, www.nkrf.org.uk.

Lindley, L., Lopot, F., Harrington, M. and Elseviers, M. (2000) Treatment of water for dialysis: a European survey. *EDTNA/ERCA Journal* **16** (4), 22–7.

Nevett, G., Nagel, C., Elseviers, M. and Lindley, L. (2000) Provision of dietary advice in selected centers across Europe. *EDTNA/ERCA Journal* **16** (4), 34–40.

Pisoni, R.L., Young, E.W., Dykstra, D.M., Greenwood, R.N., Hecking, E., Gillespie, B., Wolfe, R.A., Goodkin, D.A. and Held, P.J. (2002) Vascular access use in Europe and the United States: results from the DOPPS. *Kidney International* **61** (1), 305–316.

Roderick, P., Davies, R., Jones, C., Feest, T., Smith, S. and Farrington, K. (2002) Predicting future demand in England, a simulation model of renal replacement therapy. In: United Kingdom Renal Registry, Chapter 6. *Fifth Annual Report of the UK Renal Registry,* UK Renal Registry, Bristol, pp. 65–83.

Sesso, R. and Belasco, A.G. (1996) Late diagnosis of chronic renal failure and mortality on maintenance dialysis. *Nephrology Dialysis and Transplantation* **11** (12), 2417–20.

Stanton, J. (1999) The cost of living: kidney dialysis, rationing and health economics in Britain, 1965–1996. *Society of Scientific Medicine* **49** (9), 1169–82.

United Kingdom Renal Registry (2002) *Fifth Annual Report.* UK Renal Registry, Bristol.

Van Waeleghem, J.P. and Edwards, P. (1995) *European Standards for Nephrology Nursing Practice.* European Dialysis and Transplant Nurses Association/European Renal Care Association, Gent, Belgium.

Van Waeleghem, J.P., Elseviers, M. and Lindley, L. (2000) Management of vascular access in Europe Part 1. *EDTNA/ERCA Journal* **16** (4), 28–33.

Vora, J.P., Ibrahim, H.A. and Bakris, G.L. (2000) Responding to the challenge of diabetic nephropathy: the history of detection, prevention and management. *Journal of Human Hypertension* **14** (10/11), 667–85.

# Chapter 2
# The Physiological Basis of Renal Disease

*Peter Bentley*

## Introduction

Established renal failure has a wide range of causes, and this chapter will explore two biological aspects of renal disease that are increasingly finding interest among health care professionals, namely the effects of genetics and immunology on renal disease. The chapter will provide an overview of the underlying causes of renal disease and will then describe and evaluate the care and management of two diseases affected by genetics and altered immune responses – polycystic kidney disease (PKD) and systemic lupus erythematosus (SLE). PKD and SLE are diseases caused by altered genes and immune responses, and an understanding of both these diseases is important for those working in advanced renal practice in order to meet the needs of patients and their families.

## Anatomy and physiology

It is beyond the scope of this book to review basic anatomical and physiological principles as these can be found readily elsewhere. Chalmers (2002) provides a very good explanation of the structure and main functions of the kidney, and explores the basic renal processes of filtration, reabsorption and secretion. She also analyses the clinical features of the main conditions causing established renal failure (ERF). This and other useful texts are given as recommended reading at the end of the chapter.

## Underlying renal disease

The primary renal diagnosis of new patients on dialysis in England and Wales in 2002 is shown in Table 2.1.

**Table 2.1**  Primary renal diagnosis of new patients on dialysis in England and Wales in 2002. (Adapted from UK Renal Registry 2002 data.)

| Diagnosis | Under 65 years of age | Over 65 years of age |
|---|---|---|
| Uncertain aetiology | 15.8 | 22.8 |
| Glomerulonephritis | 13.6 | 6.1 |
| Pyelonephritis | 9.2 | 8.7 |
| Diabetes | 20.2 | 11.8 |
| Renal vascular disease | 2.4 | 11.9 |
| Hypertension | 6.1 | 7.3 |
| Polycystic kidney | 8.9 | 3.3 |
| Other | 13.3 | 13.0 |
| No data | 10.5 | 15.2 |

There are large numbers of older patients with an unknown diagnosis, whilst primary renal diseases such as polycystic kidney disease and glomerulonephritis are more common in younger patients.

Two topics that are increasingly important to renal care professionals are how genetics and immunology affect renal function. This chapter will now look at the little explored impact of genetics and altered immune responses on ERF.

# Genetics

Alterations to genes can lead to a wide range of medical disorders ranging from sickle cell disease to cancer. Genetics and how genes impact on a wide range of diseases have become more widely understood over the last decade. In 2000, the publication of the Human Genome Project saw the complete sequence of several individuals' DNA completed, heralding what was believed to lead to a genetics revolution with increased knowledge about genetics and the basis of inherited diseases. The publicity following this has led to increased public awareness, and, with it, an increased expectation of health care professionals to be knowledgeable about the role of genetics in disease processes.

However, many health care professionals lack knowledge of genetics and its impact on their patients and families. The limited genetics education of pre-registration nurses has been discussed by Kirk (1999) and the need to educate all health care professionals to increase their knowledge base has been discussed by Burton (2002), thus making the understanding of the genetics of renal disease a priority. This chapter will focus on polycystic kidney disease (PKD), which is the most common genetic disorder responsible for renal disease; 8.9% of those under 65 years old starting renal replacement therapy in 2002 in England and Wales had PKD as their underlying disease (UK Renal Registry, 2002).

# Immunology

The immune system acts as a powerful tool, fighting infections and protecting the body from a wide range of foreign antigens. Changes in the body's normal immune responses can also lead to a wide range of diseases. The kidneys are affected by altered immune responses in a number of diseases including glomerulonephritis (GN), Goodpasture's syndrome and systemic lupus erythematosus (SLE), often referred to as lupus.

SLE affects a wide range of individuals, especially those from African-Caribbean and Asian populations, making an understanding of this condition all the more important in today's multicultural society. Both PKD and SLE also affect other body systems, so whilst the focus of the chapter will be the effect on renal function, there will be brief reference to other affected organs to provide a wider understanding of the effects of the disease.

Both these topics are very complex and medical management is largely beyond the scope of this chapter; however, knowledge of the basics of genetics and immunology will help the reader understand some of the important aspects of both these conditions and the impact they have on those affected including family members. Readers wishing to read more widely on either of these topics are directed to the reference section at the end of the chapter.

# Genetics of renal disease

Genetics is the study of patterns of inheritance, which relates to features we inherit from our parents, such as the colour of eyes and blood group. The basis of this inheritance lies inside cells in a substance called deoxyribonucleic acid or DNA. Most DNA is found inside cell nuclei, but a small amount is also found inside another cellular organelle; the mitochondria. Structurally, DNA is shaped like a twisting spiral staircase or ladder which is called a double helix. On the uprights of the ladder are sugars, whilst on the rungs are chemicals called bases, and these bases are crucial to the normal function of DNA.

There are four different bases which are abbreviated to the letter they begin with; thus DNA consists of adenine (A), thymine (T), cytosine (C) and guanine (G). On each of the rungs of the ladder there are two bases, but like a jigsaw only particular bases fit together. A will always pair with T, whilst C pairs with G. Located across regions of DNA on the bases are genes. Mitochondrial DNA is much smaller in size and is a circular shape, and it contains only a small number of genes. Genes contain a code for making proteins inside cells. When the DNA is damaged or mutated this may affect the code contained in the genes and prevent a normal protein being made. This is what occurs in genetic diseases, where the normal protein may function as an enzyme important in a chemical process in the body, but is either not produced or produced in an abnormal form and is unable to function properly. There are thousands of different genes which have a wide range of different functions. Inside the cell nucleus the DNA is located on structures called chromosomes.

Humans have 23 pairs of chromosomes (or 46 in total), and one of each chromosome is received from each of our parents. The first 22 pairs are referred to by their number (e.g. chromosome 1 to 22) and are known as autosomes. The final pair of chromosomes is the sex chromosomes: females have two X chromosomes (XX), whilst males have an X and Y (XY).

As the location of genes has been gradually mapped to different chromosomes it has led to genetic diseases being classified into one of two categories. When the genes that are mutated are on one of the numbered chromosomes, the genetic disease is known as autosomal. This contrasts with genes located on the sex chromosomes which when mutated can cause sex-linked genetic diseases. Whether a disease is inherited will be due to the numbers of an individual gene that are normal or mutated.

There are two main patterns of inheritance in genetic diseases: dominant or recessive. In dominant genetic disorders, only one of the two genes needs to be mutated to lead to a genetic disease. The adult form of PKD is a good example of a dominant genetic condition. However, in contrast in recessive disorders, both genes need to be mutated.

The childhood form of PKD is an example of a recessive genetic disease. In recessive genetic disorders, individuals with one normal gene and one mutated gene tend not to suffer the effects of the disease, but act as carriers. Carriers can pass the mutated gene on to their children.

Disease processes may occur due to the impact of different genes, but can also be due to different environmental factors. Diseases that are purely due to the affects of one gene are called single gene disorders. Cystic fibrosis (CF) is a good example of a recessive single gene disorder. In contrast several genes can be responsible for a genetic disease. PKD is a good example of this, as this disease displays polygenic patterns of inheritance. Most diseases though are multifactorial, where a combination of genes and the environment may be responsible. Both hypertension and SLE are examples of multifactorial diseases.

## Polycystic kidney disease

Inherited renal disorders can be present in both adults and children. In adults about 10–15% of the causes of ERF are due to inherited diseases (Grunfeld, 1999). PKD affects between 1 in 400 to 1 in 1000 live births and is characterised by the presence of multiple cysts that damage the kidneys and eventually lead to established renal failure. Most of the cases of PKD show an autosomal dominant pattern of inheritance due to the two main genes responsible being present on two of the numbered chromosomes.

Autosomal dominant polycystic kidney disease (ADPKD), which accounts for 90% of the cases seen in Europeans, is due to a mutation of a gene known

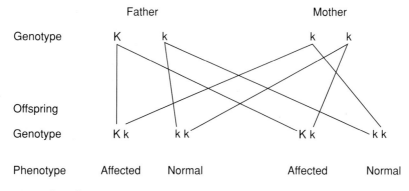

**Figure 2.1**  Genetic crossover.

as ADPKD1 which is located on chromosome 16. In contrast, the milder form of the ADPKD is due to a second gene known as ADPKD2 located on chromosome 4. Both these genes code for proteins known as polycystins, although the role of polycystins is not fully understood. It is believed that polycystins function as important cell membrane proteins and maintain normal cellular interactions. When the genes are mutated this normal cellular regulation appears to be altered and PKD develops.

The impact of having either of the forms of dominantly inherited PKD is that there is a 50% risk of the mutated gene being passed on by those suffering from PKD to their children, although equally the remaining 50% will not suffer from the disease.

A genetic crossover diagram helps illustrate the probability of the children inheriting the genetic disease; the genotype or genetic make-up of both parents needs to be known to allow this to be compiled (see Figure 2.1). This is an important consideration for those affected by ERF – those who may already have children, or those who do not yet have children but may have fertility problems as a result of their renal disease. As PKD is a dominant condition the gene for PKD is a capital letter (K), whilst the normal gene is a lower case letter (k). There is therefore a 50% chance of either of the children developing PKD.

Those affected by PKD will need to be shown great sensitivity and will need to receive genetic counselling about the risks of passing on the affected gene to their children. During pregnancy, pre-natal diagnosis is possible by amniocentesis or chorionic villi sampling (CVS) which enables DNA analysis to detect the presence of the mutated genes. Pilnick and Dingwall (2001) provide a good review of the literature on genetic counselling.

## Pathology

The pathology of PKD follows a distinct clinical course with the kidneys bilaterally affected. The cysts initially are small and affect only some parts of the nephron, but over time they enlarge and gradually impact on normal renal function. The cysts are believed to develop due to abnormal changes affecting the epithelial cells of the kidneys. It has been speculated that the normal ADPKD1 and ADPKD2 genes proteins suppress this abnormal cellular hyperplasia. The cysts cause some of the damage to the kidneys due to the pressure they cause, but also due to the fluid that is released from the cysts. High levels of epidermal growth factor have been found in some cysts and this has been implicated as a cause for the increase in size of the cysts. This fluid is rich in chemicals that are known to cause inflammatory changes and some of the abnormal fibrosis that damages the kidneys over time. The cysts can increase in size to up to 100 mm, and cumulatively their presence can have a major impact on the size of the kidney. The normal weight of an adult kidney is around 150 g (Marieb, 2001); however, PKD diseased kidneys can be up to 4 kg (Cotran et al., 1999).

## Clinical progression

Clinical progression sees the gradual deterioration in renal function occur as the cysts increase in size and damaging effects alter the normal architecture of the kidneys. The symptoms of PKD occur as the damage affects the basement membrane of the glomeruli and pressure damage affects the calyces leading to haematuria. Blood vessels in the kidneys become compressed causing ischaemia. The cysts themselves can also rupture, secreting their fluid into the renal tissues, and sometimes the fluid can cause infections such as urinary tract infections.

## Complications

Cysts can also haemorrhage, or sometimes clots can form. When these clots are cleared they can cause renal colic and abdominal pain. Hypertension is another feature seen in many patients with PKD and is common to some of the other causes of ERF occurring due to elevated levels of the enzyme renin. Hypertension is an important factor in cardiovascular mortality. Ecder et al. (2000) report on a prospective 15-year study to control blood pressure through a 10-point education programme, and show favourable results in blood pressure management.

ADPKD can develop in childhood, but most of the cases occur later in adulthood. Usually by the age of 30 years, ultrasound is able to detect cysts on the kidneys of those affected by PKD, although signs and symptoms do not usually occur until much later.

Cotran et al. (1999) describe how only around 2% of patients develop renal failure by the age of 40 years, but by 75 years of age 75% of those with PKD have developed ERF. The progression of those affected by PKD has been compared between the ADPKD1 and ADPKD2 genotypes in a detailed study by Hateboer et al. (1999). Over 30 European families from each genotype were compared for the progression and features of their PKD. Both age of onset and death occurred at an earlier age in the ADPKD1 group compared with the ADPKD2 families.

In the ADPKD1 groups there seemed to be no major differences between males and females, but this contrasted with the ADPKD2 females who presented with renal failure at a slightly later age. The ADPKD2 individuals suffered less from hypertension, haematuria and urinary tract infections. ADPKD2 disease progression tends to be seen more commonly in the African-Caribbean population, sometimes in association with sickle cell disease. Overall, ADPKD2 disease is a milder form of PKD.

In addition to ADPKD there is an autosomal recessive form of PKD (ARPKD), where both copies of the mutated gene need to be present. Grunfeld and Morgan (1998) estimate that this much rarer childhood-onset condition occurs in 1:10 000 to 40 000 births. The gene responsible for this form of PKD has not been identified, but it has been speculated to be on chromosome 6. Ward et al. (2002) describe the main features of ARPKD as dilation of collecting ducts and biliary abnormalities.

Although PKD is predominantly a condition that affects the kidneys, it can also affect other parts of the body. Cysts can be found in other organs including the liver, spleen, lungs and pancreas. Cotran et al. (1999) estimates that sub-arachnoid haemorrhage due to berry aneurysms accounts for death in 4–10% of those affected by PKD. Cardiac valve damage has also been reported in PKD; cases of valvular regurgitation and prolapse have occurred, although most cases seem to be asymptomatic and have limited effects on those with PKD. An understanding of these extra renal effects of PKD are important as they may impact on the rationale for care given to these patients and their families.

## Review of PKD

PKD is a well-known genetic disease responsible for ERF. The dominant form of the disease has an uncertain age of presentation, which may make it difficult for patients and their families to predict the likely age of onset and progression to ERF. In contrast, the rarer recessive form is often more severe and associated with higher levels of early morbidity and mortality. By understanding the different patterns of inheritance and the issues affecting patients and their families, members of the multidisciplinary team are in a position to support and care for those affected by PKD.

## The immunological basis of renal disease

The immune system provides important protective mechanisms in the body's fight against invading micro-organisms which can cause a range of diseases. It also has an important function in the recognition and targeting of abnormal tumour cells and in the body's response to allergy.

There are two main types of immunity: first, non-specific or innate immunity. Here the immune system provides a more generalised immune response to an array of foreign substances. Second, in contrast, specific immunity as its name suggests provides a more specialised and specific response to a particular foreign substance known as an antigen. Although these two forms of immunity are often discussed separately they often function together as part of the body's immune responses.

## Non-specific immunity

Non-specific immune responses include protection by the physical barriers provided by our skin and mucous membranes; also, the effects of chemicals, such as the enzyme lysozyme which damages bacterial cell walls, and the damaging effects of the acidic pH in the stomach. Processes such as phagocytosis enable immune cells to engulf and digest micro-organisms. Well-known examples of these immune cells are neutrophils and macrophages.

Inflammatory responses following tissue damage and infection facilitate the immune system's removal of micro-organisms and the early stages of tissue repair. Whilst non-specific immune responses provide an array of useful short-term and immediate immune responses, they lack the memory and specific responses that characterise specific immunity. When non-specific immune mechanisms are inadequate to destroy foreign substances, it is the turn of specific immune mechanisms to mount an immune response.

## Specific immunity

Specific immune mechanisms occur due a specific type of leukocytes known as lymphocytes. Humoral immunity is provided by the B lymphocytes; when these cells are stimulated by a foreign antigen they develop into antibodies. Antibodies are also known as immunoglobulins (Ig). A region of the Ig forms an attachment to a region on the foreign substance's antigen much like a lock and a key. Both the antigen and the Ig that is generated against it are highly specific. The combination of the antigen and Ig is known as an immune complex. The immune complex does not completely destroy the foreign substance, but in association with phagocytic cells the immune complex including the foreign antigen is phagocytosed and destroyed.

The formation of immune complexes and their subsequent phagocytosis is linked to the effects of a component of the non-specific immune system which is known as the complement cascade. Complement is a series of over 30 proteins which when activated work in a sequence to boost our immune responses. In addition to stimulating phagocytic responses, it aids the removal of the immune complexes by making them easier to degrade. The effects of complement can also increase the inflammatory response. One of the end products of the complement cascade, known as the membrane attack complex (MAC), destroys some bacteria and viruses.

Whilst the removal of immune complexes is usually a fairly efficient process, sometimes they may not always be successfully removed and cause damage to some of the body's major organs. Thus there is a classification of diseases known as immune complex diseases where the immune complexes damage organs such as the kidney, as in some forms of glomerulonephritis and in SLE.

## Cell-mediated immunity

The second type of specific immunity provided by the T lymphocytes is called cell-mediated immunity. These cells have one of two main functions; firstly, triggering the production of chemical cytokines which in association with other immune responses damage foreign antigens, and secondly, through regulation of immune responses so that the appropriate immune cells attack the correct target.

T cell activity is reduced during immunosuppression when drugs are administered to dampen down immune responses in some diseases and to prevent rejection of organs following kidney transplants. This can also make those being treated with immunosuppressive drugs vulnerable to opportunistic infections.

Although lymphocytes take several days to produce their first or primary immune responses, they do have families of cells known as memory cells. Memory cells provide surveillance to detect a subsequent second visit by a former antigen. When this occurs the secondary immune response is stronger and more rapid.

In health our immune system has an important role in destroying foreign antigens, but has the ability to distinguish our own healthy tissue. There are two main disturbances that can affect our immune system; firstly, there can be immune deficiency where a type of immune cell or immune mechanism is deficient, making those affected very vulnerable to infections. Some of these are inherited due to mutated genes. Secondly, in contrast, the immune system can be overactive where the lymphocytes are unable to distinguish between our own cells (self) and foreign antigens (non self). This results in lymphocytes incorrectly targeting the immune responses at healthy cells. This overactivity, or hypersensitivity, of the immune system leads to a group of disorders known as auto-immune diseases.

## Systemic lupus erythematosus (SLE)

SLE is an example of a complex auto-immune disease in which the abnormal immune system can cause renal damage. SLE, however, does not just affect the kidneys, but is a disease that can affect a range of different body systems in a very varied manner. As with many other auto-immune diseases there is a distinct difference between the sexes, with women, most commonly between the ages of 20 and 40 years, outnumbering males by 9:1 (Barwick, 2000).

In the UK it is estimated to affect 1:1000 of the population, which makes it a more common disease than both multiple sclerosis and leukaemia. SLE is seen across different racial groups, including Asians and African-Caribbeans where it is found at higher levels than in the Caucasian population (Janeway et al. 2001; Haq and Isenberg, 2002). African-Caribbeans are more prone to develop renal disease (Leach, 1998).

The causes of SLE are not fully understood, but it is known that environmental factors and genetics can contribute to the development of the disease. Certain tissue types have also been implicated as other risk factors for increasing the chances of developing SLE. Janeway et al. (2001) describe how those with a DR3 tissue type have over a five times greater risk of developing SLE compared with most other tissue types. Similarly to other auto-immune diseases, SLE can coexist in individuals suffering from other auto-immune diseases.

SLE is a condition that is characterised by exacerbations or 'flare ups' and periods of remission. The flare-ups often occur due to some form of trigger, which can range from stress to pregnancy. Some of the early presenting features of SLE can sometimes be vague such as fatigue, anaemia and swollen joints, which can lead to a delay in diagnosis or misdiagnosis of another disease. The most common symptoms that occur in SLE are altered haematology, with changes in the number of some of the major blood cells, swollen and often painful joints and altered appearance of the skin.

Diagnosis of SLE is based on clinical history, using the 1997 American College of Rheumatology classification criteria for SLE when 4 of the 11 criteria are documented (American College of Rheumatology, 1999). These include altered haematology, including an abnormal antibody known as anti-nuclear antibody (ANA). The skin changes have been estimated to affect up to 80% of those suffering from SLE. A classic butterfly rash can be seen on the face, and this can occur as an acute change in the skin which may only last for a few weeks. The disease follows a very varied course, with some having minimal skin changes such as erythema, whilst others have scarring.

## Renal damage in SLE

In SLE the immune complexes have a severe effect on the normal architecture and function of the kidneys, particularly the filtration membrane.

Janeway et al. (2001) describe how the immune complexes and complement damage the glomerulus, but also the podocytes, impairing their normal roles in filtration. Zimmerman et al. (2001) describe how binding by the auto-antibodies to the glomerular basement membrane alters the glomerular permeability. In addition, further damage occurs to the structures involved in filtration due to an array of cytokines, including substances that attract phagocytic cells and platelets.

Neutrophils act with MAC to damage blood vessels walls, causing a vasculitis, which can occlude the glomerular capillaries. Nephritis develops as a result of the inflammatory damage due to the effects of the neutrophils and the immune complexes. The kidneys are known to suffer some degree of alteration in SLE, and even those lacking renal disease have been shown to have changes in the kidneys on biopsy. Deterioration in renal function does occur in an estimated 50% of those affected by SLE (Cotran et al. 1999), with this group having a greater overall mortality.

The World Health Organization (WHO) has classified five possible forms of lupus glomerulonephritis (GN) (Schwartz and Lewis, 2002). These reflect the severity of renal changes seen by microscopy. Other features of renal disease may also be present such as haematuria. Some of the forms of lupus GN show some features of nephrotic syndrome. The main features of nephrotic syndrome are gross proteinuria, hypoalbuminaemia, generalised oedema, hyperlipidaemia and lipiduria.

The course of lupus GN is varied: some may remain stable whilst others with lupus may progress to more severe forms of lupus GN and thus to ERF which requires renal replacement therapy.

## Non-renal complications

There are many non-renal complications and these include joint pain, muscle pain and pulmonary damage. Ruiz Irastorza et al. (2001) have published a list of neurological problems seen in SLE. One of the most common of these are migraine-like headaches, while others include cerebrovascular disease due to the vasculitis, neuropathy and mood disorders.

Haq and Isenberg (2002) have described how coronary artery disease and carotid stenosis are double that in females between 35 and 44 years of age affected by SLE compared with healthy subjects. Whilst this can be linked to the hyperlipidaemia and hypertension, it illustrates the importance of preventing and treating such risk factors that may be present in SLE.

Some of those affected by renal disease may suffer fertility difficulties and this is compounded in SLE, as the female reproductive system can be affected with alterations to the menstrual cycle, ranging from ammenorrhoea to menorrhagia. Women with SLE who are considering having children also need a very high standard of preconception and antenatal care due to some recognised potential complications which may occur in a minority of them. These complications include increased rates of thrombosis during pregnancy.

## Medication

Although a variety of medications can be used successfully to treat lupus, as with all medication the benefits need to outweigh the side effects. Several classes of drugs are used to treat SLE, and these will be discussed shortly; however, a more detailed review of the medications used in SLE is provided by Leach (1998) and Barwick (2000).

More resistant forms of lupus can be treated using immunosuppressant drugs, with the most widely used being azathioprine, methotrexate and cyclophosphamide. However, there are well-known side effects to these drugs, so very careful consideration is given to an individual patient's history.

Haq and Isenberg (2002) have discussed how the US National Institute of Health (NIH) has shown that pulsed intravenous cyclophosphamide proved superior to sole use of steroids in long-term maintenance of renal function. The standard regime was 6-monthly pulses of $1 \, g/m^2$ followed by quarterly pulses for 2 years. Zimmerman et al. (2001) describe how this form of treatment is associated with a 50% reduced rate of relapse in those affected.

Cyclophosphamide can be used to treat lupus nephritis, severe vasculitis and in the more severe forms of cerebral lupus. Unfortunately cyclophosphamide causes alopecia, which although reversible may be a side effect some patients feel they cannot deal with. It is also contraindicated in women planning to become pregnant as it can be toxic to the ovaries and can have teratogenic effects on the developing foetus. Monitoring of side effects involves monitoring full blood counts as these drugs can affect bone marrow and hepatic function.

Other treatments used in SLE include immune-suppressing drugs; some of these have been previously used to prevent rejection following transplants, such as ciclosporin. More recently, mycophenolate mofetil (MMF) has been used, as this drug acts to reduce the activity of some of the lymphocytes and inhibits antibody production.

Intravenous immunoglobulins provide antibodies that are able to remove immune complexes and have been shown to be beneficial in treating some forms of lupus nephritis (Zimmerman et al., 2001). This treatment was seen to be effective in those who had advanced glomerulonephritis or who had shown a poor response to cyclophosphamide. However, these newer treatments tend to be used to treat the more resistant cases of SLE and they are not widely used due to their increased cost compared with some of the other treatments. Future therapies in the field of antibodies include the possible use of antibodies against some of the abnormal immune components seen in SLE and using DNAase to prevent the deposition of immune complexes containing DNA (Haq and Isenberg, 2002).

## Care and management

Vu and Escalante (1999) have found that patients with lupus nephritis who progress to established renal disease have reduced physical function and general health. Strategies to improve the quality of life of patients with SLE are needed. Nurses have an important role in the careful monitoring of the effects of medication. Barwick (2000) discusses how nurse-led clinics can help support those affected by SLE and how using a shared card system related to doses of medication can empower those affected by lupus. Voluntary societies such as Lupus UK (www.lupusuk.com) provide valuable information and leaflets which can be beneficial to those living with and affected by SLE.

# Review of SLE

SLE is a complex multisystem autoimmune disease. It follows a very variable path, and for some it has minimal effects whilst in others it can be associated with severe morbidity and early mortality. An awareness of these wider issues affecting those with SLE will facilitate high-quality individualised holistic care to meet many of the aspects of care required by these patients and their families.

# References

American College of Rheumatology (1999) Guidelines for referral and management of systemic lupus erythematosus in adults. American College of Rheumatology Ad Hoc Committee on Systemic Lupus Erythematosus Guidelines. *Arthritis and Rheumatism* **42** (9), 1785–96.

Barwick, A. (2000) Understanding lupus. *Nursing Standard* **14** (46), 47–51.

Burton, H. (2002) *Education in Genetics for Health Professionals* (Report to the Wellcome Trust). Public Health Genetics Unit, Cambridge.

Cotran, R., Kumar, V. and Collins, T. (1999) *Robbins Pathologic Basis of Disease*, 6th edn. WB Saunders, London.

Ecder, T., Edelstein, C.L., Fick-Brosnahan, G.M., Johnson, A.M., Duley, I.T., Gabow, P.A. and Schrier, R.W. (2000) Progress in blood pressure control in autosomal dominant polycystic kidney disease. *American Journal of Kidney Diseases* **36** (2), 266–7.

Grunfeld, J. (1999) Genetic abnormalities in renal disease. *Medicine* **27** (6), 56–8.

Grunfeld, J. and Morgan, S. (1998) *Inherited Disorders of the Kidney*. Oxford University Press, Oxford.

Haq, I. and Isenberg, D. (2002) Systemic lupus erythematosus. *Medicine* **30** (10), 6–12.

Hateboer, N., Dijk, M., Bogdanova, N., Coto, E., Saggar-Malik, A., San Millan, S., Torra, R., Breuning, M. and Ravine, D. (1999) Comparison of phenotypes of polycystic kidney disease types 1 and 2. *Lancet* **353**, 103–107.

Janeway, C., Travers, P., Walport, M. and Shlomchik, M. (2001) *Immunobiology, the Immune System in Health and Disease*, 5th edn. Churchill Livingston, Edinburgh.

Kirk, M. (1999) Preparing for the future: status of genetics education in diploma level training courses for nurses in the United Kingdom. *Nurse Education Today* **19**, 107–115.

Leach, M. (1998) Managing systemic lupus erythematosus. *Nursing Times* **94** (18), 58–9.

Marieb, E. (2001) *Human Anatomy and Physiology*, 5th edn. Benjamin Cummings, London.

Pilnick, A. and Dingwall, R. (2001) Research directions in genetic counselling: a review of the literature. *Patient Education and Counseling* **44** (2), 95–105.

Ruiz Irastorza, G., Khamashta, M., Castellino, G. and Hughes, G. (2001) Systemic lupus erythematosus. *Lancet* **357**, 1027–32.

Schwartz, M.M. and Lewis, E.J. (2002) Rewriting the histological classification of lupus nephritis. *Journal of Nephrology* **15** (Suppl 6), S11–9.

UK Renal Registry (2002) *Fifth Annual Report*. UK Renal Registry, Bristol.

Vu, T.V. and Escalante, A. (1999) A comparison of the quality of life of patients with systemic lupus erythematosus with and without endstage renal disease. *Journal of Rheumatology* **26** (12), 2595–601.

Ward, C., Hogan, M., Rosetti, S., et al. (2002) The gene mutated in autosomal recessive polycystic kidney disease encodes a large receptor like protein. *Nature Genetics* **30** (3), 259–69.

Zimmerman, R., Radhakrishnan, J., Valeri, A. and Appel, G. (2001) Advances in treatment of lupus nephritis. *Annual Reviews Medicine* **52**, 63–78.

# Further reading

## *General*

Chalmers, C. (2002) Applied anatomy and physiology and the renal disease process. In: *Renal Nursing* (Thomas, N., ed), 2nd edn. Baillière Tindall, Edinburgh.

Lote, C. (2000) *Principles of Renal Physiology*. Kluwer, Dordrecht.

Marieb, E. (2001) *Human Anatomy and Physiology*, 5th edn. Benjamin Cummings, London.

Martini, F., Ober, W., Garrison, C., Welch, K. and Hutchings, R. (2001) *Fundamentals of Anatomy and Physiology*, 5th edn. Prentice Hall, London.

Underwood, J. (2000) *General and Systematic Pathology*, 3rd edn. Churchill Livingstone, Edinburgh.

## *Genetics*

Nussbaum, R., McInness, R. and Willard, H. (2001) *Thompson and Thompson Genetics in Medicine*, 6th edn. WB Saunders, London.

Connor, M. and Ferguson Smith, M. (2002) *Essential Medical Genetics*, 5th edn. Blackwell Scientific, Oxford.

Mueller, R. and Young, I. (2001) *Emery's Elements of Medical Genetics*, 11th edn. Churchill Livingstone, Edinburgh.

## *Immunology*

Chapel, H., Heaney, M., Misbah, S. and Snowden, N. (1999) *Essentials of Clinical Immunology*, 4th edn. Blackwell Scientific, Oxford.

Playfair, J. and Lydyard, P. (2000) *Medical Immunology, Made Memorable*, 2nd edn. Churchill Livingstone, Edinburgh.

Wood, P. (2001) *Understanding Immunology*. Prentice Hall, London.

# Chapter 3
# Anaemia Management in Nephrology

*Karen Jenkins*

## Introduction

The aim of this chapter is to give a brief overview of the anaemia of chronic disease, to highlight possible causes and then to critically discuss the contributing factors to renal anaemia. The importance of early referral and commencement of appropriate treatments will also be explored.

The anaemia of chronic disease (ACD) may occur insidiously and is easy to overlook amid the general malaise related to the disease itself. Many of the signs and symptoms can be considered to be due to the effects of chronic disease but are also the signs and symptoms of anaemia (see Table 3.1).

Many conditions are associated with ACD, mainly because many chronic, systemic conditions lead to abnormalities in haemapoiesis (production of blood cells) (Spivak, 2000). Systemic diseases have different effects on the kidney and the bone marrow.

Successful treatment of ACD depends on targeting treatment to the individual patient. The first step is to treat the underlying disease, since this may restore normal haemoglobin. However, this is not possible in many diseases, where treatment must be directed towards improving the haemoglobin. Blood transfusion used to be the only treatment and is still necessary in some

**Table 3.1** Signs and symptoms of anaemia of chronic disease.

- Dizziness or light-headedness.
- Fatigue and weakness.
- Headache.
- Irritability.
- Less endurance in exercise.
- Shortness of breath, especially with exercise.
- Pale skin and eyes.
- Rapid heartbeat.
- Reduced cognitive function.

conditions, such as myelodysplasia and red cell aplasia. However, transfusion can cause allergic reactions and can be associated with the transmission of infection. Supplies are also often limited and treatment of blood for transfusion is increasingly complicated and expensive (Bandolier, 2001).

# Anaemia in chronic and established renal failure (ERF)

Three main factors may cause and influence renal anaemia:

- Lack of production of erythropoietin
- Iron deficiency
- Vitamin B12 and folate deficiency

Each of these factors will now be discussed in detail.

## Lack of production of erythropoietin

Erythropoietin is a glycoprotein hormone consisting of a chain of 165 amino acids and sugars, and has a molecular weight of 30 400 Da. It is very stable, resisting denaturation, and is strongly hydrophobic. The endogenous hormone is produced in the peritubular interstitial cells of the kidney. These cells are situated in the endothelial lining of capillaries adjacent to the tubules in the renal cortex. Erythropoietin cannot be stored in the body, but the hormone is always present in the plasma. Secretion into the blood is continuous, although the amount produced is increased in response to hypoxia.

Hypoxia leads to increased production of erythropoietin in the kidneys and its subsequent release into the plasma. Erythropoiesis (red blood cell formation) is thus stimulated and the number of erythrocytes entering the blood from the bone marrow becomes elevated. The increased number of erythrocytes can then carry more oxygen to the tissues and as the hypoxia resolves erythropoietin production is reduced.

In summary, erythropoiesis occurs in the bone marrow and is regulated by hormone erythropoietin and the process of regulation of erythropoiesis is shown in Figure 3.1.

It is important to know how the red cells develop and mature and at which point erythropoietin stimulation takes place. All blood cells (red cells, white cells and platelets) are derived from a single type of progenitor known as a pluripotent stem cell. These can either divide into other pluripotent stem cells or differentiate into committed progenitor cells that will develop into specific cell types. In the case of red cell production, the pluripotent stem cell differentiates first into a myeloid progenitor and then into a committed erythroid progenitor called a burst-forming unit erythroid. Although these differentiations are not influenced by erythropoietin, other cytokines are thought to be involved.

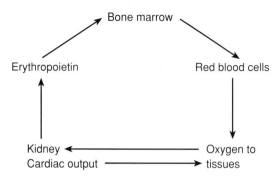

**Figure 3.1**  Regulation of erythropoiesis.

It is the burst-forming unit erythroid and the product of a further differentiation, the colony-forming unit erythroid, that are sensitive to erythropoietin. There is evidence that the hormone causes populations of these cells to clonally expand and differentiate further. It is therefore this stage of erythropoiesis that is most important in determining the final number of erythrocytes (Hoffbrand and Petit, 1985).

The erythroid cell subsequently undergoes progressive maturation to become a normoblast and it is at this stage that haemoglobin synthesis takes place. Finally, the nucleus is squeezed out and the cell becomes a reticulocyte. Reticulocytes are immature erythrocytes that mature over a period of about 30 hours. A proportion of reticulocytes complete the maturation process after they have been released into the blood from the bone marrow.

Erythropoietin deficiency is a logical consequence of damage to the renal production sites of the hormone. There is a marked decrease in the amount of erythropoietin produced in response to hypoxia and the subsequent development of anaemia. As it is well known that impaired erythropoietin production is one of the main causes of renal anaemia there is little point in measuring erythropoietin levels.

The reason for impaired red cell survival (haemolysis) is not well understood, although it is thought that uraemia plays a central role. This is when a Coombs test is useful to look at the survival of the red cells. Poor red cell production can be related to iron deficiency, hyperparathyroidism, aluminium toxicity and bone marrow failure. The production of inflammatory cytokines (common in chronic kidney disease, CKD) such as interleukin 1 and tubular necrosis factor (TNF alpha) can inhibit the maturation of the progenitor cells (Pereira et al., 1996) and lead to the reduction in production of erythropoietin.

## Iron deficiency

Iron has an essential role in supporting erythropoiesis; 65% of the iron stored in the body is used to form the haemoglobin.

*Measurement of iron status*

*Serum ferritin*: refers to the amount of iron stored in the body; 150 mg iron is required to raise haemoglobin by 1 g/dl. As red cell production increases, iron stores are depleted. Iron stores need to be adequate otherwise red cell survival is reduced.

Serum ferritin is commonly used as a standard marker for measuring iron deficiency. However, it can be falsely raised in cases of infection and inflammatory conditions. It is useful to measure the C-reactive protein (CRP) at the same time as the ferritin. If the CRP is also raised then this will indicate that there is an infection or inflammatory condition and that the raised ferritin is not a true indication of the iron status at that time.

*Transferrin saturation* (%Tsats): this is the iron transport system and needs to be more than 20% to be effective. However, this is not always a very reliable tool as %Tsats constantly alters. Therefore more than one measurement is required to ascertain an average reading.

*Hypochromic red cells*: defined as an individual cell with a haemoglobin concentration of less than 28 g/dl. Normally less than 2.5% of red cells are hypochromic. If iron stores are insufficient and/or mobilisation of iron is inadequate the number of hypochromic red cells increases and when they are greater than 10%, iron supplementation is required [European Best Practice Guidelines (EBPG), Cameron, 1999].

Using the above tests, iron deficiency can be diagnosed as follows:

(1)  *Absolute iron deficiency*: where iron stores are inadequate to support the erythropoietic needs of the bone marrow:
     —  serum ferritin is less than 100 µg/l
     —  percentage transferrin saturation is less than 20%
     —  percentage of hypochromic red cells is more than 10%.
(2)  *Functional iron deficiency*: iron stores are adequate but cannot supply the bone marrow quickly enough with the iron required to support demands of erythropoiesis
     —  normal or high serum ferritin
     —  percentage transferrin saturation is more than 20%
     —  percentage of hypochromic red cells is more than 10%.

## Vitamin B12 deficiency

Vitamin B12, also called cobalamin, is required to maintain healthy nerve cells and red blood cells, and is also needed to make DNA. Vitamin B12 is bound to protein in food. Hydrochloric acid in the stomach releases B12 from protein during digestion. Once released, B12 combines with a substance called intrinsic factor (IF) before it is absorbed into the bloodstream. Vitamin B12 deficiency is defined when B12 levels are less than 160 ng/l.

Pernicious anaemia is a form of anaemia that occurs when there is an absence of intrinsic factor. Vitamin B12 binds with intrinsic factor before it is absorbed. Absence of intrinsic factor prevents normal absorption of B12 and results in pernicious anaemia. Treatment for pernicious anaemia is by a course of intramuscular hydroxocobalamin injections of 1 mg three times a week for 2 weeks, followed by a 3-monthly maintenance injection of 1 mg (British National Formulary, 2002), which will continue indefinitely.

## *Folic acid deficiency*

Folate and folic acid are forms of a water-soluble B vitamin. Folate is essential for the production and maintenance of new red blood cells. Folate is also needed to make DNA and RNA. Those with renal disease should have a serum folate level of more than 20 µg/l. Supplementation with folic acid 5 mg once a day (British National Formulary, 2002) should be given if the serum folate level is less than 20 µg/l.

# Screening for anaemia

Screening for anaemia is essential as soon as an initial patient referral is made to the nephrologist, using the tests listed in Table 3.2.

It is important to screen for causes of anaemia in order to reach the correct diagnosis. Haematological abnormalities need to be clearly recognised and appropriate treatment given.

**Table 3.2**   Screening tests for anaemia.

- Haemoglobin
- Red cell folate concentrations
- Serum B12
- Serum ferritin
- Serum percentage transferrin saturation
- Percentage of hypochromic red cells
- Tests for haemolysis (haptoglobin, lactate dehydrogenase, Coombs test)
- Reticulocyte count
- C-reactive protein (CRP)
- Erythropoietin levels (in patients who have had a transplant)
- Assessment of occult gastrointestinal blood loss
- Nutritional status of the patient
- Bone marrow aspiration (if necessary)

**Table 3.3** Stages of chronic kidney disease (from K/DOQI, National Kidney Foundation, 2000).

| Stage | Description | GFR (ml/min/1.73 m$^2$) |
|---|---|---|
| 1 | Kidney damage with normal or higher GFR | More than or equal to 90 |
| 2 | Kidney damage with mild or lower GFR | 60–89 |
| 3 | Moderately low GFR | 30–59 |
| 4 | Severely low GFR | 15–29 |
| 5 | Kidney failure | Less than 15 (or dialysis) |

# When should renal anaemia be treated?

When to start treating anaemia in chronic kidney disease has been debated for some time. Early renal insufficiency (ERI) is a useful term to describe the stage of kidney disease before its progression to end-stage renal failure (Eknoyan and Mann, 2000).

The National Kidney Foundation has produced evidence-based clinical practice guidelines for the evaluation, classification and stratification of chronic kidney disease (CKD) [Kidney Disease Outcomes Quality Initiative (K/DOQI), National Kidney Foundation, 2000]. These guidelines suggest that presence of CKD can be established by degree of kidney damage and level of kidney function (glomerular filtration rate, GFR), irrespective of diagnosis.

CKD is defined as kidney damage or GFR of less than 60 ml/min/1.73 m$^2$ for at least 3 months. Kidney damage is defined as pathological abnormalities or markers of damage, including abnormalities in blood or urine test or imaging studies. Table 3.3 shows the specific stages of CKD.

## *Nephrology referral*

One of the major problems that faces those who care for these patients with chronic disease is late referral to a nephrologist, estimated at between 20 and 50% of cases (Arora et al., 1999). This degree of late referral (often defined as within 3 months of commencing renal replacement therapy) could be due to lack of agreement between primary care physicians and nephrologists as to which level of kidney function triggers referral. The Canadian Society of Nephrology guidelines recommend that at least 12 months are needed prior to initiation of dialysis for adequate medical and psychological preparation for renal replacement therapy (Levin, 2000).

British Renal Association Standards (Renal Association, 2002) recommend that those with a serum creatinine of more than 150 μmol/l should be referred to a nephrologist. Concerns about the high workload that this could generate have resulted in nephrologists seeking a more accurate marker of measuring reduced kidney function.

An estimation of the GFR is now being utilised alongside serum creatinine measurements. This can be achieved by using the Cockcroft–Gault (1976)

**Table 3.4**  Cockcroft–Gault calculation.

*In men:*

$$\text{Creatinine clearance} = \frac{(140 - \text{age}) \times \text{weight in kg}}{(72 \times \text{serum creatinine})}$$

*In women:*

$$\text{Creatinine clearance} = \frac{(140 - \text{age}) \times \text{weight in kg} \times 0.85}{(72 \times \text{serum creatinine})}$$

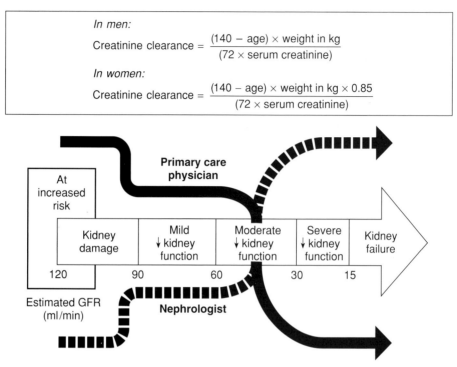

**Figure 3.2**   Referral to a nephrologist. (Adapted from Eknoyan and Mann, 2000.)

calculation. (Table 3.4), which takes into consideration weight, gender, serum creatinine and age. However, this technique tends to underestimate creatinine clearance in obese patients and overestimates it in patients who may be on a low protein diet.

As the kidney function declines, an appropriate referral needs to be made and Figure 3.2 illustrates how this could be managed. Levin (2000) suggests that a referral to a nephrologist should be made when the GFR is approximately 50 ml/min (moderate kidney damage).

Education of primary care physicians/general practitioners in the use of the Cockcroft–Gault calculations and the production of agreed local guidelines for referral would need to be established to improve the poor situation regarding late referral.

Monitoring of the GFR should continue once referral to a nephrologist has taken place to enable planned initiation of dialysis which would include timely insertion of vascular access. K/DOQI guidelines (National Kidney Foundation, 2000) suggest that vascular access should be in place when the GFR is between 29 and 15 ml/min and dialysis should be initiated when GFR is less than 15 ml/min. However, in clinical practice this is often not possible due to lack of resources for provision of haemodialysis.

Consequences of late referral include increased morbidity and mortality. There is also an impact on patients' quality of life and missed opportunities for pre-emptive transplantation. Late referral can also limit therapeutic options (Levin, 2000). Results from the ongoing Dialysis Outcomes and Practice Patterns Study (DOPPS) appear to support these findings (Lopes et al., 2003).

DOPPS is an ongoing observational study of haemodialysis patients in 12 countries, seeking to identify dialysis practices that contribute to improved mortality and morbidity rates (including hospitalisation rates, health-related quality of life and vascular access outcomes). Locatelli et al. (2000) correlated results from data collected by DOPPS that show that higher haemoglobin rates are associated with lower mortality rates and reduced hospitalisation amongst haemodialysis patients in Europe.

## Treating anaemia in early renal insufficiency

There are three sets of guidelines or standards that can be utilised to evaluate anaemia and assist in ensuring that the most appropriate treatment is given. Further discussion on definitions of targets, recommendations and standards is given in Chapter 15, but when evaluating anaemia management guidelines and standards it is important to recognise the variety of measurement instruments available to the clinician.

In summary, a *standard* is an outcome of care that is measurable, valid and realistic, a *target* is an aim that is set higher than the standard, and a *guideline* is a 'recipe' and can be used to achieve the outcome standard and may incorporate a target. A *recommendation* concerns the process or delivery of care and has an impact on workload and may involve several members of the multidisciplinary team. Recommendations can be included in guidelines.

## Guidelines and standards for anaemia management

### European Best Practice Guidelines (EBPG) for Management of Anaemia in Patients with Chronic Renal Failure (Valderrabano et al., 1999)

These have been written by a group of European nephrologists and are evidence-based and graded according to the level of evidence.

- Level A: evidence obtained from meta-analysis of several randomised controlled trials.
- Level B: evidence obtained from well-conducted clinical trials but no randomised clinical trials. Evidence may be extensive but essentially descriptive.
- Level C: evidence obtained from expert opinion and/or clinical experience of respected authorities.

### *Kidney Disease Outcomes Quality Initiative (K/DOQI) (National Kidney Foundation, 2000)*

These have been written by a working party for the National Kidney Foundation. They are evidence-based guidelines graded by level of evidence as follows:

- S: analysis of individual patient data from a single large generalised study of methodological quality.
- C: compilation of original articles (evidence tables).
- R: review of reviews and selected original articles.
- O: opinion.

### *British Renal Association Standards 3rd Edition (Renal Association, 2002)*

These have been written by the Renal Standards and Audit sub-committee on behalf of the Renal Association and the Royal College of Physicians. Chapter 7 of these Standards explores anaemia in patients with chronic renal failure. They are evidence-based guidelines graded by level of evidence as follows:

- Level A: evidence obtained from meta-analysis of several randomised controlled trials.
- Level B: evidence obtained from well-conducted clinical trials but no randomised clinical trials. Evidence may be extensive but essentially descriptive.
- Level C: evidence obtained from expert opinion and/or clinical experience of respected authorities.

The recommendations of the EBPG, K/DOQI and Renal Association are the three main sources used to assist in the management of anaemia in practice, and although quite similar there are a few small variations (see Table 3.5).

It is apparent that the treatment of anaemia should begin prior to commencement of dialysis. Guidelines and standards agree that this should start when the GFR is 30–60 ml/min, so 50 ml/min would seem an average starting point.

## The benefits of early correction of anaemia

### *Cardiovascular benefits*

Correcting anaemia in patients prior to commencing dialysis is now recognised as being beneficial. Cardiovascular complications are the leading cause of death in patients with established renal disease (ERF). Cardiac disease alone accounts for 40% of deaths (Raine et al., 1992). Left ventricular hypertrophy

**Table 3.5** Comparison of anaemia management recommendations from K/DOQI, EBPG and Renal Association.

| | K/DOQI (2002) | EBPG (1999) | British Renal Association Standards (2002) |
|---|---|---|---|
| Initial evaluation haemoglobin level | < 12 g/dl or 11 g/dl | < 12 g/dl or 11 g/dl | < 12 g/dl or 11g/dl |
| Initial evaluation of iron status | Serum ferritin > 100 µg/l %Transferrin saturation > 20% Hypochromic RBC – not mentioned as a marker | Serum ferritin > 100 µg/l %Transferrin saturation > 20% Hypochromic RBC < 10% | Serum ferritin > 100 µg/l %Transferrin saturation > 20% Hypochromic RBC < 10% |
| Initial evaluation of GFR level | 60 ml/min | < 30 ml/min or 45 ml/min in diabetes mellitus | < 30 ml/min or 45 ml/min in diabetes mellitus |
| Target haemoglobin | 11–12 g/dl Percentage of patients not mentioned | > 11 g/dl 85% patients should have Hb > 11 g/dl | 85% patients should have Hb > 10 g/dl within 6 months of seeing a nephrologist |

(LVH) is one of the most common cardiovascular changes that occur in patients with ERF and represents an independent risk factor for patient survival (London, 2001). The importance of trying to halt the progression of cardiovascular disease cannot be underestimated.

Anaemia as a contributory factor to volume and fluid overload plays an important physiological role in the development of the cardiovascular structure and functional alterations seen in patients with renal disease (Parfrey et al., 1996). Renal function and cardiac disease are inversely related. Levin (1999) reported that 36% of a cohort of chronic renal failure patients with a low GFR had LVH. Of these patients, 25% showed an increase in left ventricular mass index over a 12-month period. LVH is present in approximately 80% of patients by the time they reach dialysis (Foley et al., 1995).

Partial correction of anaemia can lead to partial regression of LVH in patients with ERF. Normalisation of haemoglobin levels may be beneficial at an early stage of the disease process, but further studies are needed to support this theory.

Left ventricular disorders progress from reversible to irreversible, with anaemia being a clear risk factor in this process. The evidence available strongly suggests that a target haemoglobin of 11–12 g/dl will benefit patients as opposed to no intervention at all (Foley et al., 2000). If the cardiovascular risks can be reduced prior to dialysis this will undoubtedly improve outcomes for the renal population.

## Quality of life improvement

Quality of life improvement has become as important as morbidity and mortality reduction in evaluating outcomes of ERF. Various tools are available to analyse the patient's perceptions of physical, psychological and social aspects of health. Tools such as the Karnofsky score and also the SF-36 questionnaire and the kidney disease quality of life (KDQOL) instruments have been developed specifically for patients with ERF (Lapaucis et al., 1992).

Anaemia is probably one of the symptoms with the most negative impact on quality of life in both pre-dialysis and dialysis patients (Valderrabano et al., 2001). Several studies have demonstrated a significant improvement in quality of life after initiation of treatment of anaemia with erythropoiesis stimulating agents in both pre-dialysis and dialysis patients (Valderrabano et al., 2001) Quality of life scores show a high correlation with haemoglobin concentration.

The majority of studies have involved the dialysis population. However, a study by Revicki et al. (1995) is one of the most conclusive performed on the pre-dialysis population. The study analysed physical function, energy, role function activity in the home, sexual dysfunction, depression and satisfaction with life. Results showed a significant improvement in haemoglobin levels and quality of life perception in the group treated with erythropoietin, whereas no change occurred in the control group other than a decrease in physical function. Further studies are needed to clearly identify what the optimum haemoglobin level should be to maximise quality of life in the pre-dialysis population.

One of the difficulties with quality of life measurements is that ethical approval is needed before they can be used in practice. K/DOQI Guideline 12 (2000) states that a patient with GFR of less than 60 ml/min/1.73 m$^2$ should undergo regular assessment of well-being in order to establish the effect of intervention on well-being. If this guideline was widely accepted in clinical practice then patients would automatically have their quality of life assessed and monitored from referral.

## Impact of anaemia on cognitive function

Cognitive function has always been associated with uraemia. There is now clear evidence that by treating renal anaemia there is an improvement in cognitive function (Stivelman, 2000). Erythropoietin receptors are found not only on erythrocyte precursor cells but also on other cells in the kidney and the central nervous system. This suggests that the role of erythropoietin is much broader than just stimulation of erythropoiesis. Immunocytochemical techniques have shown that erythropoietin receptors are present in and around the brain, which suggests that erythropoietin plays an important role in the central nervous system (Brines, 2000). Further investigations are needed, however, to ascertain the haemoglobin level most appropriate to optimise cognitive function.

## Anaemia in diabetes

Anaemia in those people with diabetes often occurs before there is any sign of renal impairment. This is thought to be due to low endogenous erythropoietin levels caused by glomerular damage, tubulo-interstitial injury [more common in type two diabetes; Winkler et al. (1999)] and autonomic neuropathy (Bosman et al., 2001). Patients with diabetic nephropathy have an even higher risk of cardiovascular complications compared with ERF patients without diabetes.

A study by Foley et al. (1996) clearly showed this when comparing the incidence of concentric LVH, ischaemic heart disease and cardiac failure in these two populations. It would be pertinent for screening for anaemia to be part of the current monitoring and screening of diabetes management, but so far it has not been universally incorporated and has not even been considered by the National Service Framework for Diabetes (Department of Health, 2001). As diabetes is now the most common cause of renal failure in some areas of the UK, collaboration between the renal and diabetes teams is essential.

## Review of anaemia

The benefits of early treatment of anaemia – prevention of progression of cardiovascular disease, improved quality of life and cognitive function – have all been shown to improve outcomes for patients with CKD. The next section will evaluate current treatment options and discuss how they can be used in practice.

# Treatment options

The correction of iron deficiency anaemia is essential before considering the use of any erythropoiesis stimulating agents.

European Best Practice Guidelines (Valderrabano et al., 1999) suggest that to achieve and maintain a target haemoglobin of 11 g/dl, serum ferritin in all patients should be more than 100 µg/l, with a percentage transferrin saturation of more than 20% or percentage of hypochromic red cells less than 10%. To achieve this guideline, two types of treatment can be used: oral iron and intravenous iron.

## Oral iron

Oral iron is sometimes poorly absorbed and the absorption can be inhibited by other drugs such as calcium-based phosphate binders and aluminium, and by taking it with food and tea. Vitamin C assists absorption and taking oral iron with a glass of orange juice may help. However, many people with renal failure have to cope with dietary changes and constraints, so this may not always be possible.

The side effects of oral iron such as constipation, diarrhoea and flatulence can often mean that patients do not take it regularly. However, oral iron is used in practice mainly for pre-dialysis and peritoneal dialysis patients where the practicalities of administering intravenous iron are limited.

## Intravenous iron

Intravenous iron is currently available in the UK as two preparations: iron dextran (Cosmofer®) and iron sucrose (Venofer®).

(1)   Iron dextran (Cosmofer®): a complex of ferric hydroxide with dextrans containing 5% (50 mg/ml) iron (British National Formulary, 2002).
— *Dose*: by intravenous slow infusion (*up to 4 hours*) calculated according to bodyweight and iron deficit. Not recommended for children under 14 years old.
— *Cautions*: facilities for cardiopulmonary resuscitation must be at hand; increased risk of allergic reaction in immune or inflammatory conditions; hepatic impairment; renal impairment; oral iron not to be given until 5 days after last injection; pregnancy.
— *Contra-indications*: history of allergic disorders including asthma and eczema; infection; active rheumatoid arthritis.
— *Side-effects*: nausea, dyspepsia, diarrhoea, chest pains, hypotension, dyspnoea, arthralgia, myalgia, pruritus, urticaria, rash, fever, shivering, flushing, headache; rarely anaphylactic reactions; injection site reactions including phlebitis reported.

There are concerns regarding risk of anaphylaxis with iron dextran. Dextran antibodies can exist, but this is unknown until iron dextran is given to the patient and within seconds an anaphylactic reaction may occur. This means that this drug must be given in an environment where there are full resuscitation facilities available. The advantage of having iron dextran is that it can be given as a single dose infusion which is advantageous if the patient has to travel long distances for treatment. It cannot be given undiluted as a bolus dose.

(2)   Iron sucrose (Venofer®): a complex of ferric hydroxide with sucrose containing 2% (20 mg/ml) of iron (British National Formulary, 2002).
— *Dose*: by slow intravenous injection (over 5–10 minutes) or by intravenous infusion, calculated according to bodyweight and iron deficit; consult product literature. Not recommended for children.
— *Cautions*: oral iron therapy should not be given until 5 days after last injection; facilities for cardiopulmonary resuscitation must be at hand; pregnancy.

— *Contraindications*: history of allergic disorders including asthma, eczema and anaphylaxis; liver disease; infection.
— *Side-effects*: nausea, vomiting, taste disturbances, headache, hypotension; less frequently paraesthesia, abdominal disorders, myalgia, fever, flushing, urticaria, peripheral oedema; rarely anaphylactoid reactions; injection site reactions including phlebitis reported.

Iron sucrose can be safely given to patients across all dialysis modalities either as an infusion or undiluted as a bolus dose via a butterfly needle. It is the most commonly used intravenous iron supplementation in renal medicine.

Haemodialysis patients are able to receive intravenous iron during dialysis without it being removed by dialysis. Therefore all haemodialysis patients who require iron supplementation can have intravenous iron rather than oral iron. The amount given will vary from unit to unit, but a standard dose is 100 mg every fortnight as a maintenance dose. Or if the patient required a course of iron 1 g would be given over a 5- to 10-week period depending on the unit protocol.

Patients in the pre-dialysis stage, or on peritoneal dialysis, may receive intravenous iron when their serum ferritin is more than 100 g/dl, %Tsats is more than 20% or percentage of hypochromic red cells is more than 10%. Patients who are intolerant of oral iron may be given maintenance intravenous iron every 6–8 weeks to maintain their serum ferritin at less than 100 µg/l.

## Monitoring iron stores

All patients who are receiving erythropoiesis stimulating agents (ESAs) require iron supplementation to support the demands made on their iron stores.

Regular monitoring of iron stores is essential during treatment. Patients with chronic renal failure with a stable haemoglobin level not being treated with ESA, should have iron stores measured every 3–6 months (EBPG Guideline 7). Patients who are being treated with ESAs should have their iron status checked every 4 weeks during the correction phase (3 months) and thereafter every 3 months.

Patients who are receiving regular intravenous iron therapy should have their iron status checked every 3 months and the intravenous therapy discontinued for at least a week prior to performing the tests. Iron toxicity needs to be avoided and if the serum ferritin is persistently above 800 µg/l and/or %Tsats is more than 50%, iron supplementation should be withheld for up to 3 months as long as there are no signs of functional iron deficiency. Iron status should be measured monthly in these situations.

Renal patients require vitamin supplementation as many of the vitamins are water soluble and can be removed during dialysis. They require folic acid 5 mg once a day and renal multivitamins (Dialyvit®) once a day. Therefore treatment for anaemia can include iron supplementation, vitamin B12 supplementation and folic acid even before ESAs are considered.

# Erythropoiesis stimulating agents

Currently three types of erythropoiesis stimulating agents (ESAs) are available:

(1)  Epoetin alfa – recombinant human erythropoietin (r-HuEPO).
(2)  Epoetin beta – recombinant human erythropoietin (r-HuEPO).
(3)  Darbepoetin alfa – novel erythropoiesis stimulating protein (NESP).

They all work in a similar way by continually stimulating the bone marrow to produce red blood cells. However, there are several pharmokinetic differences between r-HuEPO and NESP.

Table 3.6 shows a comparison between r-HuEPO and NESP. The main difference is in the number of carbohydrate chains and sialic acids. The greater the sialic-acid-containing carbohydrate content of the molecule the longer the circulating half-life (Egrie and Browne, 2001). This means that NESP has a longer half-life than r-HuEPO: 25 hours compared with 8 hours.

These differences in pharmokinetic make-up mean that there are differences in dosing and possible differences and frequency of administration. Table 3.7 shows the dosage, frequency and route of administration of ESAs.

After initial dosing the haemoglobin (Hb) level is monitored every 2–4 weeks with the aim of reaching the target Hb within 2–4 months (correction phase). The doses of r-HuEPO or NESP are titrated during this period to ensure that

**Table 3.6**  Comparison of r-HuEPO and NESP (Egrie and Brown, 2001).

| r-HuEPO | NESP |
|---|---|
| • Three N-linked carbohydrate chains | • Five N-linked carbohydrate chains |
| • Up to 14 sialic acid residues | • Up to 22 sialic acid residues |
| • 30 400 daltons | • 37 100 daltons |
| • 40% carbohydrate | • 51% carbohydrate |

**Table 3.7**  Dosage, frequency and route of administration of ESAs.

| Drug | Starting dose | Dose difference between intravenous and subcutaneous administration | Frequency | Route of administration |
|---|---|---|---|---|
| Epoetin alfa (Eprex®) | 50 iu/kg | Yes | 1–3 times a week | Intravenous only (2002) in patients with CKD |
| Epoetin beta (Neorecormon®) | 20 iu/kg | Yes | 1–3 times a week | Subcutaneous or intravenous |
| Darbepoetin alfa (Aranesp®) | 0.45 mcg/kg | No | Once a week, or once a fortnight | Subcutaneous or intravenous |

the Hb does not rise too quickly. If the Hb concentration exceeds 14 g/dl, therapy should be discontinued until the Hb falls below 13 g/dl; then the therapy should be reintroduced at a lower dose and monitored as if commencing the drug for the first time.

It is essential to have adequate iron stores prior to commencing treatment with r-HuEPO or NESP and to maintain iron stores with the use of oral or intravenous iron supplementation as discussed in the previous section.

Once the target Hb has been achieved the Hb should continue to be monitored monthly in haemodialysis patients, 6–8 times a week in peritoneal dialysis patients (EBPG, 1999) and less often in pre-dialysis patients, perhaps 2–3 times a month. Once started ESA therapy is seldom stopped (unless the Hb rises too fast). ESA therapy should not be discontinued in patients undergoing surgery, requiring blood transfusion or suffering an acute illness episode. It may be necessary to increase the dose in some cases.

## Monitoring response to treatment

Baseline blood tests will have already been done prior to commencing treatment. It is necessary therefore to carefully monitor response to treatment. The majority of patients will be receiving their ESA at home and may require support from the primary care team with administration of their injections. The primary care team are also able to assist with blood pressure monitoring and follow-up blood tests. A shared care protocol is useful in these situations to clearly outline the responsibilities of the hospital and primary care team and when and to whom abnormalities should be reported. Blood pressure is normally checked weekly for the first 6–8 weeks and then Hb levels and iron status are checked monthly during the correction phase. Long-term monitoring will depend on the treatment modality as above.

# Adverse effects of epoetin treatment

## Hypertension

A literature review in the K/DOQI guidelines (2000) showed that 23% of patients with chronic renal failure either developed or required an increase in antihypertensive medication during treatment of anaemia. This was not seen in patients with normal renal function. The causes of an increase in blood pressure are thought to be due to an increase in vasoconstrictor tone and an increase in cardiac output.

Blood pressure should therefore be monitored closely, particularly during the correction phase, perhaps weekly until the target haemoglobin has been reached. The blood pressure should be within normal range in pre-dialysis patients. British Hypertensive Society (BHS) guidelines (Ramsay et al., 1999a, b) suggest that an optimal (therapeutically treated) blood pressure for non-diabetics should be 140/85 mm Hg and 145/80 mm Hg for those with diabetes. The BHS audit standard for non-diabetics is 150/90 mm Hg and 140/85 mm Hg for those with diabetes. Parameters for intervention regarding blood pressure control and erythropoietin therapy will depend on the protocol of each unit.

Patients with uncontrolled hypertension should not be started on ESAs until the blood pressure is controlled. A single high blood pressure reading is not an indication to omit the ESA, but a trend in the rise of the blood pressure needs to be addressed and additional antihypertensive therapy considered if this occurs. If the patient develops uncontrolled hypertension the ESA should be stopped until the blood pressure is controlled and then recommenced with close monitoring.

## Access thrombosis

One of the main effects of epoetin is that it appears to improve platelet function which may be due to the effects of an increase in Hb concentration (Rivas et al., 1996). Similar changes have been noted in uraemic patients who have been transfused. Epoetin can also improve endothelial function.

As a result, patients with PTFE (polytetrafluoroethylene) grafts may be prone to an increased risk of access thrombosis if they have a higher Hb. Antiplatelet therapy may need to be considered, but aspirin is not recommended as this has been shown to increase thrombosis rates (Streedhara and Hinnelfarb, 1994). The need to observe vascular access on a regular basis and closely monitor Hb levels in patients with PTFE grafts is essential.

## Seizures

Seizures occur most frequently during the correction phase and are associated with a rapid rise in Hb and poor control of hypertension. However, this occurrence is now relatively rare due to dose titration and careful monitoring of blood pressure.

## Antibodies to epoetin

Antibodies to epoetin are rare. However, in patients who do develop antibodies, this can result in pure red cell aplasia (PRCA). PRCA is the failure to produce red cell precursors in the bone marrow and is confirmed by a bone marrow biopsy. Antibody PRCA occurs as a result of an immune response to the protein backbone of recombinant human erythropoietin. Casadevall et al. (2002) reported that antibodies were detected against the protein component of the molecule rather than the carbohydrate component. This is a very new discovery and data are currently being collected from all patients who have experienced antibody-induced PRCA due to epoetin therapy. Further details can be found later in the chapter.

## Causes of inadequate response to ESA therapy

A definition of resistance to epoetin is either failure to attain the target Hb concentration while receiving less than 300 iu/kg/week or a continued need for such dosage to maintain the target (EBPG Guideline 14).

The most common cause of an inadequate response to epoetin is *absolute or functional iron deficiency*. Another obvious reason is whether or not the patient is actually receiving the injections, particularly in those who are self-injecting.

The following also need to be considered:

- Chronic blood loss (from either gut or uterus)
- Infection/inflammation
- Diseases such as tuberculosis or systemic lupus erythematosus (SLE)
- Chronically rejecting transplants
- Hyperparathyroidism/osteitis fibrosa
- Aluminium toxicity
- Haemoglobinopathies (alpha, beta thalassaemia, sickle cell anaemia)
- Folate/vitamin B12 deficiency
- Multiple myeloma, myelofibrosis
- Malignancy
- Malnutrition
- Drug interaction such as high-dose ACE inhibitors
- Inadequate dialysis
- Antibodies to epoetin

A process of elimination should ascertain the cause of non-response to treatment. However, if none of the above is found to be positive and they have all been fully investigated, then a bone marrow test is necessary to rule out any other haematological cause of anaemia or non-response to treatment.

## Pure red cell aplasia (PRCA)

Pure red cell aplasia (PRCA) is a rare condition that means the virtual absence of red blood cell precursors confirmed by a bone marrow biopsy. It is associated with certain diseases such as parvovirus B19 infection, auto-immune disease, leukaemia or it may be drug induced (Mycophenolate, Tacrolimus, Isoniazid and others). Recently physicians have noticed rare cases of suspected PRCA in patients with kidney disease (Casadevall et al., 2002).

An antibody-mediated PRCA means that patients develop an immune response to the protein backbone of recombinant human erythropoietin. Virtually all proteins when introduced into the body can cause an immune response. PRCA seems to have been seen mainly in patients in Europe who have been exposed to subcutaneous use of Eprex®. By August 2002, 160 cases worldwide had been reported (Casadevall et al., 2002). Diagnosis of PRCA was confirmed by a bone marrow test and a test for EPO antibodies carried out by Professor Casadevall in Paris. In December 2002 the Medicines Control Agency withdrew the subcutaneous use of Eprex® for all patients with chronic renal failure. It continues to be given intravenously to haemodialysis patients. This had a huge impact in practice, resulting in vast numbers of patients being switched to either Neorecormon® or Aranesp®. Many units collected serum from these patients and have frozen the samples for possible testing for EPO antibodies at a later date. It is unknown why this problem has occurred specifically with Eprex® and research into this is continuing.

## Treatment of PRCA

Once diagnosis has been confirmed by bone marrow biopsy and the presence of EPO antibodies, all ESAs must be stopped. The patient will have a very low haemoglobin and become transfusion dependent. The use of steroids and cyclosporine has been tried in an attempt to reverse the immune response. Once the EPO has been stopped then a fall in antibodies occurs; however, the time span for this is variable. The bone marrow may recover, but this will take some time. The patient is often managed jointly by the haematologist and the nephrologist and, of course, the psychological effect of this condition needs to be taken into consideration when explaining PRCA to the patient.

# Managing anaemia

In many renal units specialist nurses are responsible for managing anaemia across all modalities. The advantage of having a dedicated team who manages anaemia means that it is managed systematically, effectively and efficiently. Other useful tools include computerised algorithms as suggested by Richardson et al. (2000). An algorithm gives a step-by-step guide to monitoring and managing anaemia following strict parameters for altering treatment.

Useful advice for managing anaemia can also be found in Table 3.8.

**Table 3.8**  Principles of anaemia management.

| |
|---|
| (1)  Set up a computerised database for all modalities using Excel or Access format. |
| (2)  Check haematinics (Hb, iron status, B12, folate) regularly across all modalities. |
| (3)  Set up protocols for anaemia management and review annually. |
| (4)  Audit and review practice annually against standards and guidelines. |
| (5)  Review ESA and iron dosage regularly. |
| (6)  Screen for non response to treatment and act accordingly. |
| (7)  Patients who are self injecting – check concordance with therapy. |
| (8)  Have dedicated persons responsible for managing anaemia and monitoring response to treatment across all modalities. |

## Prescription of ESAs

Prescribing is usually initiated by the nephrologist and then either it is taken over by the primary care physician (GP) or it continues to be prescribed by the hospital, depending on local funding issues and the acceptance of shared care protocols. As the number of patients being prescribed ESAs is increasing the Primary Care Trusts (PCTs) in the UK are moving towards providing funding for secondary care to prescribe and monitor the use of ESAs rather than the primary care physician. ESA prescribing is currently under review by the National Institute for Clinical Excellence (NICE) (2002).

To assist secondary care with ESA prescribing, each of the drug companies provides a home delivery service for patients, with the prescription generated from the hospital and the drug being delivered via a courier service. With the introduction of patient group directions and supplementary prescribing, anaemia nurse specialists are also able to undertake the responsibility of prescribing EPO, intravenous and oral iron. This may also be extended to other drugs for treating anaemia such as vitamin B12 and folic acid.

## Summary

Treating anaemia to the recommended guidelines improves morbidity and mortality. The earlier the anaemia is diagnosed and appropriately treated the better the outcome for the patient. A multiprofessional approach to managing anaemia is essential. The introduction of specialist nurses responsible for managing anaemia has enabled advanced practice within renal nursing to develop an independent role in this area. More than 50 renal units across the UK employ nurses specifically to manage anaemia across all modalities (Anaemia Nurse Specialist Association, ANSA Registry, 2001). These posts focus on anaemia in all areas within renal care and often the expertise and knowledge of these nurses is sought by other specialties such as haematology, oncology and care of the elderly with regard to the use of intravenous iron and ESAs.

The development of specialist nurses has shown to improve patient care because they are focusing on a specific patient population. Benner (2000) supports this by stating that 'astute clinical judgement increases when nurses have the opportunity to work with specific patient populations'.

Anaemia nurse specialists are responsible for screening and monitoring across all modalities, they accept direct referrals from clinicians and organise the most appropriate treatment. Many prescribe using patient group directions, which allows them to work independently. In many units the management of anaemia is solely the responsibility of these nurses, with little or no involvement from medical staff. Obviously adequate education and clinical competencies need to be in place to support this level of practice.

If there is not a designated specialist nurse in post, there is no reason why renal nurses in all areas cannot take on the responsibility of identifying the patient with anaemia and be aware of the screening tools and treatments available as part of a holistic approach to the care of the patient with kidney disease. Anaemia management is now seen as an essential part of pre-dialysis care, not only to improve quality of life but also in the prevention of the long-term complications of CKD.

Awareness of the problem of anaemia amongst other patient groups such as those with diabetes needs to be raised in order to prevent many of the cardiovascular complications as seen in those with CKD.

Patients with diabetes are not currently aware of the signs and symptoms of anaemia. A survey by the National Opinion Poll (NOP) in 2002 questioned 1054 patients with diabetes across six European countries. Most had heard of anaemia, but the causes of anaemia were not well known. Only 24% had ever been given any information about anaemia and those who had, received it from a doctor. Symptoms of anaemia such as tiredness and lethargy were associated with the disease itself and accepted by the patients as being 'part of my diabetes'. This survey clearly showed that there is a distinct lack of awareness of anaemia within this population. Information regarding anaemia was rarely given by the clinician unless asked for and nurses did not appear to have any input at all. This survey highlights one area in which anaemia of chronic disease has a large impact.

It is essential therefore to be able to differentiate between the signs and symptoms of anaemia of chronic disease and the signs and symptoms of the underlying disease so that anaemia can clearly be identified, appropriately treated and not ignored.

# References

Anaemia Nurse Specialist Association (ANSA) (2001) *Registry of Membership*. ANSA Secretariat, Woking, Surrey.

Arora, P., Obrador, G.T., Ruthazer, R., Kausz, A.T., Meyer, K.B., Jenuleson, C.S. and Pereira, B.J. (1999) Prevalence, predictors, and consequences of late nephrology referral at a tertiary care center. *Journal of the American Society of Nephrology* 10 (6), 1281–6.

Bandolier (2001) *Erythropoietin for Anaemia with Cancer Therapy*. www.jr2.ox.ac.uk/bandolier/band92/b92-5.html.

Benner, P. (2000) Shaping the future of nursing. *Nursing Management* 7 (1), 31–5.

Bosman, D.R., Marsden, J.T., Winkler, A.S., Macdougall, I.C. and Watkins, P.J. (2001) Anaemia with erythropoietin deficiency occurs early in diabetic nephropathy. *Diabetes Care* 24, 495–9.

Brines, M.L. (2000) Erythropoietin crosses the blood brain barrier to protect against experimental brain injury. *Proceedings of the National Academy of Science USA* 97, 10526–31.

British National Formulary (2002) *BNF 44: September 2002*. British Medical Association and Pharmaceutical Society of Great Britain. William Clowes, Beccles, Suffolk. www.bnf.org.index.htm.

Cameron, J.S. (1999) European Best Practice Guidelines for the management of anaemia in patients with chronic renal failure. *Nephrology Dialysis Transplantation* **14** (Suppl 2), 61–5.

Casadevall, N., Joelle, N., Teyssandier, I., et al. (2002) Pure red cell aplasia and antierythropoietin patients treated with recombinant erythropoietin. *New England Journal of Medicine* **346**, 469–75.

Cockcroft, D.W. and Gault, M.H. (1976) Prediction of creatinine clearance from serum creatinine. *Nephron* **16**, 31–41.

Department of Health (2001) *National Service Framework for Diabetes*. www.doh.gov.uk/nsf/diabetes.

Egrie, J.C. and Browne, J.K. (2001) Development and characterization of novel erythropoiesis stimulating protein (NESP). *Nephrology Dialysis Transplantation* **16** (Suppl 3).

Eknoyan, G. (2001) The importance of early treatment of the anaemia of chronic kidney disease. *Nephrology Dialysis Transplantation* **16** (Suppl 5), 45–9.

Eknoyan, G. and Mann, F.E. (2000) Benefits of early anaemia treatment in patients with renal insufficiency. *Nephrology Dialysis Transplantation* **15** (Suppl 3), 1–3.

Foley, R.N., Parfrey, P.S. and Harnett, J.D. (1995) Clinical and echocardiographic disease in patients starting end-stage renal disease therapy. *Kidney International* **47**, 186–92.

Foley, R.N., Parfrey, P.S. and Harnett, J.D. (1996) The impact of anaemia on cardiomyopathy, morbidity and mortality in end-stage renal failure disease. *American Journal of Kidney Diseases* **28**, 53–61.

Foley, R.N., Parfrey, P.S. and Morgan, J. (2000) Effects of haemoglobin levels in hemodialysis patients with asymptomatic cardiomyopathy. *Kidney International* **58**, 1325–35.

Hoffbrand, A.V. and Petit, J.E. (1985) *Essential Haematology*, 2nd edn. Blackwell Scientific Publishing, Oxford.

Lapaucis, A., Muirhead, N., Keown, P. and Wong, C. (1992) A disease-specific questionnaire for assessing quality of life in patients on haemodialysis. *Nephron* **60**, 302–306.

Levin, A. (1999) How should anaemia be managed in pre-dialysis patients? *Nephrology Dialysis Transplantation* **14** (Suppl 2), 66–74.

Levin, A. (2000) Consequences of late referral on patient outcomes. *Nephrology Dialysis Transplantation* **15** (Suppl 3), 8–13.

Levin, A., Singer, J. and Thompson, C. (1996) Prevalent left-ventricular hypertrophy in the predialysis population: identifying opportunities for intervention. *American Journal of Kidney Diseases* **27** (3), 347–54.

Locatelli, F., Pisoni, R.L., Bragg, J.L., Rayner, H.C., Piera, L., Wolfe, R.A., Young, E.W., Port, F.K. and Held, P.J. (2000) *Higher Hemoglobin Levels Are Associated with Lower Rates of Mortality and Hospitalization Among European Hemodialysis Patients. Results from the DOPPS*.

London, G.M. (2002) Left ventricular alterations and end-stage renal disease. *Nephrology Dialysis Transplantation* **17** (Suppl 1), 29–36.

Lopes, A.A., Bragg-Gresham, J.L., Satayathum, S., McCullough, K., Pifer, T., Goodkin, D., Mapes, D., Young, E., Wolfe, R., Held, P. and Port, F. (2003) Health-related quality of life and associated outcomes among haemodialysis patients of different ethnicities in the United States: The Dialysis Outcomes and Practice Patterns Study (DOPPS). *American Journal of Kidney Diseases* **41** (3), 605–15.

National Institute for Clinical Excellence (NICE) (2002) *National Institute for Clinical Excellence (NICE) Guidelines*. www.nice.org.uk.

National Institute of Diabetes and Digestive and Kidney Disease (1991) *US Renal Data*

*System Annual Report (USRDS)*. National Institute of Diabetes and Digestive and Kidney Disease, Bethesda, Maryland.

National Kidney Foundation (2000) *NKF-K/DOQI Clinical Practice Guidelines for Anemia of Chronic Kidney Disease*. www.kidney.org/professionals/kdoqi.

National Kidney Foundation (2002) Kidney disease outcomes quality initiative. *American Journal of Kidney Diseases* **39** (2) (Suppl 1), S111–69.

Parfrey, P.S., Foley, R.N., Harnett, J.D., Kent, G.M., Murray, D.C. and Barre, P.E. (1996) Outcome and risk factors for left ventricular disorders in chronic uraemia. *Nephrology Dialysis Transplantation* **11**, 1277–85.

Peirera, B.J.G., Sundaram, S., Barrett, T.W., Butt, N.K., Porat, R. and King, A.J. (1996) Cytokine production by human peripheral blood mononuclear cells stimulated by a *Pseudomonas aeruginosa* culture filtrate: role of plasma and polymyxin B. *International Journal of Artificial Organs* **5**, 276–83.

Raine, A.E., Margreiter, R., Brunner, F.P., et al. (1992) Report on management of renal failure in Europe. *Nephrology Dialysis Transplantation* **7** (Suppl 2), 7–35.

Ramsay, L.E., Williams, B., Johnston, G.O., MacGregor, G.A., Poston, L., Potter, J.F., Poulter, N.R. and Russell, G. (1999a) Guidelines for management of hypertension. Report of the third working party of the British Hypertension Society. *Journal of Human Hypertension* **13**, 569–92.

Ramsay, L.E., Williams, B., Johnston, G.O., MacGregor, G.A., Poston, L., Potter, J.F., Poulter, N.R. and Russell, G. (1999b) British Hypertension Society guidelines for hypertension management, summary. *British Medical Journal* **319**, 30–35.

Renal Association (2002) *Treatment of Adults and Children with Renal Failure: Standards and Audit Measures*, 3rd edn. Royal College of Physicians, London.

Revicki, D.A., Brown, R.E., Feeney, D.H., Henry, D., Teehan, B., Rudnick, M. and Benz, R. (1995) Health-related quality of life associated with rHu-EPO therapy for predialysis chronic renal disease patients. *American Journal of Kidney Diseases* **25**, 548–54.

Richardson, D., Bartlett, C. and Will, E.J. (2000) Intervention thresholds and ceilings can determine the haemoglobin outcome distribution in a haemodialysis population. *Nephrology Dialysis Transplantation* **15**, 2007–2013.

Rivas, J.M., Garcia, A., Möll, R. and Cervera, A. (1996) A direct action of recombinant human erythropoietin (r-HuEPO) on platelet function in uremic patients on haemodialysis. *Nefrologia* **16**, 46–53.

Spivak, J.L. (2000) The blood in systemic disorders. *Lancet* **355**, 1707–1712.

Streedhara, R. and Hinnelfarb, J. (1994) Anti-platelet therapy in graft thrombosis: result of a prospective double blind study. *Kidney International* **45**, 1477–83.

Stivelman, J.C. (2000) Benefits of anaemia treatment on cognitive function. *Nephrology Dialysis Transplantation* **15** (Suppl 3), 29–35.

Valderrabano, F., Horl, W.H., Jacobs, C., Macdougall, I.C., Parronda, I., Cremers, S. and Abraha, I.L. (1999) European best practice guidelines. *Nephrology Dialysis Transplantation* **15** (Suppl 5), S8–14.

Valderrabano, F., Jofre, R. and Lopez-Gomez, J.M. (2001) Quality of life in end stage renal disease patients. *American Journal of Kidney Diseases* **38** (3), 443–64.

Winkler, A.S., Marsden, J., Chaudhuri, K.R., Hambley, H. and Watkins, P.J. (1999) Erythropoietin depletion and anaemia in diabetes mellitus. *Diabetic Medicine* **16**, 813–19.

Young, E.W., Goodkin, D.A., Mapes, D.L., Port, F.K., Keen, M.L., Chen, K., Maroni, B.L., Wolfe, R.A. and Held, P.J. (2000) The Dialysis Outcomes and Practice Patterns Study (DOPPS): an international hemodialysis study. *Kidney International* **57** (Suppl 74), S74–81.

# Chapter 4
# Advances in Haemodialysis

*Catherine Morgan*

## Introduction

Despite considerable technical advances in haemodialysis treatment for established renal failure (ERF), the therapy can be characterised by high morbidity, mortality and poor quality of life. Ideally the treatment prescription for renal failure should closely resemble the physiology of the normal kidney that maintains the body's homeostasis. However, conventional haemodialysis does not mimic the function of the kidney well, with short intermittent dialysis schedules resulting in severe swings in solutes and water (Kjellstrand, 2001).

More recent developments in haemodialysis aim to improve tolerance of the therapy and the physiology of dialysis treatments. For example, haemodiafiltration offers improved haemodynamic stability and greater middle molecule clearance, and on-line monitoring options, like blood volume and sodium monitors, assist in reducing the incidence of haemodialysis-related hypotension. Similarly, the rationale for the resurgence of interest in the use of more frequent dialysis is to improve patient well-being by offering a treatment schedule that more closely represents normal kidney function. The following discussion incorporates a review of some of the more recent advances in haemodialysis therapy, including clinical advantages, disadvantages and cost implications.

## Daily dialysis

Intermittent haemodialysis, most commonly thrice weekly, is widely used as renal replacement therapy in patients with established renal failure (ERF). When chronic haemodialysis was first introduced the frequency was established as three times per week to avoid the development of uraemic symptoms. Sessions were generally long (up to 8 hours) due to the low efficiency of the dialysers. With the advent of the hollow fibre dialyser the efficiency of dialysis could be increased and it became common practice to shorten dialysis time. Techniques have been developed in the haemodialysis world that have allowed shorter and shorter dialysis sessions, with increasing attention being paid to the adequacy of dialysis at the expense of such parameters as volume control (Laurent and Charra, 1998; Twardowski, 2001).

However, thrice weekly dialysis is often insufficient for patients without residual renal function, with the patients suffering from uraemic symptoms, poor blood pressure control and associated co-morbidity. There is therefore a need for improvement in the current therapy offered to patients with ERF in order to reduce the high mortality rates, hospitalisations and patient symptoms. It is for this reason that in recent times interest is developing in the use of more frequent haemodialysis, either short daily (typically 1.5–2 hours, 5–7 times per week) or longer nightly sessions (typically 6–8 hours, 5–7 times per week) (Lindsay and Kortas, 2001; Twardowski, 2001).

It makes sense that patients with renal failure should be dialysed every day. Maintaining homeostasis is the main function of the kidneys and intermittent dialysis schedules that concentrate on urea clearance as a measure of adequacy fall short of mimicking the role of the kidneys. In between dialysis there are large shifts in biochemistry and fluid, often leading to oedema, hypertension and uraemia; thus the intermittent nature of dialysis is a major cause of ill effects.

## Morbidity and mortality

It is well known that more gradual haemodialysis procedures are tolerated better by patients and achieve superior control in many parameters such as blood pressure and uraemia. Laurent and Charra (1998) reported improved survival and clinical outcomes with their 8-hour, thrice-weekly haemodialysis schedules. Data from 876 patients treated at the dialysis unit in Tassin, France, between 1968 and 1996 were analysed in terms of morbidity and mortality. The use of slow ultrafiltration enabled lowering of the extracellular volume down to dry weight. In most (more than 95%) of the patients treated by this method tight control of blood pressure was achieved without the use of antihypertensive medication.

The morbidity and mortality of the patients who receive long periods of haemodialysis is reported as better than the general haemodialysis population, the major factor responsible for good long-term survival being the tight control of blood pressure. The move towards short daily or long nocturnal haemodialysis is an attempt to achieve similarly impressive results by using therapies that more closely simulate renal physiology.

A considerable body of clinical experience supports the rationale for more frequent haemodialysis (Kjellstrand, 2001; Twardowski, 2001; Vanholder et al., 2002). Many of the studies, however, have small patient numbers and therefore do not achieve statistical significance and are not representative of the haemodialysis population due to biased selection criteria. They also do not have adequate control groups in most cases and reports are limited to select parameters (Lacson and Diaz-Buxo, 2001). Despite this, the published results from the use of both short daily and nocturnal haemo-dialysis unanimously note that some improvement occurs with the imple-mentation of such therapies. These improvements include blood pressure control and tolerance of dialysis, with less intradialytic hypotension and reduced requirement for antihypertensive medication. Regression of cardiac hypertrophy (Buoncristiani et al., 1999) and better anaemia control have been achieved with less erythropoietin being used (Woods et al., 1999). Improved nutritional status has been reported, with increased serum albumin, normal-ised protein catabolic rate and dry weight (Vos et al., 2001). A better sense of well-being and quality of life, reduced fatigue and fewer hospitalisations are other positive findings of patients receiving frequent haemodialysis (Buoncristiani, 1998).

## Clinical outcomes

While for most centres the experience is more recent, some centres have long-term experience of daily dialysis. Buoncristiani (1998) reported data on 15 years of experience of multicentre daily dialysis in a total of 69 patients from six dialysis centres in Italy. Commencing in 1982, patients were switched from intermittent haemodialysis or peritoneal dialysis to daily dialysis for a variety of reasons, the majority (61%) due to patient choice; other reasons included problems with fluid overload, hypertension and cardiovascular instability. Most of the patients, 58 out of 69, were originally treated at home, with five patients returning to in-centre treatment over time; however, three continued on daily dialysis.

The reported metabolic control was greatly improved in these patients, with pH and bicarbonate remaining within normal limits and reduced swings in other electrolytes and uraemic toxins. Clinical outcomes were also significantly improved, with reduced uraemic symptoms and anaemia, improved blood pressure control (including some reversal of cardiac hypertrophy) and better quality of life that included general well-being, family and social life.

The main initial concerns of those involved in implementing the programme were vascular access survival, feasibility and patient acceptance; however, these did not prove to be limiting factors in the long term. The author also reports that the typically negative attitude of patients towards dialysis became more positive, attributing this change to improved clinical conditions and the relative shortness of the sessions.

## Cardiovascular risk

Maria et al. (2001) carried out a study to investigate the effect of daily dialysis on blood pressure control and left ventricular mass reduction in hyperten-sive patients. Twelve hypertensive patients who were stable on intermittent haemodialysis were recruited into the study. It was a prospective study and a randomised two-period crossover design was used to incorporate a control group unlike many other studies in this field.

Following a run-in period of 6 months on standard intermittent haemodialysis (12 hours per week) patients were randomised into one of two groups. Group one received intermittent haemodialysis for 6 months and then daily dialysis for 6 months, while group 2 received daily dialysis for 6 months followed by intermittent dialysis for 6 months. The hours of dialysis were unchanged as was the Kt/V, blood flow dialyser and dialysate. The results showed that daily dialysis was more effective in controlling blood pressure, with a reduction in both systolic and diastolic blood pressure in patients receiving this therapy. This was significantly correlated with a reduction in extracellular water content as measured by bioimpedance analysis. It was also noted that the majority of patients did not require pharmacological control of blood pressure whilst receiving daily dialysis. Similarly, left ventricular index mass decreased significantly in those patients receiving daily dialysis.

The prevalence of cardiovascular disease in the dialysis population is high and cardiovascular problems are the major cause of death among patients with ERF (Charra et al., 1996). This is primarily due to an increased presence of risk factors for developing such problems, for example hypertension. The pathogenesis of hypertension in haemodialysis patients is multifactorial; however, fluid retention plays a major role, as the majority of haemodialysis patients become normotensive after dialysis has been initiated and excess volume is removed (Luik et al., 1997). Therefore adequate control of volume-related hypertension and chronic volume overload represents an essential component of reducing morbidity and mortality in the dialysis population. Daily dialysis reduces extracellular water content and hence interdialytic weight gain, thereby improving blood pressure control, a factor that in itself makes more frequent dialysis worthy of consideration.

### Dialysis adequacy

There are a lack of data comparing daily nocturnal dialysis with short daily dialysis. Lacson and Diaz-Buxo (2001) reviewed published data of both these therapies and although direct comparison is not possible due to the variability in the patient population, some differences do emerge. The efficiency of nocturnal dialysis is significantly greater, offering the highest solute clearance with more time for equilibration. It can provide double the current recommended dialysis dose as measured by Kt/V and may therefore be suitable for underdialysed patients, for example those with large body mass. Superior clearance of larger solutes or middle molecules, for example, $\beta$-2 microglobulin which is commonly linked to dialysis-related amyloidosis, has been observed with nocturnal dialysis (Pierratos et al., 1998).

With regards to biochemical parameters, potassium and phosphate control is reported as similar in intermittent haemodialysis and short daily haemodialysis, although the use of pharmacological management is often reduced with the latter therapy (Woods et al., 1999; Vos et al., 2001). Nocturnal haemodialysis, however, offers improved control of serum phosphate, with patients able to maintain normal serum phosphate levels without the need for phosphate binders, and a more liberal dietary intake of phosphate is possible [up to 50% more was reported in a study by Musci et al. (1998)].

It may be argued that nocturnal haemodialysis is the more physiological of the two frequent dialysis therapies, but both demonstrate improved outcomes; therefore it may be ideal that both modalities are offered in the future so that patients may choose the most suitable option for themselves.

Several barriers exist to the adoption of daily dialysis (either short daily or slow nocturnal), the main one being cost implications. Others include the effect these therapies may have on access survival, patient acceptance of more frequent dialysis and the feasibility of implementing such programmes.

## *Patient acceptance and feasibility*

Few studies comment on patient acceptance of increasing the frequency of dialysis. Buoncristiani (1998) commented that although this was a concern initially, the majority of patients receiving daily dialysis did so through choice, with the shortness of the session compensating for the increased frequency, and that this had not been a limiting factor in the implementation of the programme.

The number of patients that dialyse at home in the UK is small, with home haemodialysis comprising only 5% of all haemodialysis in England and Wales (Renal Registry, 2001). Adoption of these new methods would require a resurgence in the home dialysis programme, with redevelopment of the support structures required (Pierratos, 2001). In the UK, recently published guidelines from the National Institute of Clinical Excellence (2002) recommend that patients should be offered the choice between home haemodialysis and unit-based haemodialysis. They also give guidance on patient suitability, for example ability and motivation to learn and carry out treatment, support, including hospital support services, the involvement of carers and suitability of the home environment.

There are unique safety issues to consider with a nocturnal dialysis programme; some centres have overcome these with the development of call centres which allow remote monitoring of haemodialysis machines and in some cases patients' vital signs, ensuring that they are responded to appropriately. For frequent home dialysis to be successful, haemodialysis machines that are easy to operate and require minimal time for set-up, take-down and cleaning need to be developed, reducing the time a patient is required to spend on the dialysis procedure. Twardowski (2001) suggests that a built-in water treatment system, a simple dialysate system and a reusable extracorporeal circuit, automatically cleaned and disinfected daily, would be necessary for frequent home haemodialysis to be practical.

*Access survival*

One of the concerns with more frequent dialysis and a potential barrier to the introduction of daily dialysis is the potential role of increased venepuncture and possible trauma to the fistula on access survival. There is little known about the effect more frequent cannulation may have on vascular access dysfunction, with daily dialysis schedules being relatively uncommon practice. Quintaliani et al. (2000) conducted an observational study comparing survival of radiocephalic, arteriovenous fistula in patients dialysing three times a week and patients undergoing daily dialysis. They reported that vascular access survival was not shortened by increased number of punctures in daily dialysis when compared to three times a week dialysis, although the number of patients in the study on daily dialysis was small (24 compared to 124 on three times a week).

Woods et al. (1999) report increased fistula survival, the vascular access failure rate falling from 0.28 per patient year to 0.05 per patient year after starting daily dialysis. The authors postulate that the reason for this could be that as the majority of patients dialyse at home, cannulation is consistently performed by one person compared to a varying number of staff for in-centre dialysis. Another suggestion is that more frequent dialysis is associated with an improvement in the condition of the fistula due to an improvement in uraemic thrombopathy that leads to a decreased tendency for formation of haematomas at the puncture site (Twardowski, 2001).

*Costs*

Another major impediment to frequent dialysis is the limited information about the economic impact that it may have in a climate where resources are limited. NICE (2002) undertook a cost analysis of home versus unit-based haemodialysis, and estimated the total cost to the NHS per year at £19 300 for home haemodialysis compared with £21 000–22 000 for hospital-based haemodialysis. However, this looked at three times a week haemodialysis at home and not frequent (daily or nocturnal) dialysis.

Mohr et al. (2001) conducted a review of the literature on costs of daily haemodialysis, comparing standard intermittent haemodialysis, short daily dialysis and nocturnal dialysis. They found that literature concerning the economics of these modalities was sparse, with the majority of reports not commenting on the financial aspects. The degree of cost alteration is dependent on several factors including whether the dialysis is at home or in-centre, the extent of reuse of dialysers and whether remote monitoring is used for nocturnal dialysis. Mohr et al. developed an economic model based on programmes at two centres in the USA (a short daily programme in California and a nocturnal programme in Virginia), which assumed reuse and no remote monitoring for home patients. They suggested that costs would increase above standard in-centre haemodialysis by 10% for nocturnal dialysis and 20% for in-centre short daily dialysis. However, others suggest that daily home haemodialysis is equivalent or even less expensive than standard in-centre haemodialysis, the cost advantages being reduced hospitalisations, a decrease in pharmacological intervention (in particular antihypertensives and erythro-poietin) and that home dialysis is less expensive than in-centre dialysis (Kooistra and Vos, 1999; Pierratos, 1999; Traeger et al., 2001). Small sample sizes, vari-ability between studies and limitations in the methods mean that further evid-ence of cost effectiveness is required. A measured demonstration of the health benefits against economic impact is necessary to enable clinicians and patients to make comparisons and choices across all treatment options.

In the majority of studies to date, numbers are small and the patients are their own controls, comparing parameters before and after conversion to fre-quent dialysis. Therefore, in the future it will be necessary that appropriate data be collected, ideally in the form of prospective randomised control trials, such that comparisons with current treatment modalities for ERF can be made. This type of study would involve large numbers of patients and take several years to complete; thus the feasibility and funding for such a project are issues as yet unresolved.

Despite the lack of robust clinical trials, results to date overwhelmingly indicate that more frequent dialysis is a superior therapy to the standard dialysis currently used in the majority of countries. It could be asserted that it is not truly ethical to wait for these large trials to be completed before patients are given the opportunity to chose daily haemodialysis therapy as a treatment option when it is likely that the health benefits, including survival, are significant.

## Alternative dialysis therapies

### *Haemodiafiltration*

An alternative strategy to combat the shortcomings of conventional haemo-dialysis treatment is haemodiafiltration (HDF). This modality combines the advantages of haemodialysis and of haemofiltration (HF) in an attempt to achieve a better therapeutic option for patients requiring long-term renal replacement therapy.

Two processes are involved in solute transport across an artificial mem-brane, diffusive and convective solute transport. Diffusive solute transport is predominant in haemodialysis and is rapid for small molecular weight solutes but decreases for increasing molecular size. Solute transport by convection or solvent drag permits increased clearance of middle molecular weight solutes and this is the mechanism of solute transfer in HF (Leypoldt, 2000). Therefore the combination of the two processes, as in HDF, provides for optimal re-moval of both small solutes and middle molecules. An additional advantage of HDF over conventional haemodialysis is improved haemodynamic stability and reduced intradialytic hypotension, due to the incorporation of convective techniques. An example of an on-line HDF machine is shown in Figure 4.1.

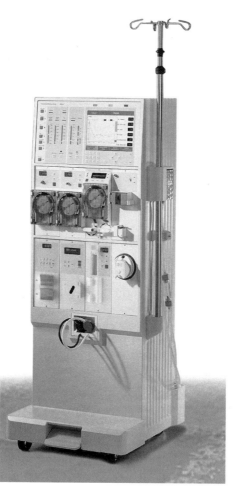

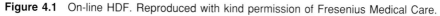

**Figure 4.1** On-line HDF. Reproduced with kind permission of Fresenius Medical Care.

Zehnder et al. (1999) carried out a prospective study evaluating the clearance of small molecules (creatinine, urea and phosphate) and middle molecules (β2 microglobulin) during high flux dialysis and HDF. Sixteen patients received 1 week of standard haemodialysis; then after a 4-week interval they received 1 week of HDF. Filters (1.6-m² polysulfone capillary filters) and duration of treatment were constant for both therapies. The results of their study demonstrated that HDF had no advantage over high flux dialysis with respect to urea and creatinine clearance; however, phosphate removal was markedly increased (from 33 to 41%) with HDF. Reduction rates for serum microglobulin were higher with HDF compared to high flux dialysis; the amount recollected in the dialysate and the ultrafiltrate, however, was unchanged. This was considered to be a consequence of increased adsorption of microglobulin by the membrane during HDF.

**Table 4.1**  Benefits of HDF over HD.

| |
|---|
| • Improved haemodynamic stability |
| • Reduced intradialytic hypotension |
| • Improved clearance of middle molecules |
| • Increased clearance of microglobulin |
| • Improved haemoglobin levels |
| • Improved patient well-being |

In a larger longer-term study, Lin et al. (2001) evaluated microglobulin levels in patients receiving high flux dialysis and HDF. They found that patients receiving HDF had reduced pre-dialysis and post-dialysis microglobulin levels and an increased microglobulin reduction rate when compared with high flux dialysis. The microglobulin reduction rate was positively correlated with the overall volume of replacement solution used per dialysis session.

The clearance of middle molecules is significantly higher during HDF than during high flux dialysis; furthermore, the clearance rate of middle molecules is increased with increased ultrafiltration. New technological advances have led to the development of on-line production of replacement fluid, in which the dialysate, free of pyrogens and toxins, is used as the replacement fluid. This allows the use of larger volumes of substitution fluid, and hence greater ultrafiltration rates and increased middle molecule clearance.

Maduell et al. (1999) evaluated the difference between on-line and conventional HDF in 37 patients who acted as their own controls. They found that tolerance of on-line HDF was good, with no observed pyrogenic reactions and no increase in haemodynamic instability. The delivered dialysis dose was increased for both small and middle molecules, with a significant increase in the microglobulin reduction ratio with on-line HDF. The investigators also found that haemoglobin and haematocrit levels increased significantly with HDF, allowing a reduction in erythropoietin doses.

Despite the known superior efficacy of on-line HDF compared to conventional haemodialysis, it is relatively expensive. Therefore before widespread adoption of HDF as an alternative renal replacement therapy is likely, the clinical advantages and cost effectiveness need to be demonstrated in larger longer-term studies. Table 4.1 summarises the possible benefits of HDF versus traditional HD.

## On-line monitoring in haemodialysis therapy

In recent years technical improvements in the equipment used for chronic haemodialysis patients have been considerable. Many of the developments have focused on improving tolerance of haemodialysis for an increasingly ageing population, with multiple co-morbidity. In order to achieve such improvements several on-line monitoring techniques have been developed. These include the following: urea sensors, to provide real-time urea kinetic measurements; temperature sensors, to target thermal balance throughout dialysis; blood volume sensors; and biofeedback systems to reduce the incidence of intradialytic hypotension.

## Urea clearance monitoring

On-line clearance monitoring is an additional option that may be used during haemodialysis to determine the average effective urea clearance, the dialysis dose (Kt/V) and the plasma sodium concentration. This tool avoids the need for blood sampling and enables real-time measurement of dialysis adequacy, such that termination of a dialysis session could be made on the basis of the Kt/V. Monitoring of other solutes, such as calcium, is also theoretically possible; therefore it is likely that the clinical uses for on-line monitoring systems will grow in the future (Yanai et al., 1998).

## Blood temperature monitoring

Blood temperature monitors (BTMs) consist of sensors that are placed on the arterial and venous lines of the extracorporeal circuit and can be used in a number of different ways during haemodialysis. BTM can be used to measure access recirculation, to improve haemodynamic stability in hypotensive-prone patients and to control thermal energy balance. One of the functions of blood temperature monitoring is to allow the thermal energy balance of a patient throughout a dialysis session to be controlled. Temperature control during haemodialysis may be used to minimise negative thermal energy balance (i.e. energy loss through the extracorporeal circuit) or for progressive cooling of a hyperthermic patient. The BTM can also be used to calculate recirculation in the vascular access using a thermodilution method. This method is based on a transient change in dialysate temperature, which changes the blood temperature returning to the patient by the venous circuit; this is compared with the arterial temperature and recirculation can be quantified (Schneditz et al., 1999). It is a more immediate and convenient method than measuring recirculation by the urea or ultrasound Doppler technique.

   There has been particular interest in blood temperature sensors for control of energy balance in critically ill patients who require renal replacement therapy. The BTM control algorithm allows the desired amount of thermal energy (in kilojoules per hour) to be fed to or withdrawn from the patient, to be programmed by the user (Rahmati et al., 2001). Additionally, temperature regulation may be used to improve haemodynamic stability during routine haemodialysis. Episodes, of intradialytic hypotension may be partly induced by changes in blood temperature in the extracorporeal circuit. Van der Sande et al. (1999) studied blood pressure and thermal energy transfer in nine patients receiving routine haemodialysis therapy, comparing standard (37.5°C) and cool (35.5°C) dialysate temperatures. Core temperature increased during standard temperature dialysis but did not change during cool temperature dialysis. Systolic blood pressure decreased to a greater extent during standard temperature dialysis compared with cool dialysis. The authors suggest that haemodialysis affects core temperature regulation, which is likely to impact on the vascular response during ultrafiltration such that the autoregulatory mechanisms related to maintaining core temperature may be responsible for the improved haemodynamic stability during cool dialysis.

In practice, blood temperature monitoring is a useful tool for gaining immediate information about access recirculation and is more accurate than the conventional urea method. For this use, purchase of one or two monitors allows recirculation measurements to be carried out on a reasonable number of patients over a relatively short period of time. Control of thermal energy balance is likely to be less useful in the chronic haemodialysis setting, but may prove of value in improving haemodynamic stability in hypotensive-prone patients. Similarly for this purpose it would not be necessary to have the BTM facility on every machine.

## Blood volume monitoring

Several devices have been recently developed to continuously monitor changes in blood volume during haemodialysis. A limit to all of the systems designed to measure blood volume is that they only supply a percentage and not an absolute blood volume. At present, absolute blood volume can only be measured by the injection of tracers into the vascular system, an invasive method that is not suitable for routine use. The non-invasive devices used for blood volume measurement during haemodialysis determine relative blood volume (RBV). RBV is the current blood volume (BV) divided by the blood volume at the beginning of the dialysis treatment, expressed as a percentage (Jaeger and Mehta, 1999):

$$\% \ RBV = \frac{current \ BV}{BV \ at \ start \ of \ treatment}$$

Recent interest has focused on blood volume monitoring (BVM) as a method to assist weight assessment and to reduce the occurrence of intradialytic symptoms. It is a method that is practical, non-invasive and relatively inexpensive, that can be used routinely for every patient during each haemodialysis session by non-specialist staff.

Techniques developed for continuous on-line measurement of BV during haemodialysis use a variety of different methods, including centrifugation, densitometry, conductivity, viscometry, optical methods and ultrasonic sound speed measurement. All of these devices make use of the fact that certain blood components, such as blood cells and plasma proteins, remain confined to the vascular compartment. Plasma water moves freely between compartments, and therefore the BV can be measured from the concentration change of the aforementioned blood constituents.

BVM has been used to detect both under- and over-hydration of patients on haemodialysis. A limitation of BVM in this setting is in the standardisation of the technique, as is particularly the case when using a blood volume monitor to reduce the incidence of dialysis-induced hypotension. Krepel et al. (2000) found considerable intra- and inter-individual variability in RBV changes in a study of 10 chronic haemodialysis patients using haematocrit measurement. The investigators found that the variability could not be explained by ultrafiltration volume alone. Different patients and disease states will result in different levels of vascular refilling, making standardisation difficult. Oliver et al. (2001) monitored intradialytic blood volume changes in a study investigating the impact of sodium and ultrafiltration profiling on haemodialysis-related symptoms. They found that neither the blood volume decrease nor the rate of decrease to be significantly associated with symptomatic dialysis sessions. The principle of its use in this context is that there is a critical level of RBV below which hypotension will occur; control of the ultrafiltration profile, for example by a closed feedback loop, so that this level is avoided may reduce the unwanted clinical side effects of ultrafiltration. The inter- and intra-patient variability of blood volume contraction means that in practice definition of the critical blood volume for each patient is difficult to attain.

Recent work has shown that BVM may also be used to detect over-hydration caused by overestimation of dry weight. Although blood volume monitors cannot be used to determine dry weight directly, continuous monitoring of blood volume can be used to detect fluid overload because changes in RBV are small in haemodialysis patients who are over-hydrated (Leypoldt and Cheung, 1998).

The RBV during haemodialysis depends on two processes, ultrafiltration and plasma refill; ultrafiltration is dependent upon the volume of fluid to be removed during that dialysis session, while plasma refill is patient specific and is affected by many variables. Plasma refill capacity depends upon several factors including dialysate buffer, plasma osmolarity and tissue hydration state (De Vries et al., 1993). It is the relationship between refill capacity and the hydration state of the tissue that is of importance when considering blood volume measurement and over-hydration of dialysis patients.

The plasma refill capacity of a patient is related to the hydration state of the interstitium. When extracellular volume is excessive, as a result of fluid overload, removal of fluid from blood will produce small changes in blood volume because of rapid refilling from the extracellular space. The more hydrated the interstitium is the more rapid and greater the capacity for refilling, resulting in a smaller decrease in BV for a given ultrafiltration rate (Steuer et al., 1996).

To date there has been little research utilising continuous blood volume monitoring as a screening tool for over-hydrated dialysis patients; however, studies that have been conducted in this field report clinically significant findings.

Steuer et al. (1998) observed blood volume profiles in 56 patients on maintenance haemodialysis; all were considered to be at dry weight by physical examination. Ten out of the 56 patients were found to have a small decrease in blood volume profile (less than 5%) during the first phase of the study. The investigators intentionally increased dialytic fluid removal in these patients in the second phase. This intervention led to an increased ultrafiltrated volume by 47% and a decreased dry weight in six out of the ten patients, with a low incidence of intradialytic symptoms. The reason for patients not being able to tolerate additional fluid removal was attributed to incompetent cardiovascular systems.

Lopot and Kotyk (1997) identified two components to blood volume reduction, a static component and a dynamic component. External factors influencing the static component of blood volume reduction during haemodialysis include the ultrafiltrated volume and the degree of over-hydration. The dominant internal or patient factor is compliance of the cardiovascular system. In patients with low cardiovascular compliance (for example those with diabetes and congestive cardiac failure), the blood volume could not diminish substantially. Patients with high cardiovascular compliance will accommodate part of their interdialytic water load in the intravascular space, whereas those with low cardiovascular compliance will keep the whole interdialytic load in their interstitial space.

Despite the difficulties of standardisation, employment of continuous blood volume monitoring as part of routine haemodialysis treatment may assist in the recognition of patients who may be over-hydrated and may improve tolerance of treatment by reducing the incidence of intradialytic hypotension.

## Sodium and ultrafiltration profiling

Despite technical advances in the field, the combination of short efficient haemodialysis sessions and an ageing population requiring renal replacement therapy means that patients are still symptomatic on dialysis. These typical haemodialysis-related side effects include symptomatic hypotension, cramps, thirst and osmotic disequilibrium syndrome, which is characterised clinically by headache, high blood pressure, nausea and vomiting (Mann and Stiller, 2000). Symptomatic hypotension occurs when the rate of ultrafiltration exceeds the rate of plasma refilling (Jaeger and Mehta, 1999). The unwanted side effects of osmotic disequilibrium syndrome can be explained by shifts of water during dialysis between blood and dialysis fluid and between the intracellular and extracellular fluid compartments. It is said to occur when the plasma sodium concentration decreases by more than 7 mmol/l (Guerich et al., 1980).

One technique which can minimise the occurrence of these side effects is profiled dialysis, which consists of the use of dialysis profiles aimed at maintaining stable intradialytic plasma osmolality by modulation of sodium and water removal during dialysis treatments (Splendiani et al., 2001).

There is much practical experience concerning ultrafiltration (UF) profiling, which shows that patients better tolerate higher rates of ultrafiltration at the beginning of dialysis. If the UF rate is low at the end of dialysis then the risk of symptomatic hypotension is reduced; however, even with profiled UF, hypotension will still occur if the UF rate exceeds the plasma-refilling rate (Mann and Stiller, 1996). A variety of UF profiles are available including linear decreasing, stepwise decreasing and intermittent high UF rates with UF pauses. Donauer et al. (2000) followed up 188 dialysis sessions in 53 patients and evaluated the incidence of symptomatic hypotension. They found that a linear decreasing profile showed a reduced incidence of hypotension (5.7%) compared with a constant UF rate (10.6%). The UF profiles using intermittently high UF pulses led to an increased incidence of hypotension (18.4%).

Sodium profiling aims to minimise osmotic disequilibrium by avoiding acute declines in plasma osmolality and to improve plasma refilling, thereby reducing the side effects of UF of large amounts of fluid. During sodium profiled dialysis the sodium content of the dialysis fluid is varied throughout the course of the treatment. A wide variety of sodium profiles have been used, for example decreasing, increasing and alternating, with different forms including linear, stepwise and exponential. Decreasing profiles have most commonly been utilised, taking advantage of using high sodium concentrations at the beginning of dialysis to enhance plasma refilling when ultrafiltration is highest.

There are also different profiles with respect to sodium balance: balance neutral profiles do not change the net sodium shift at the end of dialysis, sodium positive profiles result in increased plasma osmolality and sodium negative profiles lead to sodium loss (Stiller et al., 2001). The risks associated with sodium profiling are related to sodium accumulation, which may lead to thirst, increased interdialytic weight gain and hypertension (Sang et al., 1997). Song et al. (2002) investigated the relationship between time-averaged concentration of dialysate sodium (TACNa) and sodium load during profiled dialysis. They found that TACNa was a factor in determining sodium load and interdialytic complications such as interdialytic weight gain, blood pressure and thirst.

In a review of 22 clinical studies by Stiller et al. (2001) the majority of studies were of insufficient length to give insight into the long-term effect of sodium profiling. Only eight of the 22 studies were for periods of more than 2 weeks and of these all had positive sodium balances: two reported an increase in dry weight, four found patients had increased thirst and two reported an increase in serum sodium. The positive effects of sodium profiling that were suggested in these studies included: a reduced incidence of intradialytic hypotension, less reduction in relative blood volume, increased plasma refilling and less intradialytic saline infusions.

Oliver et al. (2001) reported positive effects of combined sodium and ultrafiltration profiling with significantly reduced haemodialysis-related symptoms. Twenty nine patients completed the study protocol and were randomised to a two-treatment crossover protocol of either standard or profiled dialysis. The profiled dialysis consisted of an exponential decrease in dialysate sodium from 152 mmol/l to 142 mmol/l, with an exponentially decreasing UF rate. The standard dialysis protocol consisted of constant dialysate sodium at 142 mmol/l and a constant UF rate. They found a significant reduction in the occurrence of hypotension in the profiled treatments compared with the standard treatments (20.4% and 30.6% respectively). The patients also reported significantly less intradialytic symptoms during the profiled treatments. Negative effects of profiled dialysis were also reported: post-dialysis serum sodium was significantly increased and pre-dialysis weight was significantly increased by a mean of 0.3 kg. There was, however, no difference in post-dialysis weight and pre- or post-dialysis blood pressure.

Splendiani et al. (2001) trialed a new model of sodium profiled dialysis, which they termed as the 'bell pattern'. Eight patients were observed for two periods of 4 weeks, each comparing standard dialysis (constant ultrafiltration and dialysate sodium) with profiled dialysis (progressive decrease of ultrafiltration and variable dialysate sodium). The dialysate sodium profile was individualised and varied from 140±3 mmol/l in the first hour to 145±4 mmol/l in the second hour and then to 138±4 mmol/l at the end of dialysis. Despite the small sample size, clinically important results were reported. The investigators found that during profiled dialysis the mean arterial pressure was more stable, plasma refilling occurred during the second and third hour of dialysis and significantly fewer hypotensive episodes occurred.

It is worth noting that the effect of sodium profiling on the extracellular fluid volume is small when compared to the reduction caused by ultrafiltration. For example, a rise of 1 mmol/l in the sodium concentration of the extracellular space will only result in an expansion of 130 ml, only 30 ml of which is in the intravascular compartment (Stiller et al., 2001). Hence sodium profiling will not entirely overcome intradialytic symptoms caused by UF of large fluid volumes, but if conducted correctly by maintaining a neutral sodium balance in the long term, it may be effective in alleviating some symptoms in hypotensive-prone patients. Mathematical models are now available to assist in the prediction of plasma sodium levels that may result from the use of various sodium profiles. In addition, the technology now exists to enable monitoring of sodium flux on-line, based on conductivity measurements of plasma and dialysate fluid (Splendiani et al., 2001; Stiller et al., 2001). In the future, biofeedback systems integrated with technology that accurately monitors sodium flux and profile may facilitate more precise and effective use of the concept of a more physiological dialysis.

## Summary

Many of the technical and practical developments discussed go some way to offering improvements to the patient experience of haemodialysis and may assist in improving morbidity and mortality in haemodialysis patients. For example, use of blood volume monitoring to detect inadequately high dry weight may reduce the incidence of chronic volume overload, hypertension and cardiovascular morbidity. Blood temperature monitoring allows for convenient accurate measurement of access recirculation and access blood flow, and therefore enables early intervention for problematic access, which may reduce the use of temporary access and increase access longevity.

Practical implications for many of the developments discussed revolve around finance and education. Staff education is required alongside implementation of these technical developments such that safe and effective use is ensured. Some cost implications may be offset in the long term by improved patient health, for example in frequent haemodialysis, but in many areas further evidence is required before investment in new technology is realistic.

# References

Buoncristiani, U. (1998) Fifteen years of clinical experience with daily dialysis. *Nephrology Dialysis Transplantation* **13** (Suppl 6), 148–51.

Buoncristiani, U., Fagugli, R., Ciao, G., Ciucci, A., Carobi, C., Quintaliani, G. and Pasini, P. (1999) Left ventricular hypertrophy in daily dialysis. *Mineral Electrolyte Metabolism* **25**, 90–94.

Charra, B., Laurent, G., Chazot, C., Calemard, E., Terrat, J.-C., Vanel, T., Jean, G. and Ruffet, M. (1996) Clinical assessment of dry weight. *Nephrology Dialysis Transplantation* **11**, 16–19.

De Vries, J.-P., Bogaard, H.-J., Kouw, P., Oe, L., Stevens, P. and De Vries, P. (1993) The adjustment of post-dialytic dry weight based on non-invasive measurement of extracellular fluid and blood volumes. *ASAIO Journal* **39**, M368–72.

Donauer, J., Kolbin, D., Bek, M., Krause, A. and Bohler, J. (2000) Ultrafiltration profiling and measurement of relative blood volume as strategies to reduce haemodialysis-related side effects. *American Journal of Kidney Diseases* **36** (1), 115–23.

Guerich, W., Mann, H. and Stiller, S. (1980) Sodium elimination and change in the EEG during dialysis. *Artificial Organs* **3** (Suppl 3), 94–8.

Jaeger, J. and Mehta, R. (1999) Assessment of dry weight in haemodialysis. An overview. *Journal of the American Society of Nephrology* **10** (2), 1046–66.

Kjellstrand, C.M. (2001) Rationale for daily haemodialysis. *ASAIO Journal* **47** (5), 438–42.

Kooistra, M. and Vos, P. (1999) Daily home haemodialysis: towards a more physiological treatment of patients with ESRD. *Seminars in Dialysis* **12**, 424–30.

Krepel, H., Nette, R., Akcahuseyin, E., Weimar, W. and Zietse, R. (2000) Variability of relative blood volume during haemodialysis. *Nephrology Dialysis Transplantation* **15**, 673–9.

Lacson, E. and Diaz-Buxo, J. (2001) Daily and nocturnal haemodialysis: how do they stack up? *American Journal of Kidney Diseases* **38** (2), 225–39.

Laurent, G. and Charra, B. (1998) The results of an eight-hour thrice weekly haemodialysis schedule. *Nephrology Dialysis Transplantation* **13** (Suppl 6), 125–31.

Leypoldt, J. (2000) Solute fluxes in different treatment modalities. *Nephrology Dialysis Transplantation* **15** (Suppl 1), 3–9.

Leypoldt, J. and Cheung, A. (1998) Evaluating volume status in haemodialysis patients. *Advances in Renal Replacement Therapy* **5** (1), 64–74.

Lin, C.C., Yang, C.W., Chiang, C.C., Chang, C.T. and Huang, C.C. (2001) Long-term haemodiafiltration reduces pre-dialysis beta-2-microglobulin levels in chronic haemodialysis patients. *Blood Purification* **19**, 301–307.

Lindsay, R. and Kortas, C. (2001) Hemeral (daily) haemodialysis. *Advances in Renal Replacement Therapy* **8** (4), 236–49.

Lopot, F. and Kotyk, P. (1997) Computational analysis of blood volume dynamics during haemodialysis. *International Journal of Artificial Organs* **29** (2), 91–5.

Luik, A., Kooman, J. and Leunissen, K. (1997) Hypertension in haemodialysis patients: is it only hypervolaemia? *Nephrology Dialysis Transplantation* **12**, 1557–9.

Maduell, F., Pozo, C., Garcia, H., Sanchez, L., Hdez-Jaras, J., Albero, M., Calvo, C., Torregrosa, I. and Navarro, V. (1999) Change from conventional haemodiafiltration to on-line haemodiafiltration. *Nephrology Dialysis Transplantation* **14**, 1202–1207.

Mann, H. and Stiller, S. (1996) Urea, sodium and water changes in profiling dialysis. *Nephrology Dialysis Transplantation* **11** (Suppl 8), 10–15.

Mann, H. and Stiller, S. (2000) Sodium modelling. *Kidney International* **58** (Suppl 76), 79–88.

Maria, R., Reboldi, G., Quintaliani, G., Pasini, P., Ciao, G., Cicconi, B., Pasticci, F., Kaufman, J.M. and Buoncristiani, U. (2001) Short daily haemodialysis: blood pressure control and left ventricular mass reduction in hypertensive haemodialysis patients. *American Journal of Kidney Diseases* **38** (2), 371–6.

Mohr, P., Neumann, P., Franco, S., Marainen, J., Lockridge, R. and Ting, G. (2001) The case for daily dialysis: its impact on costs and quality of life. *American Journal of Kidney Diseases* **37** (4), 777–89.

Musci, I., Hercz, G., Uldall, R., Ouwendyk, M., Francoeur, R. and Pierratos, A. (1998) Control of serum phosphate without any phosphate binders in patients treated with nocturnal haemodialysis. *Kidney International* **53** (5), 1399–1404.

National Institute for Clinical Excellence (NICE) (2002) *National Institute for Clinical Excellence (NICE) Guidelines.* www.nice.org.uk.

Oliver, M., Edwards, L. and Churchill, D. (2001) Impact of sodium and ultrafiltration profiling on haemodialysis related symptoms. *Journal of the American Society of Nephrology* **12**, 151–6.

Pierratos, A. (1999) Nocturnal home haemodialysis: an update on a 5-year experience. *Nephrology Dialysis Transplantation* **14**, 2835–40.

Pierratos, A. (2001) Introduction: entering the era of daily haemodialysis. *Advances in Renal Replacement Therapy* **8** (4), 223–6.

Pierratos, A., Ouwendyk, M., Francoeur, R., Vas, S., Raj, D.S., Ecclestone, A.M., Langos, V. and Uldall, R. (1998) Nocturnal haemodialysis: three year experience. *Journal of American Society of Nephrology* **9** (5), 899–900.

Quintaliani, G., Buoncristiani, U., Fagugli, R., Kuluriani, H., Ciao, G., Rondini, L., Lowenthal, D. and Reboldi, G. (2000) Survival of vascular access during daily and three times a week haemodialysis. *Clinical Nephrology* **53** (5), 327–77.

Rahmati, S., Ronco, F., Spittle, M., Morris, A., Schleper, C., Rosales, L., Kuafman, A., Amerling, R., Ronco, C. and Levin, N. (2001) Validation of the blood temperature monitor for extracorporeal thermal energy balance during in vitro continuous haemodialysis. *Blood Purification* **19**, 245–50.

Renal Registry (2001) *Fourth Annual Report.* UK Renal Registry, Bristol.

Sang, G.L., Kovithavongs, C., Ulan, R. and Kjellstrand, C.M. (1997) Sodium ramping in haemodialysis: a study of beneficial and adverse effects. *American Journal of Kidney Diseases* **29**, 669–79.

Schneditz, D., Wang, E. and Levin, N. (1999) Validation of haemodialysis recirculation and access blood flow measured by thermodilution. *Nephrology Dialysis Transplantation* **14**, 376–83.

Song, J.H., Lee, S.W., Suh, C.K. and Kim, M.J. (2002) Time-averaged concentration of dialysate sodium relates with sodium load and interdialytic weight gain during sodium-profiling haemodialysis. *American Journal of Kidney Diseases* **40** (2), 291–301.

Splendiani, G., Costanzi, S., Passalacqua, S., Fulignati, P. and Sturniolo, A. (2001) Sodium and fluid modulation in dialysis: a new approach. *Nephron* **89** (4), 377–80.

Steuer, R., Bell, D. and Conis, J. (1996) Incidence of high prescribed dry weights and intradialytic morbidity as detected by continuous volume monitoring. *Nephrology Dialysis Transplantation* **11**, A197.

Steuer, R., Germain, M., Leypoldt, J. and Cheung, A. (1998) Enhanced fluid removal guided by blood volume monitoring during chronic haemodialysis. *Artificial Organs* **22** (8), 627–32.

Stiller, S., Bonnie-Schorn, E., Grassman, A., Uhlenbusch-Kower, I. and Mann, H. (2001) A critical review of sodium profiling for haemodialysis. *Seminars in Dialysis* **14** (5), 337–47.

Traeger, J., Galland, R. and Arkouche, W. (2001) Short daily haemodialysis: a four-year experience. *Dialysis and Transplant* **30**, 76–86.

Twardowski, Z. (2001) Daily dialysis: is this a reasonable option for the new millennium? *Nephrology Dialysis Transplantation* **16**, 1321–4.

Van der Sande, F.M., Kooman, J.P., Burema, J.H., Hammeleers, P., Kerkhos, A.M., Barendregt, J.M. and Leunissen, K.M. (1999) Effect of dialysate temperature on energy balance during haemodialysis: quantification of extracorporeal energy transfer. *American Journal of Kidney Diseases* **33** (6), 1115–21.

Vanholder, R., Veys, N., Van Biesen, W. and Lameire, N. (2002) Alternative timeframes for haemodialysis. *Artificial Organs* **26** (2), 160–162.

Vos, P., Zilch, O. and Kooistra, M. (2001) Clinical outcome of daily dialysis. *American Journal of Kidney Diseases* **37** (Suppl 2), S99–102.

Woods, J., Port, F., Orzol, S., Buoncristiani, U., Young, E., Wolfe, R. and Held, P. (1999) Clinical and biochemical correlates of starting daily haemodialysis. *Kidney International* **55**, 2467–76.

Yanai, M., Kihara, K., Yamada, A., Takahashi, S. and Sugino, N. (1998) A newly developed on-line monitoring system for the determination of serum electrolytes and urea during haemodialysis. *Artificial Organs* **22** (12), 1010–13.

Zehnder, C., Gutzwiller, J.P. and Renggli, K. (1999) Haemodiafiltration – a new treatment option for hyperphosphataemia in haemodialysis patients. *Clinical Nephrology* **52** (3), 152–9.

# Chapter 5
# Advances in Peritoneal Dialysis

*Althea Mahon*

## Introduction

In the UK, peritoneal dialysis (PD) is a well-established therapy option and is used for approximately 35% of new patients requiring dialysis. PD provides a treatment option for a wide variety of patients, with patient survival for PD equivalent to that for haemodialysis over the first 2–4 years (Fenton, 1997; Keshaviah et al., 2002). This chapter will discuss and outline the current trends and innovations in PD.

## PD catheters

Since the development of the Tenckhoff catheter (Tenckhoff et al., 1968), there have been further developments in both the design and insertion techniques of PD catheters. The main focus has been on the reduction of the incidence of exit site infections and peritonitis, the provision of efficient dialysate flow, and the prevention of catheter migration and malfunction. There are many catheter variations such as the arcuate swan neck, straight or coiled Tenckhoff, the Toronto-Western, the use of one or two cuffs, and a straight or curled intraperitoneal section to the catheter.

Placement of catheters has also evolved and current techniques used include via surgical laparotomy (with a paramedium or median incision) and percutaneous or laparoscopic insertion. Laparoscopic techniques have also been successfully used to rescue malfunctioning catheters (Ogunc, 2002). Exit sites which are traditionally located in the abdomen can also be located in the thoracic region, which is especially effective for obese patients. The use of the pre-sternal swan-neck peritoneal catheter (which is made up of two silicone rubber catheters joined together by a titanium connector when implanted and with the exit site situated in the chest region) has been studied. The results of 974 catheters implanted worldwide and followed over 130 patient months found that, not surprisingly, the dialysate flow was slower due to the increase in catheter length, they tended to have fewer exit site and tunnel infections and they were ideal for the overweight, incontinent patients or those with a stoma. The authors also suggest that it is a better catheter for those patients who are at risk of psychological problems related to altered body image (Twardowski, 2002).

The T-fluted (Ash Advantage) PD catheter, which has segments with long flutes as the fluid ports rather than the standard 1-mm-diameter holes, is also under clinical trial. Initial results show that outflow rates were higher than that of the Tenckhoff catheter. Further data are required, but a recent study carried out on 18 patients with a follow-up of 8.4 months suggests that this catheter may reduce omental attachment, catheter extrusion, peri-catheter hernias and leaks (Ash et al., 2002).

Lastly, the Moncrief-Popovich catheter and implantation technique involves embedding the external segment of the catheter in the tunnel for 6–8 weeks before use and results suggest a reduction in peri-catheter and exit site infections. This is due to the healing of the catheter cuffs prior to creation of an exit site (Dasgupta, 2002b).

The LifeSite® PD access system is currently under trial within the UK; however, no results have been published to date. In principle it is the same as the haemodialysis version, which involves the implantation of a stainless-steel/titanium valve and silicone cannula, which is placed in the subcutaneous tissue pocket. The patient can choose the site, which varies from abdomen to chest. The device is then cannulated and the standard PD or APD (automated peritoneal dialysis) system can be connected via an adaptor (Haynes et al., 2002). An ongoing study (Steele at al., 2001) has shown that patient acceptance of the LifeSite® PD access system is very positive and no patient has yet to decline to participate in the study ($N = 19$) because of the requirement to self-cannulate as part of the procedure (see Figure 5.1).

## New catheter material

Along with different types of catheter insertion are the new developments in catheter material, which continue to aim at reducing biofilm formation and the associated complications with silastic catheters. Among the new materials are hydroxyapatite and silver-coated catheters. Silver-coated catheters are biocompatible and prevent colonisation as they possess antibacterial activity. However, in animal studies it was found that the silver was released from the catheter and as a result they are not safe for patients (Dasgupta, 1997, 2000a). There are also limited data on hydroxyapatite-coated catheters. Both of these new catheter materials are still in the clinical trial phase, but there may be developments in the future.

## Exit site care

The Renal Association (2002) recommends the use of mupirocin 2% ointment for regular exit site care. It is widely accepted that nasal and peri-catheter

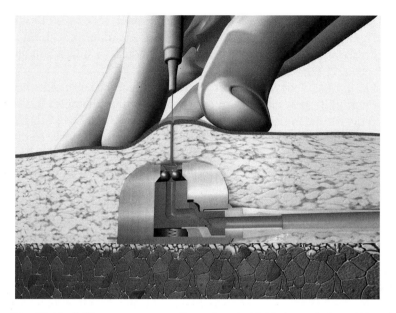

**Figure 5.1**   LifeSite® PD access system. Reproduced with kind permission of VascA Inc.

colonisation by *Staphylococcus aureus* (*S. aureus*) is associated with an increased risk of peritonitis and exit site infections in patients on PD (Piraino, 2000; Ritzau et al., 2001).

The use of a topical application of mupirocin has become the treatment of choice in the management of *S. aureus* carriage in PD patients and has demonstrated its efficacy at eradicating this bacterium. However, recolonisation is common and patients often require further treatments (Perez-Fontan et al., 1993). Although the current recommendations are to use mupirocin prophylactically, many UK units are failing to do this due to concerns regarding the development of antimicrobial resistance, which have been reported in recent papers (Annigeri et al., 2001; Perez-Fontan et al., 2002). Although evidence is available that mupirocin can cause resistance, it should not be excluded as an option, so long as adequate strategies are in place such as identifying and monitoring the cases of resistance to ensure early detection (Conly and Vas, 2002).

## *Biofilms*

Biofilm bacterial infections are common in patients undergoing PD and are responsible for recurrent peritonitis, with the subsequent loss of catheter and technique failure (Dasgupta and Costerton, 1989). Factors that regulate biofilm formation are skin bacteria which colonise catheters, the catheter material itself which may allow bacteria to adhere to it, and the PD environment that provides optimal conditions for growth of biofilm bacterial colonies. Further clinical studies have indicated that biofilms are associated with recurrent peritonitis and catheter-related infections. As biofilms tend to be resistant to antibiotic therapy they are frequently associated with technique failure (Dasgupta et al., 1991).

Unfortunately, few drugs penetrate the biofilm layer, which is needed for them to act directly on the biofilm bacteria. The current recommended antibiotics are rifampicin, which is effective against staphylococcal biofilms, and which has a synergistic effect with other antibiotics, such as vancomycin and ciprofloxacin; there has also been some success with the use of thrombolytic agents such as urokinase and streptokinase to lyse biofilms; this in turn allows the antibiotic to penetrate and has been used for recurrent peritonitis (Worland et al., 1998). However, the use of streptokinase and urokinase can be associated with adverse effects and may not be easily available. Tissue plasminogen activators (tPA) can be used as an alternative and have been used successfully (Dutch and Yee, 2001).

Endoluminal brushes to re-establish flow in PD catheters have been used by some units and have been suggested as an alternative to urokinase to improve the flow of the catheter. They have also been used to remove the biofilm in patients with recurrent peritonitis. The endoluminal brush is a metal wire with a brush tip of nylon bristles, which is inserted into the lumen of the catheter to remove debris. However, there are few studies of large enough patient numbers to validate this as an effective treatment (Figueiredo et al., 2000; Tranter, 2002).

## PD solutions

Glucose-based solutions are widely accepted and used as osmotic agents in the prescription regime of patients requiring PD. For many years they were the preferred choice of osmotic agent due to the low level of toxicity, free availability and low cost. However, the long-term disadvantages of using conventional glucose-based solutions are becoming more evident, and these include the fast absorption of glucose through the peritoneal membrane, which can result in the loss of ultrafiltration and the metabolic complications of hyperglycaemia, hyperinsulinaemia, hyperlipidaemia and obesity. Glucose-based solutions are acidic, with a pH of approximately 5.3, which is kept low to prevent caramelisation of the glucose during the heat sterilisation process. These solutions have a high osmolality of 340–486 mOsm/kg, and a high glucose concentration of between 1.36 and 4.5%. All of these factors have been shown to affect the viability of the peritoneal macrophages and mesothelial cells.

Conventional PD fluid contains acidic lactate buffering solution. The lactate concentration of 40 mM required as the buffering system and the high glucose concentration and high osmolality are necessary to provide an osmotic gradient required for ultrafiltration. So, although the components may have a long-term negative effect at cellular level, they are essential for ultrafiltration and stability of the solution.

The result of the heat sterilisation process of the glucose-containing solutions is that they contain bioactive metabolites known as glucose degradation products (GDPs). These occur as a result of the breakdown of glucose during this process, which has been shown to affect cell function, and are responsible for the formation of advanced glycation end products (AGEs), which have been shown in both in-vitro and in-vivo studies. AGEs are formed during the non-enzymatic reaction of sugars and protein together. The long-term use of these glucose-based solutions has been linked to the structural and functional changes that occur in peritoneal membranes, such as the progression of interstitial fibrosis and vascular sclerosis, increased glucose absorption and the subsequent loss in ultrafiltration capacity (Henderson et al., 1986; Tauer et al., 2003).

The use of a high lactate concentration in a solution combined with a low pH may lead to impaired cellular function (Mackenzie et al., 1998) and also be the cause of infusion pain during dialysis (Mactier et al., 1998). If a more biocompatible solution is being sought, it should not affect the structure and/ or function of the peritoneum. This is the ideal solution that most companies are searching for. In other words, a solution that is identical to the body's extracellular composition is required.

Data from recent clinical trials using PD-Bio® and Physioneal® suggest true in-vivo effects, although more evidence is required of the long-term benefits of these solutions. The idea is to replace the current lactate-based solutions such as Dianeal® and glucose concentrations with alternative osmotic agents, e.g. icodextrin (polyglucose) and amino acid solutions. The aim is for new solutions to provide a neutral or near-neutral pH; this is achieved by either replacing the lactate as a buffer and/or using dual-chamber bags. In this case the glucose can be sterilised separately. Solutions such as bicarbonate, bicarbonate in combination with glycyl-glycerine or lactate, or conventional lactate solutions are at a pH of 6.8. Physioneal® maintains a normal intraperitoneal pH whereas conventional lactate solutions require up to 120 minutes for the intraperitoneal pH to reach 7.4 or physiologic level (Heimburger et al., 1998). Its use is associated with a significant reduction of inflow pain and/or discomfort in sensitive patients (Coles et al., 1998; Mactier et al., 1998) and it has a high potential for improved long-term preservation of the peritoneal membrane. This then provides the advantage of lower GDP levels as the need to sterilise glucose at a low pH is removed. So, as mentioned before, the formation of GDPs is strongly related to the pH of the fluid, and this can be counterbalanced by the development of new PD fluid using double chamber bags.

The bag itself is easy to use and comes as a two-chambered format. The top chamber contains a solution of dextrose, calcium chloride and magnesium chloride, and the bottom chamber contains a solution of sodium bicarbonate, sodium lactate and sodium chloride. When the frangible seal between the chambers is broken, both solutions are mixed together and can then be infused into the patient.

## Icodextrin

Although icodextrin 7.5% has been around for many years and is commonly used, it is worthwhile reviewing its properties. It is a glucose polymer and has been used successfully in both PD and APD patients for long dwells (12–16 hours), with the effect of sustained ultrafiltration (Mistry et al., 1994; Woodrow et al., 1999). This is an iso-osmolar solution (284 mOsm/kg), has a pH of 5.3 and provides an equivalent ultrafiltration (UF) capacity to a high-glucose dialysate bag. UF by colloid osmosis is achieved due to the high molecular and reflection coefficient, with the transport of water occurring through the small pore and ultra-small pore system. However, glucose solutions are believed to act on the ultra-small transcellular pores (Mistry et al., 1987; Krediet et al., 1997). Some of the icodextrin is absorbed and metabolised to smaller oligosaccharide breakdown products, such as disaccharide maltose. The normal metabolism of maltose to glucose occurs in the kidney and in the diseased kidney maltose cannot be metabolised. A steady state of maltose occurs after 2 weeks and is removed by the use of non-icodextrin dialysis exchanges. This solution has no side effects; however, it is only licensed for one exchange per day to prevent maltose buildup. There are also lower levels of AGE formation than with glucose solutions and this has allowed for an extension of time on PD therapy for those patients with UF failure (Dawnay and Millar, 1997; Wilkie et al., 1997; Posthuma et al., 2001).

The nursing consideration with this solution is the need to reduce or alter insulin regimes, especially if the solution is used as an overnight exchange. There have been reports of patients experiencing hypoglycaemic episodes, although their glucometer reads a normal blood sugar level. Some glucometer systems that do not use a glucose dehydrogenase enzyme will detect maltose and produce false positive readings (Mehmet et al., 2001).

Recent publications have highlighted the problems of sterile peritonitis associated with the use of icodextrin solutions. Patients may complain of mild abdominal pain and allergic and hypersensitivity reactions, including misty dialysate bags (Fletcher et al., 1998; Lam-Po-Tang et al., 1997). Many units stop the icodextrin solution if sterile peritonitis is suspected and then re-trial at a later date. If the problem persists, stopping icodextrin altogether is advised.

## Amino acid solutions

Although these solutions have existed for some time, there are many mixed views on whether they are effective. Many patients who commence PD are already malnourished. PD patients lose approximately 3–4 g/day of amino acids and 8–15 g/day of protein, and this is further increased during an episode of peritonitis. Taylor et al. (2002) studied the use of an amino-acid solution on 22 patients over a 30-month period and found that it was safe to use for extended periods, and was associated with a reduced incidence of peritonitis and mortality rate. The use of amino acids in conjunction with glucose solutions is possible and safe for use in APD therapy (Canepa et al., 2001).

# Ultrafiltration failure (UFF)

One of the major complications of PD is UFF. This is responsible for a large proportion of patients requiring transfer to haemodialysis, although it is well recognised that UFF is underestimated in the PD population.

There are three types of UFF: rapid solute transport (membrane failure), a combination of poor UF and small solute transport failure, normal solute transport with catheter malfuntion or leakage of dialysate.

## Type 1: rapid solute transport (also known as membrane failure)

This is the most common of the three types, and is characterised by increased peritoneal transport of low molecular weight solutes, rapid absorption of glucose, loss of the osmotic gradient and the presence of a large vascular surface area. As there are a large number of perfused peritoneal capillaries, they provide the ability for high levels of water transport. A large number of small pores and water channels are present. The rapid absorption of glucose counters the high levels of water movement, in effect negating the osmotic effect.

The decrease in UF correlates directly with the length of time on PD therapy, with an increase in the effective peritoneal surface area. This is caused by an increase in the number of microvessels in the peritoneum. Impaired aquaporin-mediated water transport can be responsible for loss of UF and is seen in patients with sclerosing peritonitis. This can also occur during peritonitis, due to the increased transport of low molecular weight solutions, with an increase in the number of capillaries that are perfused during the inflammatory response. However, this response in acute peritonitis is different from what is seen in chronic UFF, because of the effects of the inflammatory response. Here the pores become large in size, hence the increased loss of proteins, although it is usually reversible.

## Type 2: a combination of poor UF and small solute transport failure

This is uncommon and is seen in a small number of patients with sclerosing peritonitis and is associated with impaired solute transport. It is also seen after a severe episode of peritonitis, with associated adhesion formation or after intraperitoneal bleeding. The overall decrease in solute transport and fluid removal is related to a reduction in peritoneal surface area with reduced functional capacity.

## Type 3: normal solute transport with catheter malfunction or leakage of dialysate

With this type of UFF, there needs to be clarification of whether the problem is technical or due to lymphatic absorption. This can be diagnosed by the use of a macromolecular marker such as dextran, which is added to the dialysate and can allow the absorption rate to be calculated. The loss of UF to high effective lymphatic absorption is rare.

## Diagnosis of UFF

Measurement of ultrafiltration capacity is necessary within clinical practice. Inadequate ultrafiltration should be suspected in those patients who ultrafiltrate less than 200 ml per exchange or have high solute transport. Some units use the standard permeability analysis (SPA) test, which uses a 3.86% glucose dwell over 4 hours and defines UF failure as a net UF of less than 400 ml, in the absence of any catheter leaks or mechanical problems (Ho-dac-Pannekeet et al., 1997; Davies, 2001). Measuring sodium dialysate/plasma (D/P) ratio at 1 hour will provide an estimate of the sodium sieving that occurs across the peritoneal vasculature. By using a strong hypertonic solution, providing an osmotic pull and water influx via the aquaporins, there is a resultant decline in sodium in the dialysate. If this is absent it indicates poor ultrafiltration (Mujais et al., 2000; Pride et al., 2002).

Current evidence suggests that patient survival and technique failure are worse for high transporters and they require more intense fluid management (Churchill et al., 1998; Davies et al., 1998). Low transporters on APD may do poorly unless they have good residual renal function. These patients tend to do well on continuous ambulatory peritoneal dialysis (CAPD) as they UF well over longer dwells and have fewer problems with fluid overload.

## Ultrafiltration management

With the introduction of the peritoneal equilibration test (PET), nurses have become reliant on computer programs such as Adequest 2.0® for profiling the optimal dialysis regime for patients. In the initial phase of The TARGET™ program, the 4-hour dwells of 396 patients were simulated. The PET data and long dwell data on all of these patients were known, which are required to estimate the kinetic parameters. The findings were that patients with high or high average transporter status developed a negative ultrafiltration volume within 4–6 hours with a 1.5% dextrose bag, unlike the low and low average transporters who took 8–12 hours. This means that the high/high average transporter will absorb on a long dwell using a 1.5% bag. The UF was calculated for 1.5, 2.5, 4.25 and 7.5% icodextrin solutions (see Figures 5.2–5.5).

Within clinical practice the use of such graphs provides the ability to predict the UF and plan exchange regimes. Not all patients who are high or high average transporters can be converted to APD. There is a need to be more creative with the timing of exchanges and the use of icodextrin as the long dwell solution.

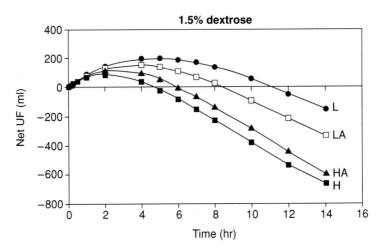

**Figure 5.2**  Temporal profile of net ultrafiltration in the four standard transport categories with the use of 1.5% dextrose solution. Abbreviations: *L* low transport; *LA* low average transport; *HA* high average transport; *H* high transport group. [Reproduced with kind permission of Salim Mujais MD, Baxter Healthcare Corporation, taken from Mujais et al. (2002).]

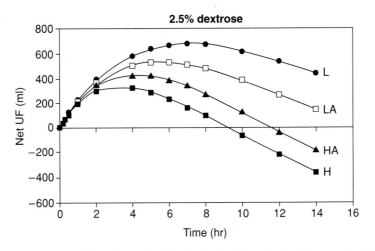

**Figure 5.3**  Temporal profile of net ultrafiltration in the four standard transport categories with the use of 2.5% dextrose solution. For abbreviations see Figure 5.2. [Reproduced with kind permission of Salim Mujais MD, Baxter Healthcare Corporation, taken from Mujais et al. (2002).]

## Adequacy of dialysis

Adequacy of dialysis has become one of the most controversial issues within renal care. For many years targets have been based on the outcomes of the CANUSA study, which were the basis of the 1997 National Kidney Foundation Dialysis Outcomes Quality Initiative (K/DOQI) clinical practice guidelines

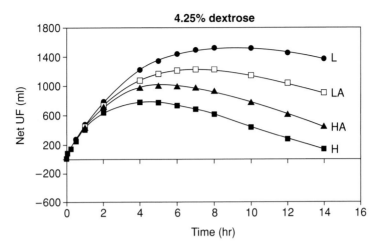

**Figure 5.4**   Temporal profile of net ultrafiltration in the four standard transport categories with the use of 4.25% dextrose solution. For abbreviations see Figure 5.2. [Reproduced with kind permission of Salim Mujais MD, Baxter Healthcare Corporation, taken from Mujais et al. (2002).]

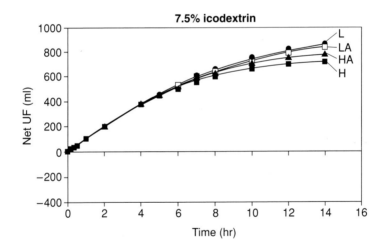

**Figure 5.5**   Temporal profile of net ultrafiltration in the four standard transport categories with the use of 7.5% icodextrin solution. For abbreviations see Figure 5.2. [Reproduced with kind permission of Salim Mujais MD, Baxter Healthcare Corporation, taken from Mujais et al. (2002).]

for total target of small solute clearances. These targets are the result of the interpretation of the CANUSA study [Canada-USA (CANUSA) Peritoneal Dialysis Study Group, 1996; Churchill, 1998]. The CANUSA study suggested that the higher the small solute clearance the better the survival. However, on review of the CANUSA data it has been suggested that the degree of residual renal function and the urine volume are the main effect on mortality (Bargman et al., 2001).

The Renal Association (2002) recommends the following standards for PD adequacy:

- A total weekly creatinine clearance (CrCl) (dialysis + residual renal function) of more than $50\,l/week/1.73\,m^2$
  and/or
- a total weekly dialysis Kt/V urea of more than 1.7

The search for the right target dose of dialysis has continued. The ADEMEX (ADEquacy of PD in MEXico) study is the largest international PD study examining the effects of increased peritoneal small solute clearances on mortality rates among patients on CAPD. This was a prospective, randomised, active-controlled clinical trial with a follow-up of at least 2 years in the Mexican population. This study found that increases in peritoneal solute clearances have a neutral effect on patient survival. They found no clear survival advantage by increasing small solute clearance (Paniagua et al., 2002). The study aimed at a CrCl of $60\,l/week/1.73\,m^2$ in the intervention group and the control group had a set prescription of four exchanges of 2-l fill volumes. However, the patients excluded from the study were those with HIV infection, malignancy or cardiac failure. The overall mortality rate was similar in the two groups, with a 2-year survival of 69% in both groups. This is similar to the results of the CANUSA study and reiterated that small solute clearance did not affect the patients' survival, even in the anuric group of patients.

The European APD Outcome Study (EAPOS) was a 2-year, prospective, multicenter study of 177 anuric automated peritoneal dialysis patients (APD). The findings from this study are the association between poor UF and reduced survival. The dialysis prescription was altered on these patients throughout the study to achieve a UF target of more than $750\,ml/24$ hours and creatinine clearance of more than $60\,l/week/1.73\,m^2$. This study has shown that it is possible to successfully manage anuric APD patients. The survival predictors were age, diabetes, malnutrition and UF; survival was not influenced by small solute clearance (Brown et al., 2003).

These results as with those of the ADEMEX study add to the debate as to whether emphasis on targets such as creatinine clearance has distracted clinical care from more important aspects of care such as ultrafiltration.

## Maintenance of residual renal function (RRF)

Not enough emphasis can be placed on maintenance of RRF, as it has a positive effect on patient outcomes (Bargman et al., 2001). Good blood pressure control and preserving RRF will lower the cardiovascular risk. The target blood pressure should be 125/75 mm Hg if RRF is present as per the Modification of Diet in Renal Disease (MDRD) study, especially if proteinuria is also present, and below 130/80 mm Hg in all other PD patients (Renal Association, 2002).

The use of ACE inhibitors should be considered unless the patient has renal vascular disease. Loop diuretics can be used to maintain urine output, and avoidance of nephrotoxic agents such as contrast medium, non-steroidal anti-inflammatory agents and aminoglycosides is necessary (Rocco et al., 2002). Preservation of RRF is crucial.

## Cardiovascular disease

Cardiovascular disease, such as ischaemic heart disease and heart failure, is the most common cause of death in PD patients. In the recent ADEMEX study, myocardial infarction was the major cause of death (Paniagua et al., 2002; Abu-Alfa, 2003). Many patients already have existing cardiac disease when commencing PD treatment and this is associated with a lower survival on dialysis [Lupo et al., 1994; Canada-USA (CANUSA) Peritoneal Dialysis Study Group, 1996]. Ganesh et al. (2003) found that new patients with coronary artery disease commencing PD, irrelevant of diabetes status, had a significantly poorer survival rate when compared with haemodialysis patients. Factors that are related to cardiovascular outcomes are inadequate dialysis, such as refractory hypertension, hypercatabolism and malnutrition, hyperphosphataemia and susceptibility to infections. Another common factor is the existence of fluid overload associated with left ventricular dilatation and left ventricular hypertrophy. The main risks for PD patients are the use of high glucose concentration dialysate and the related obesity, atherogenic lipid profile and risk of fluid overload.

The common lipid abnormality associated with PD patients is hypertryglyceridaemia with low HDL (high density lipoprotein) levels. Treatment of hyperlipidaemia in patients on PD should commence with dietary control and this includes effective glycaemic control in those with diabetes, which is effective for elevated triglycerides. The use of statins to reduce the total LDL (low density lipoprotein) cholesterol and increase the HDL is important. Fibrates can be used to reduce the triglycerides level, but low doses are required to avoid any incidence of myopathy. However, there is no evidence that improving lipid levels leads to a reduction in cardiovascular events in patients on PD (Fried et al., 1999). The aim should be to keep the plasma cholesterol below 5.0 mmol/l (Little et al., 1998; Renal Association, 2002).

Although a number of physical effects need to be considered when caring for those on PD, important issues are sometimes forgotten that have a more detrimental effect on an individual's life quality. Sleep disturbance is one of these.

## Sleep

A high incidence of sleep disorders is associated with end stage renal failure and this may affect from 20–80% of patients (Stepanski et al., 1995; Wadhwa and Akhtar, 1998). Lack of sleep and/or disturbed sleep can lead to sleepiness during the day, affecting functional capacity, quality of life and even causing increased mortality rates (Benz et al., 2000). A questionnaire was given to 201 patients on PD in order to assess the quality of sleep. The most common complaints were daytime sleepiness, frequent awakening at night, insomnia and restless leg symptoms (Hui et al., 2000).

There is evidence to suggest that both sleep apnoea and restless leg syndrome may have a role in essential hypertension and the secondary hypertension of those with chronic renal failure (Silverberg et al., 1997). The causes of sleep disorders are multifactorial and include male gender, higher age, caffeine intake, depression, worry, medications and primary sleep disorders such as sleep apnoea.

Sleep apnoea is difficult to diagnose due to the similarities between uraemic symptoms and sleep apnoea. Sleep apnoea is associated with periods where the person stops breathing whilst sleeping and is caused by repeated episodes of upper airway obstruction and lowered oxygen saturation blood levels. However, if metabolic disorders and adequate dialysis are excluded, then diagnosis is required by the use of polysomnography. The main treatment for sleep apnoea is the use of continuous positive airway pressure (CPAP) and some patients' symptoms improve after transplantation.

Restless leg syndrome (RLS) is also common and the symptoms are of an 'odd', 'creepy-crawly' feeling in the legs (sometimes the arms), which causes them to move involuntarily. Treatments include the use of carbemazepine and gabapentin. Both drugs are anticonvulsants, and in a study by Thorp et al. (2001), gabapentin was shown to be effective for RLS in haemodialysis patients. If the patient is complaining of nocturnal cramps, which are different from RLS, the use of quinine sulphate can be effective.

Sleep disorders can be associated with anxiety, depression, poor sleep hygiene and medications such as steroids, some antihypertensive medications, diuretics, clonidine, cimetidine and thyroxine. Treatments should firstly exclude any medications that are exacerbating poor sleep, before addressing the issues of anxiety and depression. This may involve possible referral for counselling, and the use of mild sedatives or antidepressants. Correcting bad sleep habits is also very important and these include avoiding watching the television in bed, stopping daytime sleeping and avoiding exercise before going to bed.

Although, the discussion of sleep may seem inconsequential, it is important to consider that lack of sleep or inability to sleep can cause poor functioning and performance during the day, irritability and may affect the relationship and quality of life of the patient and partner.

## Patient education

Most renal units educate their patients/carers on how to perform their own PD at home. Some units utilise the private sector to provide the initial patient teaching programme for various reasons such as resources and space. On reviewing the literature, there is no formal research into the effectiveness of such educational programmes on patient outcomes. There are also no guidelines on the qualifications the nurse who is responsible for teaching the patient should have. With all that is known about learning styles and needs, a formal approach to educating patients should also be used. Although we are aware of the importance of using adult learning theories, such as those proposed by Knowles (1970), for our own teaching these are not always reflected in the clinical education of patients. The importance of teaching adult patients to be self-caring does not always take into consideration the uniqueness of the individual and there is minimal emphasis placed on the humanistic approach to education. This is an area that requires further research and education of staff involved in teaching patients, to ensure that the use of effective teaching methods, such as identifying learning needs and barriers to learning, is included in the process.

## The National Service Framework (NSF)

The first part of the Renal NSF, Dialysis and Transplantation was published in January 2004. It identifies five standards and markers of good practice. This document should be used in conjunction with the Renal Association Guidelines (2002) for PD. An example of the relevance of this document is Standard Four: Dialysis. The key element in clinical care is the prevention of peritonitis. The overall aim is to ensure that patients receive quality care and are involved throughout the decision-making process.

## Summary

Innovative ideas often bring new challenges. This may be through the development of new technology such as more biocompatible solutions or improved systems. Alongside these challenges there is constant striving to provide patients with better care, so that clinical practice now needs to be supported by sound evidence/research. For many it is difficult to constantly keep up with the latest studies and clinical practices in PD, so it is hoped that this chapter provides both a taster for exploring the trends in PD and a discussion on some current clinical topics.

## References

Abu-Alfa, A. (2003) The ADEMEX study: expanding the boundaries of peritoneal dialysis adequacy beyond small solute clearances. *Dialysis and Transplantation* **32** (3), 115–121.

Annigeri, R., Conly, J., Vas, S., Dedier, H., Prakashan, K., Bargman, J., Jassal, V. and Oreopoulos, D. (2001) Emergence of mupirocin-resistant *Staphylococcus aureus* in chronic peritoneal dialysis patients using mupirocin prophylaxis to prevent exit site infection. *Peritoneal Dialysis International* **21**, 554–9.

Ash, S.R., Sutton, J.M., Mankus, R.A., Rossman, J., De Ridder, V., Nassvi, M.S. and Ross, J. (2002) Clinical trials of the T-fluted (Ash advantage) peritoneal dialysis catheter. *Advances in Renal Replacement Therapy* **9** (2), 133–43.

Bargman, J.M., Thorpe, K.E., Churchill, D.N. and CANUSA Peritoneal Dialysis Study Group (2001) Relative contribution of residual renal function and peritoneal clearance to adequacy of dialysis: a reanalysis of the CANUSA study. *Journal of the American Society of Nephrology* **12** (10), 2158–62.

Benz, R.L., Pressman, M.R., Hovick, E.T. and Peterson, D.D. (2000) Potential novel predictors of mortality in end-stage renal disease patients with sleep disorders. *American Journal of Kidney Diseases* **35**, 1052–60.

Brown, E., Davies, S., Rutherford, P., Meeus, F., Borras, M., Riegal, W., Divino Filho, J., Vonesh, E. and Van Bree, M. on behalf of the EAPOS Group (2003) Survival of functionally anuric patients on automated peritoneal dialysis: the European APD Outcome Study. *Journal of the American Society of Nephrology* **14**, 2948–57.

Canada-USA (CANUSA) Peritoneal Dialysis Study Group (1996) Adequacy of dialysis and nutrition in peritoneal dialysis: association with clinical outcomes. *Journal of the American Society of Nephrology* **7**, 198–207.

Canepa, A., Carrea, A., Menoni, S., Verrina, E., Trivelli, A., Gusmano, R. and Perfumo, F. (2001) Acute effects of simultaneous intraperitoneal infusion of glucose and amino acids. *Kidney International* **59**, 1967–73.

Churchill, D.N. (1998) Implications of the CAN-USA (CANUSA) study of the adequacy of dialysis on peritoneal dialysis schedule. *Nephrology Dialysis Transplantation* **13** (Suppl 6), 158–63.

Churchill, D.N., Thorpe, K.E., Nolph, K.D., et al. (1998) Increased peritoneal membrane transport is associated with decreased patient and technique survival for continuous peritoneal dialysis patients. *Journal of the American Society of Nephrology* **9**, 1285–92.

Coles, G., O'Donoghue, D., Pritchard, N., et al. (1998) A controlled trial of two bicarbonate-containing dialysis fluids for CAPD – final report. *Nephrology Dialysis Transplantation* **13**, 3165–71.

Conly, J. and Vas, S. (2002) Increasing mupirocin resistance of *Staphylococcus aureus* in CAPD – should it continue to be used as prophylaxis? *Peritoneal Dialysis International* **22**, 649–52.

Dasgupta, M.K. (1997) Silver coated catheters in peritoneal dialysis. *Peritoneal Dialysis International* **17** (Suppl 2), 142–5.

Dasgupta, M.K. (2000) Exit site and catheter-related infections in peritoneal dialysis. Problems and progress. *Nephrology* **5**, 17–25.

Dasgupta, M.K. (2002a) Biofilms and infection in dialysis patients. *Seminars in Dialysis* **15** (5), 338–46.

Dasgupta, M.K. (2002b) Moncrief-Popovich catheter and implantation technique: the AV fistula of peritoneal dialysis. *Advances in Renal Replacement Therapy* **9** (2), 116–24.

Dasgupta, M.K. and Costerton, J.W. (1989) Significance of bio-film-adherent bacterial microcolonies on Tenckhoff catheters of CAPD patients. *Blood Purification* **7**, 144–55.

Dasgupta, M.K., Kowalewska-Grochowska, K., Larabie, M. and Costerton, J.W. (1991) Catheter biofilms and recurrent CAPD peritonitis. *Advances in Peritoneal Dialysis* **7**, 169–72.

Davies, S. (2001) Monitoring of long-term peritoneal membrane function. *Peritoneal Dialysis International* **21** (2), 225–30.

Davies, S.J., Phillips, L. and Russell, G.I. (1998) Peritoneal solute transport predicts survival on CAPD independently of residual renal function. *Nephrology Dialysis Transplantation* **13**, 962–8.

Dawnay, A. and Millar, D.J. (1997) Glycation and advanced glycation end-product formation with icodextrin and glucose. *Peritoneal Dialysis International* **17**, 52–8.

Department of Health (2004) *The National Service Framework for Renal Services. Part One: Dialysis and Transplantation.* www.doh.gov.uk/nsf/renal.

Dreyden, M.S., Ludlam, H.A., Wing, A.J. and Phillips, J. (1991) Active intervention dramatically reduces CAPD-associated infection. *Advances in Peritoneal Dialysis* **7**, 125–8.

Dutch, J.M. and Yee, J. (2001) Successful use of recombinant tissue plasminogen activators in a patient with relapsing peritonitis. *American Journal of Kidney Diseases* **37**, 149–53.

Fenton, S.S.A., Schaubel, D.E., Desmeules, M., et al. (1997) Hemodialysis versus peritoneal dialysis: comparison of adjusted mortality rates. *American Journal of Kidney Diseases* **30**, 334–42.

Figueiredo, A., Tettamanzy, F., Vercoza, A. and Figueiredo, C. (2000) Endoluminal brush for clearing peritoneal dialysis catheter obstruction. *Peritoneal Dialysis International* **20** (6), 805.

Fletcher, S., Stables, G.A. and Turney, J.H. (1998) Icodextrin allergy in a peritoneal dialysis patient. *Nephrology Dialysis Transplantation* **13**, 2656–8.

Fried, L., Hutchison, A., Stegmayr, B., Prichard, S. and Bargman, J. (1999) ISPD guidelines/recommendation: recommendations for the treatment of lipid disorders in patients on peritoneal dialysis. *Peritoneal Dialysis International* **19** (1) , 7–16.

Ganesh, S., Hulbert-Shearon, T., Port, F., Eagle, K. and Stack, A. (2003) Mortality differences by dialysis modality among incident ESRD patients with and without coronary artery disease. *Journal of the American Society of Nephrology* **14**, 415–24.

Haynes, B.J., Walker Quarles, A., Vavrinchik, J., White, J. and Pedan, A. (2002) The LifeSite haemodialysis access system: implications for the nephrology nurse. *Nephrology Nursing Journal* **29** (1), 27–33.

Heimburger, O., Waniewski, J., Wang, T., Widstam, U., Lindholm, B. and Tranaeus, A. (1998) Peritoneal transport with lactate 40 mmol/L vs. bicarbonate/lactate 25/15 mmol/L dialysis fluids. *Journal of the American Society of Nephrology* **9**, 192A.

Henderson, I.S., Couper, I.A. and Lumsden, A. (1986) Potentially irritant glucose metabolites in unused CAPD fluid. In: Maher, J.F. and Winchester, J.F. (eds) *Frontiers in PD*, pp 261–4. Field Rich and Associates, New York.

Ho-dac-Pannekeet, M.M., Atasever, B., Struijk, D.G. and Krediet, R.T. (1997) Analysis of ultrafiltration failure in peritoneal dialysis patients by means of standard peritoneal permeability analysis. *Peritoneal Dialysis International* **17**, 144–50.

Hui, D.S., Wong, T., Fanny, W., Thomas, S., Choy, D., Wong, K., Szeto, C., Lui, S. and Li, P. (2000) Prevalence of sleep disturbances in Chinese patients with end-stage renal failure on continuous ambulatory peritoneal dialysis. *American Journal of Kidney Diseases* **36** (4), 783–8.

Johnson, D.W., Herzig, K.A., Purdie, D.M., Chang, W., Brown, A.M., Rigby Campbell, S.B., Nicol, D.L. and Hawley, C.M. (2000) Is obesity a favourable prognostic factor in peritoneal dialysis patients? *Peritoneal Dialysis International* **20** (6), 715–21.

Keshaviah, P., Collins, A.J., Ma, J.Z., Churchill, D.N. and Thorpe, K.E. (2002) Survival comparison between hemodialysis and peritoneal dialysis based on matched doses of delivered therapy. *Journal of the American Society of Nephrology* **13** (Suppl 1), S48–52.

Kidney Alliance (2001) *End-Stage Renal Failure – A Framework for Planning and Service Delivery.* www.kidneyalliance.org.uk.

Knowles, M.S. (1970) *The Modern Practice of Adult Education.* Association Press, New York.

Krediet, R.T., Ho-dac-Pannekeet, M.M., Imholz, A.L.T. and Struijk, D.G. (1997) Icodextrin's effect on peritoneal transport. *Peritoneal Dialysis International* **17**, 35–41.

Lam-Po-Tang, M.K.L., Bending, M.R. and Kwan, J.T. (1997) Icodextrin hypersensitivity in a CAPD patient. *Peritoneal Dialysis International* **17**, 82–4.

Little, J., Phillips, L., Russell, L., et al. (1998) Longitudinal lipid profiles on CAPD: their relationship to weight gain, comorbidity, and dialysis factors. *Journal of the American Society of Nephrology* 9, 1931–9.

Lupo, A., Tarchini, R., Cancarini, G., et al. (1994) Long-term outcome in continuous ambulatory peritoneal dialysis: a 10 year survey by the Italian Cooperative Peritoneal Dialysis Study Group. *American Journal of Kidney Diseases* 24, 826–37.

Mackenzie, R.K., Holmes, C.J., Moseley, A., et al. (1998) Bicarbonate/lactate- and bicarbonate-buffered peritoneal dialysis fluids improve ex vivo peritoneal macrophage TNF α secretion. *Journal of the American Society of Nephrology* **9**, 1499–506.

Mactier, R.A., Sprosen, T.S., Gokal, R., et al. (1998) Bicarbonate and bicarbonate/lactate PD solutions for the treatment of infusion pain. *Kidney International* 53, 1061–7.

Mehmet, S., QWuan, G., Thomas, S. and Goldsmith, D. (2001) Important causes of hypoglycaemia in patients with diabetes on peritoneal dialysis. *Diabetic Medicine* 18, 679–82.

Mercer, T.H., Crawford, C., Gleeson, N.P. and Naish, P.F. (2002) Low-volume exercise rehabilitation improves functional capacity and self-reported functional status of dialysis patients. *American Journal of Physical Medical Rehabilitation* **81** (3), 162–7.

Miller, T.E. and Findon, G. (1997) Touch contamination of connection devices in peritoneal dialysis – a quantitative microbiologic analysis. *Peritoneal Dialysis International* **17**, 560–67.

Mistry, C.D., Mallick, N.P. and Gokal, R. (1987) Ultrafiltration with an isosmotic solution during peritoneal dialysis exchanges. *Lancet* **2**, 178–81.

Mistry, C.D., Gokal, R., Peers, E. and The Midas Study Group (1994) A randomized multicenter clinical trial comparing isosmolar icodextrin with hyperosmolar glucose solutions in CAPD. *Kidney International* **46**, 496–503.

Mujais, S. and Vonesh, E. (2002) Profiling of peritoneal ultrafiltration. *Kidney International* **62**, S17–22, S81.

Mujais, S., Nolph, K., Gokal, R., et al. (2000) Evaluation and management of ultrafiltration problems in peritoneal dialysis. *Peritoneal Dialysis International* **20** (Suppl 4), S5–21.

National Kidney Foundation Dialysis Outcomes Quality Initiative (1997) Clinical practice guidelines for peritoneal dialysis adequacy. *American Journal of Kidney Diseases* **30**, S67–136.

Ogunc, G. (2002) Malfunctioning peritoneal dialysis catheter and accompanying surgical pathology repaired by laparoscopic surgery. *Peritoneal Dialysis International* **22** (4), 454–62.

Paniagua, R., Amato, D., Vonesh, E., Correa-Rotter, R., Ramos, A., Moran, J. and Mujais, S. (2002) Effects of increased peritoneal clearances on mortality rates in peritoneal dialysis: ADEMEX, a prospective, randomized, controlled trial. *Journal of the American Society of Nephrology* 13, 1307–20.

Perez-Fontan, M., Garcia Falcon, T., Rosales, M., Rodriguez-Carmona, A., Adeva, M., Rodriguez-Lozano, M.I. and Moncalian, J. (1993) Treatment of *Staphylococcus aureus* nasal carriers in CAPD with mupirocin: long-term results. *American Journal of Kidney Diseases* 22, 708–12.

Perez-Fontan, M., Rosales, M., Rodriguez-Carmona, A., Falcon, T. and Valdes, F. (2002) Mupirocin resistance after long-term use of *Staphylococcus aureus* colonization in patients undergoing chronic peritoneal dialysis. *American Journal of Kidney Diseases* **39** (2), 337–41.

Piraino, B. (2000) *Staphylococcus aureus* infections in dialysis patients. Focus on prevention. *American Society of Artificial Internal Organs* **46**, S13–17.

Posthuma, N., Wee, P., Niessen, H., Donker, A., Verbrugh, H. and Schalkwijk, C. (2001) Amadori albumin and advanced glycation end-product formation in peritoneal dialysis using icodextrin. *Peritoneal Dialysis International* **21**, 43–51.

Pride, E., Gustafson, J., Graham, A., Spainhour, L., Mauck, V., Brown, P. and Burkart, J. (2002) Comparison of a 2.5% and a 4.25% dextrose peritoneal equilibration test. *Peritoneal Dialysis International* **22**, 365–70.

Renal Association (2002) *Treatment of Adults and Children with Renal Failure: Standards and Audit Measures*, 3rd edn. Royal College of Physicians, London.

Ritzau, J., Hoffman, R. and Tzamaloukas, A. (2001) Effect of preventing *Staphylococcus aureus* carriage on rates of peritoneal catheter-related staphylococcal infections. Literature synthesis. *Peritoneal Dialysis International* **21**, 471–9.

Rocco, M.V., Frankenfield, D.L., Prowant, B., Frederick, P. and Flanigan, M.J. (2002) Risk factors for early mortality in U.S. peritoneal dialysis patients: impact of residual renal function. *Peritoneal Dialysis International* **22** (3), 371–9.

Silverberg, D., Iaina, A. and Ocksenberg, A. (1997) Sleep-related breathing disturbances: their pathogenesis and potential interest to the nephrologist. *Nephrology Dialysis Transplantation* **12**, 680–83.

Steele, M., Goodwin, S., Kwan, J.T.C., Chawdhery, M.Z., Moran, J. (2001) *A New Subcutaneous Device for Peritoneal Dialysis Access*. Oral presentation at 9th Congress of the International Society for Peritoneal Dialysis, June 2001, Montreal.

Stepanski, E., Faber, M., Zorick, F., Basner, R. and Roth, T. (1995) Sleep disorders in patients on continuous ambulatory peritoneal dialysis. *Journal of the American Society of Nephrology* **26**, 751–6.

Tauer, A., Zhang, X., Schaub, T., Zimmerick, T., Niwa, T., Passlick-Deetjen, J. and Pischetsrieder, M. (2003) Formation of advanced glycation end products during CAPD. *American Journal of Kidney Diseases* **41** (3) (Suppl 1), S57–60.

Taylor, G.S., Patel, V., Spencer, S., Fluck, R.J. and McIntyre, C.W. (2002) Long-term use of 1.1% amino acid dialysis solution in hypoalbuminemic continuous ambulatory peritoneal dialysis patients. *Clinical Nephrology* **58** (6), 445–50.

Tenckhoff, J. and Schechter, H. (1968) A bacteriologically safe peritoneal access device. *Trans American Society of Artificial Internal Organs* **14**, 181–7.

Thorp, M., Morris, C. and Bagby, S. (2001) A crossover study of gabapentin in treatment of restless legs syndrome among hemodialysis patients. *American Journal of Kidney Diseases* **38** (1), 104–108.

Tranter, S. (2002) Re-establishment of flow in peritoneal dialysis catheters using the endoluminal FAS brush (editorial). *Peritoneal Dialysis International* **22**, 275–6.

Twardowski, Z.J. (2002) Presternal peritoneal catheter. *Advances in Renal Replacement Therapy* **9** (2), 125–32.

Wadhwa, N.K. and Akhtar, S. (1998) Sleep disorders in dialysis patients. *Seminars in Dialysis* **11**, 287–97.

Wilkie, M., Plant, L., Edwards, L. and Brown, C.B. (1997) Icodextrin 7.5% dialysate solution (glucose polymer) in patients with ultrafiltration failure: extension of CAPD technique survival. *Peritoneal Dialysis International* **17**, 84–7.

Woodrow, G., Stables, G., Oldroyd, B., Gibson, J., Turney, J. and Brownjohn, A. (1999) Comparison of icodextrin and glucose solutions for the daytime dwell in automated peritoneal dialysis. *Nephrology Dialysis Transplantation* **14**, 1530–35.

Worland, M.A., Radabaugh, R.S. and Mueller, B.A. (1998) Intraperitoneal thrombolytic therapy for peritoneal dialysis associated peritonitis. *Annals of Pharmacotherapy* **32**, 1216–20.

# Further reading

Gokal, R., Khanna, R., Krediet, R. and Nolph, K. (2000) *Textbook of Peritoneal Dialysis*, 2nd edn. Kluwer, Dordrecht.

# Chapter 6
# Advances in Renal Transplantation

*Ray Trevitt*

## Introduction

This chapter describes and analyses some of the issues currently influencing thoughts and practice in the field of renal transplantation. The main challenges facing the transplant team are the increasing number of patients waiting for a kidney, the rate of graft loss and patient death and improving patient quality of life. The introduction and best use of new immunosuppressants and technologies such as xenotransplantation and stem cells, and the ethical concerns raised as a result of these challenges, are also important.

The role of the transplant nurse has become increasingly specialised over the years and is often now the lynchpin of any renal transplant clinic and ward service (Rochera Gaya, 1999). The transplant nurse plays a key role in pre- and post-transplant inpatient care, maintenance of the transplant list, pre- and post-transplant education, live donor work-up, management of outpatient clinics and audit. These are interesting and exciting times and a proactive approach to learning and developing practice will pay dividends, both professionally and in terms of patient outcome.

## Waiting lists

In the UK in 2002, 5000 people were on the waiting list for a cadaveric kidney transplant. The total number of cadaveric kidney transplants was 1385 (UK Transplant, 2003). Table 6.1 shows the continued increase in list size contrasted with the decrease in cadaveric transplants carried out. The increasing number of living donor transplants has not compensated for the increased numbers waiting for a kidney.

A comparison with other European countries is shown in Table 6.2. The rise in numbers waiting for a kidney has not been met by an increase in donation, except in Spain.

The Spanish model, beginning in 1989 with the creation of the National Transplant Organisation (ONT), involved heavy investment and continues to

**Table 6.1**  Kidney-only transplants and active waiting list at year-end in the UK, 1992–2001 (UK Transplant, 2003).

| Year | Cadaveric transplants | Living donor transplants | Waiting list (active) |
|------|------|------|------|
| 1992 | 1622 | 100 | 3748 |
| 1993 | 1555 | 142 | 3918 |
| 1994 | 1588 | 135 | 3910 |
| 1995 | 1615 | 155 | 4032 |
| 1996 | 1499 | 183 | 4304 |
| 1997 | 1487 | 179 | 4412 |
| 1998 | 1330 | 252 | 4584 |
| 1999 | 1311 | 270 | 4691 |
| 2000 | 1324 | 347 | 4822 |
| 2001 | 1333 | 358 | 4846 |

**Table 6.2**  Donor and transplant activity in Europe, 2001 (per million population, pmp).

| | Euro transplant[1] | France | Italy | Scandia transplant[2] | Spain | UK[3] |
|------|------|------|------|------|------|------|
| Cadaveric donors | 14.3 | 17.8 | 17.1 | 13.8 | 32.5 | 13.1 |
| Cadaveric transplants | 25.9 | 32.0 | 25.0 | 25.0 | 46.1 | 23.4 |
| Living donor transplants | 5.1 | 1.7 | 1.7 | 10.4 | 0.8 | 6.1 |

[1] Euro transplant includes Germany, Austria, Belgium, Luxembourg, The Netherlands and Slovenia.
[2] Scandia transplant includes Denmark, Norway, Sweden and Finland.
[3] Figures taken from National Transplant Database, February 2002 (maintained on behalf of transplant services in the UK and Republic of Ireland by UK Transplant). All others are provisional figures taken from Organización Nacional de Tranplantes (ONT) data (www.msc.es/ont/esp).

give outstanding results (Matesanz et al., 1996). The Spanish explored the identification of potential donors, the legal framework surrounding certification of death, consent, education and information and the organisation of recipient registration and organ allocation. Transplant co-ordinators were placed in every hospital and the donation rate rose to 33.6 pmp within 10 years. In the UK and Germany, the number of organ donors remained at about 13 pmp. A second initiative increased investment in neurosurgical facilities, which increased the number of potential donors available. A third step invested in public and health care worker education concerning the benefits of increasing cadaver donation. An opt-out law was introduced, but in practice the consent of families is always sought.

In Britain, UK Transplant is the NHS organisation responsible for matching and allocating donated organs. One of the steps taken to improve donation rates is the formation of the UK Organ Donor Register, which allows individuals to register as willing to be considered as an organ donor after their death. The usefulness of this register has been questioned, and there is no evidence yet that shows an increase in donation rates attributed to it. This is called 'opting in'. Even in 'opting out' and 'required request' systems the wishes of the next of kin remain paramount. The opt-out system presumes consent unless the individual has specifically registered as unwilling to donate. Next of kin are still contacted. The opt-out system has received little political support but is supported by the British Medical Association (BMA) and by population surveys (British Medical Association, 2000).

Belgium introduced an opt-out system in 1982 and the number of donors increased. Germany and Italy introduced it in 1997 and 2000 respectively. France was forced to modify its opt-out law in 1996 after adverse publicity, and since then donation rates have improved. Spain has an opt out law, but consent is always sought. UK Transplant has set up a patients' forum to ensure patients' views are taken into account when policy decisions are made, and encourages any debate that raises the profile of transplantation, thereby increasing the supply of organs.

The practice of being active in more than one transplant pool is not usually accommodated within Europe, but, as the system is not policed throughout, the resourceful patient could be on more than one waiting list. This reduces equal access to cadaveric organs, but there is no evidence of significant abuse. New York State in 1990 banned multiple listing within its jurisdiction, but those patients on two or more lists waited significantly less time for a transplant (White et al., 1998). However, most patients lack the financial resources and wherewithal to do this. In regions or countries not sharing organs, there is little motivation to prevent a patient from trying to receive an organ from a separate source and patients may indeed move from a country with a long waiting list to one with improved chances of transplantation, for example from the UK to Spain.

## Donation

The response by the UK government, through UK Transplant, to the challenge of increasing kidney donation has been to target extra resources to employ more cadaver transplant co-ordinators in intensive care units and living donor co-ordinators in transplant units. Since 2002, additional funds have been invested in the NHS to boost the number of organ transplants. UK Transplant is funding 35 donor liaison schemes, 25 living donation programmes, a further 11 transplant co-ordinators and six non-heart-beating programmes. Organ donor rates are being included in health authority performance indicators for the first time, a new web site has been launched and local councils are being encouraged to send out details of the NHS Organ Donor Register with electoral registration forms. About 9 million people have registered so far.

UK Transplant and the Unrelated Live Transplant Regulatory Authority (ULTRA) are moving to have accredited third parties for the ULTRA application process, to ensure both consistency and that parties undergo a period of training, and to improve efficiency. Currently the system relies on the goodwill of consultants willing to cooperate.

## Compensation for cadaveric donation

The American Medical Association is looking into whether paying for organs from cadaveric donors would increase rates, for example to cover funeral expenses (Arnold et al., 2002). Compensation for cadaveric donation need not be financial, as people who opt-in to become cadaver donors could be awarded points towards receiving an organ themselves should they ever need one. More indirectly, institutions can be encouraged to maximise cadaveric donation by use of funding-based performance indicators, publicising results (league tables) and being given adequate resources to cover the work involved.

## Living donation

Living donation would not be accepted if there were better alternatives. Living donor transplantation is accepted practice because, in view of the shortage of cadaveric organs, potential donors and recipients wish to benefit from the good results achieved. It will only stop when alternatives are available, for example from xenotransplants or organs grown from stem cells, or perhaps if cadaver organs can be made to last a lifetime. In Norway, 38% of transplants are from live donors and this has seen a reduction in waiting list size. In the UK about 20% of transplants are from live donors.

Considerable investment is required in a live donor programme as there is a high drop out rate of about 50–90% (depending on when first measured) for a variety of medical, social and immunological reasons (Saunders et al., 2000). It is recommended that simple, inexpensive screening is carried out at the earliest stage, such as medical history, blood pressure, urine dipstick and basic blood count and chemistry (Trevitt et al., 2001). Dialysis patients often turn down an offer of living donation for social, emotional and ethnomedical reasons (Gordon, 2001).

There is much debate over who should be allowed to donate, and under what conditions. The person who gives consent to be a live organ donor should be competent, willing to donate, free from coercion, medically and psychosocially suitable, fully informed of the risks and benefits as a donor, and fully informed of the risks, benefits and alternative treatment available to the recipient. The benefits to both must outweigh the risks associated with it (Abercassis et al., 2000).

How can we be sure that a potential donor is acting autonomously and whether they have a right to donate? Informed consent is a universal requirement but may not be achievable or necessary. When a recipient is very dear to a donor, the donor may base the decision on care and concern rather than weighing up risk/benefits (Spital, 2001).

Free and informed consent is generally acknowledged as the legal and ethical basis for living organ donation, but assessments of live donors are not always easy (Biller-Andorno et al., 2001).

Some authors have discussed the question of gender bias in live donation, as women donate more kidneys. This issue is tied up in the general question of choice within a cultural and family dynamic; should culture-based gender bias in living donor renal transplantation be discouraged on ethical and graft survival grounds (Donnelly et al., 2001)?

Centres differ markedly in their rates of live donor transplants. There are differences in appreciation of medical risk and what constitutes ethical selection, so some donors may be inappropriately denied and others inappropriately selected. Steiner and Gert (2000) identify three fundamental obligations: to recognise that it is often ethical to participate in acts of individual risk and sacrifice that are performed to benefit others; to not deny a transplant without good reason to donors and recipients who apply; and to neutralise, but not overreact to, centre self-interest which stems from the professional benefit of transplantation and the centre's desire to help potential recipients. The basic facts must be understood by all as part of ethical decision-making, using national statistics as a baseline of risk (Steiner and Gert, 2000).

## Kidney exchanges

Ross et al. (1997) proposed to increase the number of living kidney donations by using kidneys from living ABO-incompatible (or crossmatch-incompatible) donors through an exchange arrangement between two living kidney donor–recipient pairs. Only a small proportion of potential live donor pairs would be eligible for an exchange on the basis of blood group incompatibility or crossmatch incompatibility. There are three variations: altruistically unbalanced live donor–recipient exchanges, an indirect exchange between a live donor–recipient pair with a cadaveric donor–recipient pair on the basis of positive crossmatch, and an indirect exchange on the basis of ABO incompatibility. The goal of kidney paired exchange programmes is to increase the supply of kidneys available for transplantation. Ross et al. (1997) acknowledge that all exchanges increase the potential for coercion and currently rejects the proposal of altruistically unbalanced exchanges because of this. However, voluntary consent could be achieved for indirect exchanges. The indirect ABO-compatible exchange creates no new ethical concerns to the original living paired exchange programme and is supported by the authors.

The indirect ABO-incompatible exchange, however, does create a new ethical concern because it may disadvantage group O recipients. If mechanisms could be developed to avoid increasing the waiting time for group O recipients (as group O donors will always be blood group compatible), there could be support for the implementation of indirect ABO-incompatible exchange. Such systems would require endorsement from national bodies that oversee organ allocation. This has happened in a small number of areas in the USA, who have set up a pool of potential live donors. If a suitable organ is not available, the patient is given priority on the cadaver list. This remains controversial (Ross and Woodle, 2000), and in the UK may constitute offering an inducement for a person to donate a kidney, which contravenes the Human Organ Transplant (HOT) Act of 1989.

A shortage of cadaveric donor kidneys has created waiting lists for patients on chronic dialysis. It may be said that organ acquisition has moved sequentially from cadaveric, then to living relatives, then to living emotionally related donors, and now we see altruistic living donation to strangers. These developments have evolved with improvements to regulation and safety, and the issues of living donation continue to be debated by health care professionals and ethicists. Some authors have argued that patients should have more of a say in what is acceptable practice to them, for example to encourage living, non-directed altruistic donation (Kaplan and Polise, 2000). However, we also need to protect potential donors' freedom of choice, the option to say no. This can be done with appropriate measures (Kinnaert et al., 1999), but we must not forget that the emotional imperative and sense of duty to offer a kidney would not exist if a suitable cadaveric kidney was available.

## Cadaver donation

### Definition of death

There remains some debate over the definition of death, as the definition of experimental animal death is that the heart has stopped beating – otherwise the animal must be anaesthetised for surgery or invasive procedures. Cadaver donors are not defined in this way and to do so may affect public willingness to accept brain stem death. Sensationalised media reports of patients coming back from the dead may discourage people from registering as donors. Truog (1997) points out that a rigorous definition of brain and brain stem function death implies loss of vasomotor tone, temperature control and diabetes insipidus, and not all countries have the same criteria for organ donation. The UK uses brain stem death, whereas Sweden requires brain death, which is a stage further on from the UK definition.

Kerridge et al. (2002) stated that the public distrust the concept of, and criteria for, whole brain death and the equation of this new concept with death of a human being. They suggest that irreversible loss of circulation be reinstated as the major defining characteristic of death, but that brain-dead, heart-beating entities should remain suitable for organ donation despite being alive. Brain-dead people are suitable because of irreversible loss of personhood, accurately and robustly defined by current brain stem death criteria.

### Marginal donors

Grafts from older donors are associated with reduced nephron mass, increased susceptibility to cold ischaemic time (CIT) and impaired long-term survival.

Similarly, very young donors are associated with inadequate nephron mass and a high incidence of technical failure. In practice, centres should inform potential recipients of any sub-optimal kidneys, including young/old kidneys, long ischaemia time, diabetes, vascular injury, impaired function, anatomical abnormality, hypertension, prolonged illness before death and non-heart-beating donors.

Sola (2001) found that patient survival is influenced by patient age, whereas donor age is reflected post-transplant only in higher serum creatinine readings. However, recipient comorbidities at time of transplant can only be worsened by prolonged non-function or treatment for rejection.

## Non-heart-beating donors

A small number of kidneys are retrieved from donors without an active circulation. Rapid retrieval is necessary to minimise warm ischaemic damage. The retrieval team needs to be immediately available, requiring considerable investment, but this practice is thought to have the potential to increase the donation rate by 20–40%, and funding has begun in the UK to expand this. Asystolic donors are declared dead on cardiac arrest criteria: the heart has ceased to function and cannot be restored despite vigorous cardiopulmonary resuscitation. The retrieval team would then restart cardiac massage and ventilation. The time between cardiac arrest and in-situ cooling should not exceed about 30 minutes. As a crude guide, 1 minute of warm ischaemia is equal to 1 hour of CIT (Kootstra, 1997).

The non-heart-beating cadaver donor comes from a variety of situations: dying after unsuccessful resuscitation, for example, in a coronary care unit, with otherwise good kidneys; brought in dead to an Accident & Emergency department; people knowing they will die and deciding to be a donor after a natural death; or withdrawal of life-support so that natural death occurs. These types of donor give results comparable to other cadaver donors (Kootstra et al., 1997).

It may not be ethically acceptable to subject the body to arterial catheterisation to cold-perfuse the kidneys before relatives' consent is obtained, and this has caused problems in some UK units, who, after discussion with the coroner, have stopped the practice. It does, however, preserve the right of the family to be able to donate. Potential donors may be attached to a mechanical thoracic pump resuscitator to maintain circulation until relatives can be approached, but this again raises ethical questions. Coroners do not have legal power to authorise either preservation or removal of organs, but they can agree to the process going ahead as long as it would not jeopardise any of their investigations into a death, and if it has been clearly established that it was the wish of the deceased and those close to him or her. The 'Human Bodies Human Choices' consultation report (Department of Health/Welsh Assembly Government, 2002) recognises that the present framework of law in these areas is uneven and in places unclear. In future, coroners are likely to be asked more frequently about organ donation. Clarification is needed on whether, and if so in what circumstances, they would be prepared to agree to organ perfusion being started before specific consent has been obtained from those close to the deceased.

UK Transplant data show that between 1990 and 1998, 347 kidneys were transplanted (into 345 recipients) from asystolic donors. 1-year transplant survival was 72% (84% heart beating) and 5-year survival 59% (69% heart beating). The main difference in outcome is due to the poorer survival of asystolic donor transplants during the first 6 months. However, the asystolic donor transplants were less well matched than the heart-beating donor transplants and it is not clear how fit the recipients were, which makes comparisons difficult. The results are good enough to continue to invest in this source of kidneys.

## Xenotransplantation

The United Kingdom Xenotransplantation Interim Regulatory Authority (UKXIRA) was formed in 1997 to advise the government on actions necessary to regulate tissue or organ transplants between species.

The breeding of pigs for food is widely acceptable; they are easy to breed and produce large litters. Many religions, including Judaism and Islam, have issued statements accepting the use of porcine tissue for medical purposes, including xenotransplantation (First, 1997).

Successful xenotransplantation would enable planned, timely transplantation. Although considerable obstacles remain, advances have been made towards crossing the pig-to-human barrier. Hyperacute rejection, the first major barrier, has been largely overcome in the experimental setting. Control of acute vascular rejection is now required. Ciclosporin, cyclophosphamide and corticosteroids limit acute vascular rejection in pig-to-primate transplantation, allowing graft survival of 78 days using transgenic kidneys (Cozzi et al., 2000). Recipients in this study required erythropoietin, presumably related to the incompatibility of porcine erythropoietin.

Three criteria must be fulfilled before the clinical phase of research can be commenced: reproducible and sustained graft function using an acceptable immunosuppressive regime, evidence of adequate graft function and maintenance of physiological homeostasis, and evidence of adequate safety, particularly in relation to zoonotic disease transmission (Soin and Friend, 2001). The widespread introduction of clinical renal xenotransplantation is not imminent.

There is concern over the risk of porcine endogenous retroviruses, which are incorporated in the porcine genome and cannot readily be eradicated. They have been shown to infect human cell lines in culture (Patience et al., 1997). Many patients have been exposed to porcine tissue with skin grafts, pancreatic islet cells, liver and splenic extracorporeal perfusions. In a study of 160 patients exposed directly to porcine tissues, they showed no evidence of infection with porcine endogenous retrovirus after 12 years, but there was evidence of microchimerism in 23 patients (Paradis et al., 1999).

# Selling of kidneys

## *Compensation for donation*

A gift, compensation for pain and loss of earnings, expenses: these sound reasonable if not laudable. It could work like the compensation for injuries system. If it is great to give a kidney for free, why is it abominable to do it for money? We prefer patients to die rather than sanction kidneys for sale. Health professionals are not allowed to encourage or be involved in the buying and selling of organs, but donors may be compensated by the recipient's purchasing authority. If funding is found to fly over a relative from a poor country, is this different? Are we aiding and abetting the buying of kidneys by giving patients a copy of their blood group and tissue type – does it belong to them? In some parts of the USA the case for compensation for cadaveric donor families, such as for funeral expenses, is being considered (Arnold et al., 2002).

The sale of human organs is against the law in virtually every country and has been condemned by all of the world's medical associations. Yet, in countries such as Israel, Turkey, India, China, Russia and Iraq organ sales are conducted with only token efforts at secrecy. In Israel, it is even possible to claim back costs from the national health insurance system for kidney transplants paid for and carried out abroad (Scheper-Hughes, 2001). Patients may prefer to purchase a kidney from a stranger than accept a kidney from a loved one. Israel and the UK have a national body that is responsible for ensuring no impropriety with live donor transplants, but the USA depends on hospital committees to police them.

Payment to living donors is part of the transplant process in many developing countries, even if there are laws forbidding it, and these patients would otherwise die when they can no longer pay for regular dialysis. In the western world we do not know how much indirect or covert compensation occurs to living donors. By preventing a legislated and regulated framework for the purchase of living kidneys, it could be argued that we are just protecting our own sensibilities while patients have their best option taken from them (Radcliffe-Richards et al., 1998).

## *The case for legalisation*

This would introduce quality control and regulate the practice. One study from Israel reports that 300 patients transplanted abroad from bought kidneys have better kidney function than the rest of the transplant population (Friedlaender, 2002). This contrasts with other reports of less favourable outcomes – perhaps because of the way in which the transplants are organised. In Turkey one report found a 5-year graft survival of kidneys bought in India of 66%, compared with a local living unrelated graft survival rate of 78% (Sever et al., 2001). In the UK a survey of those transplanted abroad found that of 23 patients, 8 had subsequently died (Inston and Ready, 2002).

Medically, there is no evidence that donating a kidney endangers a person's health in any significant way. Currently, a kidney is allowed to be given up for no payment at all, but the patient, the hospital, the purchaser of care and the professionals all profit. If it was legalised, more money would flow to the sellers. There could be a national regulatory body, which would screen and allocate donors in a similar way to how cadaver organs are allocated now, and arrange payment via government or health purchasers. Although sellers would come from the poor, recipients would include both rich and poor. It can be argued that depriving sellers of the opportunity is not justified, the implication being that they cannot make an informed, rational decision. It is legal to sell ova, semen and blood. It is legal to become a surrogate mother. Radcliffe-Richards et al., point out that if the well-off are entitled to play dangerous sports for pleasure, or dangerous jobs for high pay, it is difficult to see why the poor who take the lesser risk of selling a kidney for greater rewards – perhaps saving a life or extricating themselves from poverty and debt – should be thought so misguided as to need saving from themselves.

## The case against organ sales

Involvement in organs for sale violates the Hippocratic Oath to do no harm. The utilitarian approach would have the benefit to the recipient offsetting the risk to the donor. However, long-term follow-up studies on donors have been carried out in wealthy, developed nations only. People who sell kidneys often live in conditions of poverty and under threats to health from diet, drinking water and lack of health care. Only a more rigorous enforcement of existing laws can protect these people (Scheper-Hughes, 2001).

Even in developed countries, however, living donor follow-up is not always thorough. In the USA, 56 people who had been living donors were found to subsequently require a kidney transplant themselves (Ellison et al., 2002). The reasons for this are unclear.

George Soros, the infamous free-marketeer, noted that the spread of global capitalism has eroded social values and social cohesion in the face of anti-social market values. Markets, by their nature, are indiscriminate and reduce everything to the status of commodities, which can be bought, sold, traded and stolen (Soros, 1998). This global market has outstripped the development of a mediating global society. Local and religious beliefs and laws have given way to the weight of market demands due to the scarcity of organs and abundance of poverty.

A recent study in a city in India looked at 305 sellers of kidneys and found a largely negative outcome for the donors; 87% reported a deterioration in health and on average experienced a one-third reduction in family income post-nephrectomy. Of the 292 donors who had sold their kidneys to pay off debts, 74% still had debts 6 years later and those in poverty had increased from 54% to 71%; furthermore, 9% would not recommend selling a kidney (Goyal et al., 2002).

## Recipients

### UK Transplant and equity

UK Transplant ensures that organs are matched and allocated in a fair and unbiased way. Allocation is based on human leucocyte antigen (HLA) matching, but other considerations include the need for a short cold ischaemic time, age of recipient, age matching, time on transplant list and level of sensitisation. The most common blood group in the UK is O, but in Asians and Afro-Caribbeans group B is the most prevalent. These ethnic groups have a higher incidence of end-stage renal disease (ESRD), and in recent years there has been an accumulation of blood group B patients on transplant lists in areas of high Asian and Afro-Caribbean populations. This led to UK Transplant, in July 2002, altering the system for allocation of kidneys so that now some group O kidneys will be offered to group B patients. There is also less good matching in ethnic recipients because of differences in tissue types, but it has not been shown that this in itself reduces graft survival.

Rates of graft or patient survival are lower in some sub-groups such as in those with diabetes, older people and those with focal segmental glomerulosclerosis (FSGS), but transplantation improves quality of life and life expectancy for all groups. Patients are not generally transplanted before being established on dialysis, but there is good evidence that pre-emptive transplantation is associated with lower morbidity and improved long-term outcome.

Donor families cannot impose conditions regarding the potential recipient, except of course in the case of biologically or emotionally related living donation. ULTRA has yet to be tested by an altruistic donation from a stranger.

So should dialysis and transplantation be preferentially given to younger, healthier, contributing patients? There is no facility to put patients in dire medical need of a transplant at the top of the list. Should non-compliant patients be transplanted? Should they be forced to demonstrate compliance with dialysis, be educated as to what to expect with treatment, and what a donor family somewhere has gone through to allow them to receive an organ?

## Improvements in quality of life, patient and graft survival

To improve quality of life it is important to reduce the side effects of immunosuppression and complications during the first few months, reduce the long-term side effects of treatment and prolong the life of the graft and of the patient. Major side effects are associated with ciclosporin, steroids and polyclonal antibodies. The advent of newer immunosuppressants means that it is possible to reduce or avoid these side effects with an equal or improved anti-rejection effect. Many approaches are being used and it will be some time before there is a consensus regarding immunosuppression. It is undoubtedly true that patients vary as to the immunological risk involved at transplant, for instance according to age, transplant history, antibody level and matching, and that some donor organs carry a higher risk than others, for example, according to age of donor and cold ischaemic time. A tailored approach to immunosuppression would stratify patients according to immunological or non-immunological risk. The high incidence of post-transplant diabetes mellitus in groups such as Asians, or those with a strong family history of diabetes, should preclude use of tacrolimus as a first choice unless a steroid-tapering regime is used. Elderly recipients need less severe treatment, while young or high antibody titre patients will need more. There is evidence that African-Americans should receive a higher 3-g dose of mycophenolate mofetil to reduce their rejection problems to levels comparable with Caucasian and Asian groups (Neylan, 1997; Hricik, 2001).

## Reduction of long-term side effects

Skin problems remain a cause of concern for patients and health care workers. It remains to be seen whether the dermatological side effects of the newer immunosuppressant regimes are better or worse than ciclosporin, steroids and azathiaprine. Patients should be taught how to reduce the risk of skin cancer caused by exposure to strong sunlight and to be screened by a dermatologist for skin lesions and for risks associated with skin type and exposure to sunlight (Venning, 1998).

Osteoporosis occurs soon after transplantation, so treatment needs to be started early. The risk of fracture depends on pre- and post-transplant variables, but the risk is highest in post-menopausal women. Steroid-sparing immunosuppression may offer the best hope (Hollander et al., 1997). Bone density is ascertained with dual energy X-ray absorptiometry (DEXA) scanning and newly transplanted patients can be given osteoporosis prophylaxis to reduce the risk of long-term bone loss, pain and fractures. Treatment with 1 mg/kg pamidronate IV in weeks 1 and 4 and with oral calcium/vitamin D supplement daily long-term has been found to be of benefit (Fan et al., 2000).

Post-transplant infection is minimised by tailoring immunosuppression and use of Cytomegalovirus (CMV) prophylaxis for high-risk patients. Some patients have risk factors at the time of assessment of suitability for transplantation, or develop them while on dialysis. Each unit must decide how thoroughly to screen suitability for transplantation and what the limits of suitability are. Additionally, those kidney diseases that have a risk of recurrence in the transplant kidney must be considered.

# Infection

Most infections are from common pathogens, although more serious opportunistic infections occur frequently enough to justify a careful approach.

Bacterial infections that occur early affect the urinary tract, respiratory tract, wound and vascular access sites, and can lead to septicaemia. Pneumococcal vaccination is recommended but is generally ineffective in immunosuppressed or uraemic patients (Shapiro and Clemens, 1984). Recurrent or chronic urinary tract infection (UTI) is reasonably common in women and this is always investigated, but usually the only recourse is long-term antibiotic prophylaxis.

CMV remains the most important infection affecting transplant recipients. The severity of all infections is related to the degree of immunosuppression. With the advent of ganciclovir, CMV prophylaxis is now widely used for recipients deemed at risk, although in a proportion of patients the active disease is only postponed, and a course of treatment is then required. CMV disease, especially graft-invasive disease, is associated with rejection and reduced renal function (Akposso et al., 1997).

The BK virus is a polyomavirus, a member of the papovavirus group, which includes papillomaviruses, and about 70% of adults in the USA are positive for BK or its close relative the JC virus (Gardner, 1977). BK nephropathy is now being reported more, which may be related to the changes in immunosuppressive regimes or may be because it is only now being identified properly. Overall, about 60% of renal transplant recipients show evidence of infection or reactivation at some time after transplantation. Most BK virus infections are asymptomatic, but it is implicated in ureteric stenoses and late haemorrhagic cystitis, and thought to be a significant cause of tubulointerstitial nephritis and allograft dysfunction in renal transplant patients (Randhawa et al., 1999; Nickeleit et al., 2000; Reploeg et al., 2001). There is yet no proven antiviral therapy, although cidofovir appears to have a role (Held et al., 2000; Gonzalez-Fraile et al., 2001), but some centres have reported stabilised but impaired graft function after reduction of immunosuppression.

Hepatitis C virus (HCV)-positive recipients have an increased risk of acute allograft glomerulopathy compared to HCV-negative recipients (55% vs 6%) within 6 months. HCV-negative recipients who received an HCV-positive kidney also had a high incidence (40%) of glomerulopathy. There is also increased rejection and thrombotic micrangiopathy (Cosio et al., 1996).

Depending on a patient's age at transplant, skin type, exposure to the sun and immunosuppressive therapy, there is an escalation in the number of cutaneous malignancies. Human papillomaviruses cause squamous cell proliferation. The ratio of squamous cell carcinomas to basal cell cacinomas is 15:1 (Barr et al., 1989). Topical imiquimod is a local immune modulator and may improve the therapeutic efficacy of fluorouracil therapy in treatment of squamous cell carcinomas (Smith et al., 2001). Imiquimod has also been used to treat perianal warts (Gayed, 2002).

Post-transplant lymphoproliferative disorder (PTLD), usually associated with the Epstein-Barr virus, is a well-known consequence of immunosuppression, albeit at low incidence. A large study in the USA is exploring the effects of specific immunosuppressants and other risk factors on PTLD and effect of treatment regimes (Funch et al., 2002). Median time to disease is 268 days and incidence is 0.7%. The most common single site is the graft, and this study has noticed no increase in incidence with newer immunosuppressants.

In the USA it is usual practice to give aciclovir prophylaxis to EBV-negative recipients receiving an EBV-positive graft. Birkeland et al. (1999) found a reduction in primary or reactivated EBV, and PTLD, using ciclosporin, antilymphocyte globulin (ALG) and mycophenolate mofetil (MMF) in combination with aciclovir, apparently due to both direct viral prophylaxis and better rejection control.

Most units will not transplant human immunodeficiency virus (HIV)-infected patients (Zeier and Ritz, 2002). Swanson et al. (2002) looked at 10 years of registry data in the USA and found that only 32 patients (0.05%) were reported as HIV-positive at time of transplant. These patients were younger, with younger donors, and had better matching than the general transplant population, but patient and graft survival was 53% and 83% respectively at 3 years, compared to an overall rate of 73% and 88%. It remains to be seen how the use of highly active anti-retroviral therapy will improve outcomes, but preliminary reports are encouraging (Kumar et al., 2002).

Recipients with evidence of previous hepatitis B virus (HBV) infection may reactivate the virus (Dhedin et al., 1998). Lamuvidine has been shown to remove HBV DNA from the blood and improve liver function in this group (Jung et al., 1998).

## Overall survival/long-term care

### Long term

*Cardiovascular disease (CVD) and diabetes mellitus (DM)*

In the medium term after transplantation, outcomes are so good that it is difficult to improve the survival of patients or grafts. Rejection rates have been falling and this is now an uncommon cause of early graft loss. The main issues are the inadequate supply of donor organs, equity of access and the side effects of treatment, especially cardiovascular disease. The latest generation of immunosuppressive drugs offers hope for improved graft survival, but this is not the only way that graft survival can be improved.

Graft survival can be improved by exploring the kidney itself and also looking at the general health of the patient to see if any improvements can be made to reduce risk factors.

Cardiovascular death (CVD) with a functioning transplant is one of the major causes of graft loss and it is in this area that the greatest potential for improved outcomes and graft survival lies. In a study of long-term outcomes, Arend et al. (1997) found a standardised mortality ratio for recipients of a first transplant of 14 times the population average. CVD accounted for 32% of all deaths.

Persons with established renal failure (ERF) have an accelerated risk of cardiovascular morbidity and mortality; unfortunately this risk persists even after transplantation and is associated with pre- and post-transplant vascular disease, number of rejections, use of high-dose steroids, prolonged use of immunosuppressants, co-existing conditions, male gender and family history. Martin et al. (2001) found that in men the risk of myocardial infarction increased with smoking, with higher systolic blood pressure and with advancing age. The risk of stroke was, however, associated with higher body mass index, but not of heart attacks. Obviously, the renal team should aim to lessen those risks that are modifiable (Martin et al., 2001).

Hypertension, hyperlipidaemia and smoking were found to be predictive of CVD in renal transplant recipients, as were two or more acute rejection episodes in the first year. Lower risk was associated with pre-transplant nephrectomy, and high serum albumin reduced the risk of ischaemic heart events (Kasiske, 2001).

Carotid arteriosclerotic lesions were found in 24.6% of renal transplant patients compared with 6.2% of age and gender matched controls. Age and hypertension were the main predictors of atherosclerosis in transplant patients in this study, and no association was found between plaques and high density lipoproteins (HDLs) in patients (Barbagallo et al., 1999).

Hypertension is a common feature amongst renal transplant recipients. The major causes of this are impaired renal function, use of calineurin inhibitors (CNIs), uncontrolled renin secretion by native kidneys, stenosed renal arterial supply, polycythaemia and donor factors. Even a small degree of hypertension has a significant impact on the recipient, through CVD, graft survival and amplification of vascular injury. Angiotensen converting enzyme (ACE) inhibitors are indicated for hypertension; they improve left ventricular hypertrophy and vessel wall and endothelial dysfunction; they are also indicated for their nephro-protective effect. However, given the causal role of sodium retention and graft vasoconstriction, diuretics and calcium channel blockers remain the mainstays of antihypertensive treatment (Schwenger et al., 2001).

ACE inhibitors have been shown to slow the progression of renal failure in patients with chronic disease; this effect correlates with the reduction of proteinuria. In transplanted patients, they have been shown to reduce urinary protein excretion. This is presumed to be due to the prevention of glomerular hyperfiltration (Hausberg et al., 2001). The British Hypertension Society advocates a blood pressure of less than 125/75 mm Hg for those with type 1 diabetes with 1 g or more of proteinuria, and a blood pressure of less than 130/80 mm Hg for those with type 1 diabetes with nephropathy. Most units are now aiming for this level, which is lower than the target in previous years. Recent guidance from the USA suggests lowering the target even further by defining hypertension as a blood pressure of more than 120/80 mm Hg (Chobanian et al., 2003).

Massy et al. (1998) found an increased risk of cardiovascular events with increasing carotid plaques. Other, modifiable risk factors should be monitored as only serum cholesterol and the presence of diabetes mellitus could be identified as risk factors; serum lipoprotein and homocysteine could not. Patients should also be given lifestyle advice concerning dietetic modification, weight control, exercise and smoking. An awareness of relevant family history may also offer opportunities to intervene.

Anaemia and hyperhomocysteinaemia may contribute to cardiovascular disease following poor graft function (Ponticelli and Villa, 2002).

Routine screening will show up risk factors such as hypertension, obesity, high cholesterol, smoking and high blood sugar, and these can be modified by lifestyle changes and aggressive treatment. The prophylactic use of low-dose aspirin, statins and ACE inhibitors following renal transplantation is now widespread. Those with diabetes should be seen regularly in a specialist clinic to help ensure tight glycaemic control. HbA1c should be monitored regularly in the transplant clinic and poorly controlled diabetes re-referred to a diabetologist. Anaemia should be investigated and treated appropriately according to Renal Association (2002) guidelines.

## Increasing the life of the transplant

### Cold ischaemic time

UK Transplant aims to keep cold ischaemic time as short as possible, ideally under 20 hours, to minimise damage to the graft, which has an adverse effect on outcome. Transplant co-ordinators assess and record any other aspects of the donor history that may affect outcome, such as a history of hypertension or prolonged hypotension in intensive care, and offer help in best management of potential cadaver donors.

## Chronic allograft nephropathy

Chronic allograft nephropathy is the appearance on biopsy of permanent damage, characteristically seen in long-standing grafts that have begun to deteriorate. Halloran (2002) proposed a structured approach to this often-seen eventual deterioration in graft function, to more accurately define what may be encompassed by the term *chronic rejection*. The status of the graft can be determined by the presence and extent of rejection (T-cell mediated or antibody mediated), allograft nephropathy (parenchyma atrophy, fibrosis, fibrous intimal thickening in arteries), transplant glomerulopathy, specific diseases and factors that could accelerate progression. The level of function and the rate of loss of function should be determined to facilitate any use of corrective interventions. Much work is currently in progress to establish the extent of the role of CNIs, particularly ciclosporin, in chronic allograft nephropathy (CAN). Dudley (2002) has so far found a beneficial effect in stopping ciclosporin and switching to mycophenolate mofetil.

## Multi-professional working

The multiplicity of management and treatment options surrounding transplantation mean that the use of written guidelines and protocols is essential for meaningful practice. A considered and consistent approach based on these allows audit of outcomes, a structure for logical decision making and problem solving, and an educational resource for staff.

Members of the multidisciplinary team must work together to provide a comprehensive service and also forge links with services in diabetes, obstetrics and gynaecology, urology and dermatology. Patient groups, counsellors and general practitioners also play an important role in providing a patient-centred approach to care.

Nurses have had to work hard to keep up with the changes in transplantation, interactions with patients are much more than a therapeutic act and there is increasing specialisation (Rochera Gaya, 1999). Nurse roles are often extended, accepting tasks previously carried out by doctors, and expanded, moving forward the fundamental role to help and enable patients (Holder, 1989; Wright, 1998).

## The future

### Stem cells

Following the major breakthrough when J.A. Thomson et al. (1998) obtained stem cells from pre-implantation blastocysts following in-vitro fertilisation, new findings are being published at an extraordinary rate. Embryonic stem cells have a quasi-infinite capacity for self-renewal and the ability to give rise to one or more differentiated cell types (Lovell-Badge, 2001).

Researchers in the USA have fabricated, and implanted, primitive artificial kidneys using tissue from a cloned animal embryo. The kidney units were implanted into the same animal, a cow, from which the tissue was cloned. The units were not rejected and mimicked the action of a real kidney. This suggests that growing human kidneys for transplantation, cloned from a patient's own cells, could become a reality. This study also had success with the cloned heart and muscle cells implanted into the same cow. Ethically it would be impossible to grow human embryos until 8 weeks old and then destroy them to remove the growing kidney cells. The UK has legislated to allow research on human embryos but has banned experiments beyond the blastocyst stage. To satisfy moral objections, we first need to learn how to reliably clone a human embryo, extract stem cells from it in the first few days of existence, then nurture and guide the development of these human stem cells into kidney cells (Lanza et al., 2001).

## Tolerance

In kidney transplantation we are often used to thinking in one direction only, that is, a response from the recipient immune system to the donor organ. However, we can also look at the donor immune response to the recipient. Tolerance occurs when there are reciprocally modulating immune responses of co-existing immune-competent cell populations. The donor organ, despite losing most of its passenger leukocytes, apparently remains an important site for donor precursor and stem cells (Ichikawa et al., 2000).

The donor kidney carries leucocytes and dendritic cells which continue to develop in the host. Chimaeric immune system cells can be found in the host blood long after transplantation. The recipient and donor immune cells interact to neutralise one another.

A key requirement for maintaining tolerance is the persistence of donor antigen. This has been shown in experimental models. The source of the antigen can be donor-derived cells introduced before transplantation, as is the case in models of mixed chimaerism (Khan et al., 1996), or the graft itself after transplantation (Hamano et al., 1996). In the absence of antigen the tolerance is lost because the mechanisms responsible for maintaining it are no longer stimulated.

Surgeons from the University of Pittsburgh's Starzl Institute transfused donor stem cells 3 days after transplanting a kidney from a patient's brother in January 2002 (peripheral blood stem cell transplantation, a technique used in some cancer treatments). Priming the patient's body with donor peripheral stem cells may protect the transplanted kidney from being rejected by inducing chimaerism. After several months a decision on weaning-off drugs can be made, perhaps allowing an immunosuppression-free regime. As well as no drug side effects this would stop chronic rejection (Millan et al., 2002; Shapiro et al., 2002; Starzl, 2002).

Stem cells from bone marrow can change into kidney cells and may provide a new method to treat kidney disease. Researchers at the Imperial Cancer Research Fund showed that kidney cells can be derived from stem cells in bone marrow. This opens up the possibility of mobilising a patient's own stem cells to repair or replace kidney cells destroyed through disease or injury. It could also provide a way of using stem cells containing a gene to protect against cancer or other diseases in order to protect the kidney from further damage. In mice, they found kidney cells, derived from donated male bone marrow, in female mice whose bone marrow had been destroyed by radiation. In humans, biopsies from male kidney transplant patients, who had received a kidney from a female donor, showed male kidney cells among the female ones, showing that the recipient's bone marrow cells had transformed into kidney tissue in the graft (Poulsom et al., 2001).

The explanation of organ engraftment by immunosuppression only – assuming donor leukocytes had been destroyed – was not challenged until small numbers of multilineage donor haematopoietic cells (chimaeric cells) were shown in 1992 in the blood or tissue of 30 long-surviving kidney or liver recipients (Starzl et al., 1992, 1993). Bone marrow and solid organ transplants appear to be mirror images.

A degree of tolerance develops in most allograft recipients, who require less immunosuppression over time, and a small number of patients become completely tolerant to their graft, requiring no immunosuppression. The therapeutic future for stem cells is promising, although non-renal transplant applications are likely to lead the way, for example, a patient's own stem cells have already been used to regenerate cardiac tissue damaged after a heart attack and injected into the damaged heart muscle (Strauer et al., 2001).

At the Third Annual Conference on Regenerative Medicine, December 2002, Dr David Humes presented preliminary results of a biohybrid kidney used to treat patients suffering from acute renal failure (Humes, 2002). This Renal Assist Device from the University of Michigan relies on renal stem and precursor cells to replace kidney function, enhancing conventional haemodialysis treatments. Initial results of phase I and II of the clinical trials show improved patient outcome.

## Summary

This chapter has explored the major issues affecting renal transplantation and has analysed the problems in order to identify how transplantation may move forward in the coming years. Continued improvements in immunosuppression, and in maintaining the health and quality of life of the recipient, are currently overshadowed by the spectre of organ shortages. By continuing to invest more in both cadaveric and living donor programmes and in new technologies we are moving slowly towards the day when a kidney will be available to any person with ERF fit enough to receive one.

## References

Abercassis, M., Adams, M., Adams, P., et al. (2000) Consensus statement on the live organ donor *JAMA* **284** (22), 2919–26.

Akposso, K., Rondeau, E., Hayman, J.P., et al. (1997) Long-term prognosis of renal transplantation after pre-emptive treatment of cytomegalovirus infection. *Transplantation* **63**, 974.

Arend, S.M., Mallat, M.J., Westendorp, R.J., van der Woude, F.J. and van Es, L.A. (1997) Patient survival after renal transplantation; more than 25 years follow-up. *Nephrology Dialysis Transplantation* **12** (8), 1672–9.

Arnold, R., Bartlett, S., Bernat, J., et al. (2002) Financial incentives for cadaver organ donation: an ethical reappraisal. *Transplantation* **73** (8), 1361–7.

Barbagallo, C.M., Pinto, A., Gallo, S., et al. (1999) Carotid atherosclerosis in renal transplant recipients: relationships with cardiovascular risk factors and plasma lipoproteins. *Transplantation* **67** (3), 366–71.

Barr, B.B.B., Benton, E.C., McLaren, K., et al. (1989) Human papillomavirus infection and skin cancer in renal allograft recipients. *Lancet* **1** (8630), 124–9.

Biller-Andorno, N., Agich, G.J., Doepkens, K. and Schauenburg, H. (2001) Who shall be allowed to give? Living organ donors and the concept of autonomy. *Theoretical Medicine and Bioethics* **22** (4), 351–68.

Birkeland, S.A., Anderson, H.K. and Hamilton-Dutoit, S.J. (1999) Preventing acute rejection, Epstein-Barr virus infection, and posttransplant lymphoproliferative disorders after kidney transplantation: use of aciclovir and mycophenolate mofetil in a steroid-free immunosuppressive protocol. *Transplantation* **67**, 1209–14.

British Medical Association (2000) BMA Policy (Transplant of Human Organs). www.bma.org.uk.

Chobanian, A.V., Bakris, G.L., Black, H.R., et al. (2003) National Heart, Lung, and Blood Institute Joint National Committee on Prevention, Detection, Evaluation, and Treatment of High Blood Pressure; National High Blood Pressure Education Program Coordinating Committee (2003). Seventh report of the Joint National Committee on Prevention, Detection, Evaluation, and Treatment of High Blood Pressure: The JNC 7 Report. *JAMA* **289** (19), 2560–72.

Cosio, F.G., Roche, Z., Agarwal, A., Falkenhain, M.E., Sedmak, D.D. and Ferguson, R.M. (1996) Prevalence of hepatitis C in patients with idiopathic glomerulopathies in native and transplant kidneys. *American Journal of Kidney Diseases* **28** (5), 752–8.

Cozzi, E., Bhatti, F., Schmoeckel, M., et al. (2000) Long-term survival of non-human primates receiving life-supporting transgenic porcine kidney allografts. *Transplantation* **70** (1), 15–21.

Department of Health/Welsh Assembly Government (2002) 'Human Bodies Human Choices'. Consultation report on the law on human organs and tissues in England and Wales. HMSO, London.

Dhedin, N., Douvin, C., Kuentz, M., et al. (1998) Reverse seroconversion of hepatitis B after allogenic bone marrow transplantation: a retrospective study of 37 patients with pretransplant anti-HBs and anti-HBc. *Transplantation* **66** (5), 616–19.

Donnelly, P., Oman, P. and Opelz, G. (2001) Should culture-based gender bias in living donor renal transplantation be discouraged on ethical and graft survival grounds? *Transplantation Proceedings* **33** (1–2), 1882–3.

Dudley, C.R.K. (2002) (The creeping creatinine study group.) MMF replacing ciclosporin A reverses the creeping creatinine of renal transplant recipients of a multicentre randomised controlled trial. *Transplantation* **74** (Suppl 4), 162–3.

Ellison, M.D., McBride, M.A., Taranto, S.E., Delmonico, F.L. and Kauffman, H.M. (2002) Living kidney donors in need of kidney transplants: a report on the organ procurement and transplantation network. *Transplantation* **74** (9), 245–67.

Fan, S.L., Almond, M.K., Ball, E., Evans, K. and Cunningham, J. (2000) Pamidronate therapy as prevention of bone loss following renal transplantation. *Kidney International* **57**, 684–90.

First, M.R. (1997) Xenotransplantation: social, ethical, religious and political issues. *Kidney International* **58** (Suppl), 46.

Friedlaender, M.M. (2002) The right to buy or sell a kidney: are we failing our patients? *Lancet* **359**, 971–3.

Funch, D.P., Brady, J., Ko, H.H., Dreyer, N.A. and Walker, A.M. (2002) Methods and objectives of a large US multicentre case-control study of PTLD in renal transplant patients. Recent results. *Cancer Research* **159**, 81–8.

Gardner, S.D. (1977) The new human papovaviruses: their nature and significance. In Watson, A.P. (ed.) *Recent Advances in Clinical Virology*. Churchill Livingstone, Edinburgh, p. 93.

Gayed, S.L. (2002) Topical imiquimod cream 5% for resistant perianal warts in a renal transplant patient. *International Journal of STD and AIDS* **13**, 349–51.

Gonzalez-Fraile, M.I., Canizo, C., Caballero, D., et al. (2001) Cidofovir treatment of human polyomavirus-associated acute haemorrhagic cystitis. *Transplant Infectious Disease* **3** (1), 44–6.

Gordon, E.J. (2001) 'They don't have to suffer for me': why dialysis patients refuse offers of living donor kidneys. *Medical Anthropology Quarterly* **15** (2), 245–67.

Goyal, M., Mehta, R.L., Schneiderman, L.J. and Segal, A.R. (2002) Economic and health consequences of selling a kidney in one Indian city. *JAMA* **288**, 1589–93.

Halloran, P.F. (2002) Call for revolution: a new approach to describing allograft deterioration. *American Journal of Transplantation* **2** (3), 195–200.

Hamano, K., Rawsthorne, M., Bushell, A.R., Morris, P.J. and Wood, K.J. (1996) Evidence that the continued presence of the organ graft and not peripheral donor microchimerism is essential for the maintenance of tolerance to alloantigen in anti-CD4 treated recipients. *Transplantation* **62** (6), 856–60.

Hausberg, M., Kosch, M., Hohage, H., Suwelack, B., Barenbrock, M., Kisters, K. and Rahn, K.H. (2001) Antihypertensive treatment in renal transplant patients – is there a role for ACE inhibitors? *Annals of Transplantation* **6** (4), 31–7.

Held, T.K., Biel, S.S., Nitsche, A., Kurth, A., Chen, S., Gelderblom, H.R. and Siegert, W. (2000) Treatment of BK virus-associated hemorrhagic cystitis and simultaneous CMV reactivation with cidofovir. *Bone Marrow Transplant* **26** (3), 347–50.

Holder, S. (1989) Expanding role. *Nursing Standard* **38** (3), 52.

Hollander, A.A., Hene, R.J., Hermans, J., van Es, L.A. and van der Woude, F.J. (1997) Late prednisone withdrawal in ciclosporin-treated kidney transplant recipients: a randomized study. *Journal of the American Society of Nephrology* **8**, 294.

Hricik, D.E. (2001) Safety and efficacy of TOR inhibitors and other immunosuppressive regimens in African-American renal transplant patients. *American Journal of Kidney Disease* **38** (4) (Suppl 2) S11–5.

Humes, D. (2002) *Preliminary Results of a Biohybrid Kidney Used to Treat Patients Suffering Acute Renal Failure*. Proc 3rd Annual Conference on Regenerative Medicine, December 2002.

Ichikawa, N., Demetris, A.J., Starzl, T.E., Ye, Q., Okuda, T., Chun, H.J., Liu, K., Kim, Y.M. and Murase, N. (2000) Donor and recipient leukocytes in organ allografts of recipients with variable donor-specific tolerance: with particular reference to chronic rejection. *Liver Transplantation* **6** (6), 686–702.

Inston, N. and Ready, A. (2002) The right to buy or sell a kidney. *Lancet* **360**, 948–9.

Jung, Y.O., Less, Y.S. and Yang, W.S. (1998) Treatment of chronic hepatitis B with Lamivudine in renal transplant recipients. *Transplantation* **66** (6), 733–7.

Kaplan, B.S. and Polise, K. (2000) In defence of altruistic kidney donation by strangers. *Pediatric Nephrology* **14** (6), 518–22.

Kasiske, B.L. (2001) Epidemiology of cardiovascular disease after renal transplantation. *Transplantation* **72**, S5–8.

Kerridge, I.H., Saul, P., Lowe, M., McPhee, J. and Williams, D. (2002) Death, dying and donation: organ transplantation and the diagnosis of death. *Journal of Medical Ethics* **28**, 89–94.

Khan, A., Tomita, Y. and Sykes, M. (1996) Thymic dependence of loss of tolerance in mixed allogeneic bone marrow chimeras after depletion of donor antigen. *Transplantation* **62**, 380.

Kinnaert, P., Abramowicz, D., De Pauw, L., Jansenn, F., Hall, M., Wissing, M. and Hooghe, L. (1999) What degree of freedom is there for living donors? *Revue Medicale de Bruxelles* **20** (4), A279–82.

Kootstra, G. (1997) The asystolic, or non-heart beating donor. *Transplantation* **63**, 917.

Kootstra, G., Kievit, J.K. and Heineman, E. (1997) The non-heart beating donor. *British Medical Bulletin* **53**, 844.

Kumar, M.S.A., Damask, A.M. and Roland, M. (2002) Kidney transplantation in HIV positive end stage renal disease (ESRD) patients – a prospective study. *American Journal of Transplantation* **2**, 174 (Abstr).

Lanza, R.P., Cibelli, J.B., Faber, D., Sweeney, R.W., Henderson, B., Nevala, W., West, M.D. and Wettstein, P.J. (2001) Cloned cattle can be healthy and normal. *Science* **294** (5548), 1893–4.

Lovell-Badge, R. (2001) The future for stem cell research. *Nature* **414**, 88–91.

Martin, J.C., Hathaway, D.K., Egidi, M.F. and Gaber, A.O. (2001) Lifestyle behaviours affect cardiovascular risk status in men one year after transplantation. *Clinical Transplantation* **15** (Suppl 6), 41–5.

Massy, Z.A., Mamzer-Bruneel, M.F., Chevalier, A., et al. (1998) Carotid atherosclerosis in renal transplant recipients. *Nephrology Dialysis Transplantation* **13** (7), 1792–8.

Matesanz, R., Miranda, B., Felipe, C. and Naya, M.T. (1996) Continuous improvement in organ donation. The Spanish experience. *Transplantation* **61** (7), 1119–21.

Millan, M.T., Shizuri, J.A., Hoffman, P., et al. (2002) Mixed chimerism and donor specific unresponsiveness without graft versus host disease after MHC-mismatched haemopoietic stem cell infusion and kidney transplantation. *Transplantation* **74** (Suppl 4), 37.

Neylan, J.F. (1997) Immunosuppressive therapy in high-risk transplant patients: dose dependent efficacy of mycophenolate mofetil in African-American renal allograft recipients. *Transplantation* **64** (9), 1277–82.

Nickeleit, V., Klimkait, T., Binet, I.F., Dalquen, P., Del Zenero, V., Thiel, G., Mihatsch, M.J. and Hirsch, H.H. (2000) Testing for polyomavirus type BK DNA in plasma to identify renal-allograft recipients with viral nephropathy. *New England Journal of Medicine* **342** (18), 1309–15).

Paradis, K., Langford, G., Long, Z., et al. (1999) Search for cross-species transmission of porcine endogenous retrovirus in patients treated with living pig tissue. *Science* **285** (5431), 1236–41.

Patience, C., Takeuchi, Y. and Weiss, R.A. (1997) Infection of human cells by an endogenous retrovirus of pigs. *Nature Medicine* **3**, 282.

Ponticelli, C. and Villa, M. (2002) Role of anaemia in cardiovascular mortality and morbidity in transplant patients. *Nephrology Dialysis Transplantation* **17** (Suppl 1), 41–6.

Poulsom, R., Forbes, S.J., DilkeHodivala, K., et al. (2001) Bone marrow contributes to renal parenchymal turnover and regeneration. *Journal of Pathology* **195** (2), 229–35.

Radcliffe-Richards, J., Daar, A.S., Guttman, R.D., Hoffenburg, R., Kennedy, I., Lock, M., Sells, R.A. and Tilney, N. (1998) The case for allsowing kidney sales (International Forum for Transplant Ethics). *Lancet* **351**, 1950–52.

Randhawa, P.S., Finkelstein, S., Scantlebury, V.P., Shapiro, R., Vivas, C., Jordan, M., Picken, M.M. and Demetris, A.J. (1999) Human polyoma virus-associated interstitial nephritis in the allograft kidney. *Transplantation* **67** (1), 103–109.

Renal Association (2002) *Treatment of Adult Patients with Renal Failure*, 3rd edn. Royal College of Physicians, London.

Reploeg, M.D., Storch, G.A. and Clifford, D.B. (2001) BK virus: a clinical review. *Clinical Infectious Diseases* **33** (2), 191–202.

Rochera Gaya, A. (1999) The evolution of kidney transplantation in Spain: role of the nurse. *EDTNA/ERCA Journal* **25** (1), 15.

Ross, L.F. and Woodle, E.S. (2000) Ethical issues in increasing living kidney donations by expanding kidney paired exchange programmes. *Transplantation* **69** (8), 1539–43.

Ross, L.F., Rubin, D.T., Siegler, M., Josephson, M.A., Thistlethwaite, J.R. and Wordle, E.S. (1997) Ethics of a paired-kidney-exchange program. *New England Journal of Medicine* **336** (24), 1752–5.

Saunders, R.N., Elwell, R., Murphy, G.J., Horsburgh, T., Carr, S.J. and Nicholson, M.L. (2000) Workload generated by a living donor programme for renal transplantation. *Nephrology Dialysis Transplantation* **15** (10), 1667–72.

Scheper-Hughes, N. (2001) *The New Cannibalism: The Global Traffic in Human Organs.* Report for the International Operations and Human Rights Congressional Sub-committee hearings, First Session, 27 June, 107th Congress Serial no. 107–29. US Government Printing Office, Washington, pp 73–452. www.publicanthropology.org/timespast/scheper-hughes.htm.

Schwenger, V., Zeier, M. and Ritz, E. (2001) Hypertension after renal transplantation. *Annals of Transplantation* **6** (4), 25–30.

Sever, M.S., Kazancioglu, R., Yildez, A., et al. (2001) Outcome of living unrelated (commercial) renal transplantation. *Kidney International* **60** (4), 1477–83.

Shapiro, E.D. and Clemens, J.D. (1984) A controlled evaluation of the protective efficacy of pneumococcal vaccine for patients at high risk of serious pneumococcal infections. *Annals of International Medicine* **101**, 325.

Shapiro, R., Scantlebury, V. and Yeager, A. (2002) www.augustachronicle.com 2/5/2002, www.univ-relations.pitt.edu/utimes/issues/34/020207/research.html.

Smith, K.J., Germain, M. and Skelton, H. (2001) Squamous cell carcinoma in situ (Bowen's disease) in renal transplant patients treated with 5% imiquimod and 5% 5-fluorouracil therapy. *Dermatologic Surgery* **27** (6), 561–4.

Soin, B. and Friend, P.J. (2001) Renal xenotransplantation. In: Morris, P.J. (ed.) *Kidney Transplantation: Principles and Practice*, 5th edn. W.B. Saunders, Philadelphia, pp 751–2.

Sola, R. (2001) Proc 2nd International Congress of Nephrology for Internet 2001. www.uninet.edu/cin2001.

Soros, G. (1998) *The Crisis of Global Capitalism.* Public Affairs, New York.

Spital, A. (2001) Ethical issues in living organ donation: donor autonomy and beyond. *American Journal of Kidney Disease* **38** (1), 189–95.

Starzl, T.E. (2002) A tolerogenic strategy for organ transplantation. *Transplantation* **74** (Suppl 4), 147.

Starzl, T.E., Demetris, A.J., Murase, N., Ildstad, S., Ricordi, C. and Trucco, M. (1992) Cell migration, chimerism, and graft acceptance. *Lancet* **339** (8809), 1579–82.

Starzl, T.E., Demetri, A.J., Trucco, M., et al. (1993) Cell migration and chimerism after whole-organ transplantation: the basis of graft acceptance. *Hepatology* **17** (6), 1127–52.

Steiner, R.W. and Gert, B. (2000) Ethical selection of living donors. *American Journal of Kidney Disease* **36** (4), 677–86.

Strauer, B.E., et al. (2001) Myocardial regeneration after intercoronary transplantation of human autologous stem cells following acute myocardial infarction. *Deutsche Medizinische Wochenschrschrift* **126** (34–35), 932–8.

Swanson, S.J., Kirk, A.D., Ko, C.W., Jones, C.A., Agodoa, L.Y. and Abbott, K.C. (2002) Impact of HIV seropositivity on graft and patient survival after cadaveric renal transplantation in the United States in the pre-highly active antiretroviral therapy (HAART) era: an historical cohort analysis of the United States Renal Data System. *Transplant Infectious Disease* **4**, 144–7.

Thomson, J.A., Itskovitz-Eldor, J., Shapiro, S.S., Waknitz, M.A., Swiergiel, J.J., Marshall, V.S. and Jones, J.M. (1998) Embryonic stem cell lines derived from human blastocysts. *Science* **282** (5391), 1145–7.

Trevitt, R., Whittaker, C., Ball, E.A. and FitzGerald, L. (2001) Drop-out rate during living donor selection. *EDTNA/ERCA Journal* **17** (2), 88–91.

Truog, R.D. (1997) Is it time to abandon brain death? *Hastings Center Report* **27**, 29.

UK Transplant (2003) *UK Transplant yearly statistics.* www.uktransplant.org.uk/statistics/statistics.htm.

Venning, V. (1998) Renal transplantation and the skin. *Lancet* **1**, 294.

White, A.J., Ozminkowski, R.J., Hassol, A., Dennis, J.M. and Murphy, M. (1998) The effects of New York State's ban on multiple listing for cadaveric kidney transplantation. *Health Services Research* **33** (2, part 1), 205–222.

Wright, S. (1998) Modelling excellence: the role of the consultant nurse. In: Butterworth, T., Faugier, J. and Burnard, P. (1998) *Clinical Supervision and Mentorship in Nursing.* Stanley Thornes, Cheltenham, pp 205–214.

Zeier, M. and Ritz, E. (2002) Preparation of the dialysis patient for transplantation. *Nephrology Dialysis Transplantation* **17**, 552–6.

# Chapter 7
# Care of Older People on Dialysis

*Jane Bentley*

## Introduction

As highlighted in Chapter 1, there has been a global rise in the number of older patients making use of renal services in recent years. Within the UK, for example, 47% of patients accepted onto renal replacement therapy were over 65 in 1999, compared with 37% in 1992 (UK Renal Registry, 2000). Factors contributing to this rapid rise include a worldwide growth in the older population and a relaxation of age-related acceptance criteria (Grapsa and Oreopoulos, 1996). Furthermore, advances in dialysis techniques have made it easier for older people to tolerate renal replacement therapy, so that once they have started dialysis, they are living longer (Bhatnagar, 1998).

A key problem for renal staff adapting to such changes in user population profile is that (as in the case of many other acute and specialist health care settings) their services were originally configured around the needs of younger age groups. Renal failure (and related treatment) in itself commonly results in a high incidence of health, social and emotional problems amongst sufferers of all ages (Harries, 1996); therefore many aspects of developed services will already be suitable for both younger and older patients' needs. Nevertheless, it is likely that a higher number of older patients will present with complex needs, leading to a greater demand for specialist skills and resources within renal units as the proportion of older renal patients grows. Staff also need to take into account that needs amongst the older group are likely to be more multifaceted, because of additional exacerbating factors commonly associated with ageing. For example, older people are more likely to have concurrent co-morbidities, to be affected by physical, sensory, communication and memory deficits and more likely to be living alone with little support [Standing Nursing and Advisory Committee (SNMAC), 2001].

So far, little research appears to have been conducted as to how well renal services are meeting the needs of this population group. However, studies in other acute settings have found that older people and their carers are often less than satisfied with care. Specific problems have been identified relating to the suitability of the physical environment, to inadequacies in communication between staff and patients, to a lack of relevant resources and equipment, to deficiencies in staff awareness of needs and to a lack of specific nursing skills (Health Advisory Service, 1998; Davies et al., 1999; Meyer et al., 1999; Royal College of Physicians, 2000).

Some emerging evidence from renal studies would also support such findings and suggest that many service providers are presently falling short of providing older patients with care fully appropriate for their needs (Oreopoulos, 1997; Meyer and Bentley, 2002). As a result of concerns over older patients' care within the UK, the National Service Framework (NSF) for Older People (Department of Health, 2001) has been introduced to try to raise standards of care provision across health and social care settings. As throughout the health service, therefore, renal units will be required to evaluate the appropriateness of care provided for older patients and to put in place initiatives to meet any deficiencies in service provision for this group. To assist with this process, this chapter will therefore aim to highlight some key issues and recommendations relating to ways that current care of older renal patients might be improved.

## Key issues and recommendations for the improvement of renal services to better meet older dialysis patients' needs

Six key areas of recommendation for the improvement of older dialysis patients' care are outlined in this chapter. These areas are synthesised directly from findings from a recent study in this area (Meyer and Bentley, 2002), supported by issues highlighted both in other renal studies and in recent policy targeting the care of older patients by the National Health Service generally. The areas recommended are as follows:

(1)  Promote a planned entry onto dialysis in a greater proportion of older patients.
(2)  Base older patients' care on co-ordinated multidisciplinary assessment of holistic needs.
(3)  Ensure service provision for older renal patients is based on a multidisciplinary and preventative approach to care.
(4)  Ensure renal units have access to the right mix of specialists and resources to address the holistic needs of older renal patients.
(5)  Promote better awareness of the particular needs of this age group and ensure staff have the appropriate skills and resources to meet these needs.
(6)  Encourage greater openness and reflection amongst staff to address ageist attitudes towards older dialysis patients.

### *Promote a planned entry onto dialysis in a greater proportion of older patients*

It is well recognised that a planned start to dialysis treatment (where possible) is the best option for patients of all ages (Jungers, 2002). In this case, patients can be prepared mentally and physically for the start of treatment and the physical complications associated with renal failure reduced. Earlier commencement of dialysis has also been found to be linked to improved survival rates and decreased morbidity (Levin et al., 1997; Schrag et al., 1999). Even so, the Kidney Alliance concludes that too high a proportion of older patients in particular commence dialysis acutely, rather than in the co-ordinated and 'seamless' way recommended in its National Service Standards (Kidney Alliance, 2001). Late referral from primary and secondary care may undoubtedly be one reason for acute entry to dialysis care (Khan et al., 1994; Oreopoulos, 1997; Ifudu, 1999). However, Hines et al. (1997) also express concern that, whilst clinically it should be possible to predict the need for dialysis a minimum of 1 year in advance in all but around 10% of people with kidney failure, late referral occurs in some cases even with patients who are regularly monitored by nephrologists.

Doctors do face a number of difficulties in determining when end-stage renal failure is imminent, due to the individuality of patients' symptom responses to rising uraemia and other biochemical changes. Specific factors relating to ageing, such as some of the physiological changes and reduced dietary protein intake that may occur, may also mask signs of renal failure in the older group (Latos, 1996; Winchester and Rakowski, 1998). In addition, the early symptoms of established renal failure (ERF), such as weakness, fatigue and anorexia, may easily be attributed to other conditions or to 'age' (Latos, 1996). Nevertheless, judgements about quality of life, ageism and personal bias based on a perceived lack of resources or poor prognosis are also thought to play a part (Oreopoulos, 1997).

It seems apparent, therefore, that more needs to be done to explore and address this issue, from primary care through to nephrology departments. One means of further clarifying factors associated with this issue for the older renal population may be through the introduction of regular audits by service commissioners of the number of patients entering dialysis as 'late' uraemic emergencies (Kidney Alliance, 2001). This, in turn, may assist renal units in the development of mechanisms to reduce this number and to promote the timely commencement of dialysis in older patients.

## Base older patients' care on co-ordinated multidisciplinary assessment of holistic needs

Once older patients have been identified as likely to progress to end-stage, it is important that they receive assessment of their holistic needs as part of the process of identifying the most appropriate form of modality for their health and circumstances. Use of a comprehensive assessment for older people within renal care is also suggested as a means of improving the diagnosis of commonly experienced health problems of older adults and of enhancing care planning and referral (Kutner, 1996). Furthermore, ensuring that medical, social and psychological factors are explored through a co-ordinated multidisciplinary assessment of these areas is well recognised as highly beneficial for the ongoing care of older patients (Health Advisory Service, 1998; Winchester and Rakowski, 1998; Hazzard, 1999; Stack and Messana, 2000; Department of Health, 2001).

As part of the NSF for Older People (Department of Health, 2001), a single assessment process is to be introduced across health and social care within the UK from June 2002. In the further documentation that supports this introduction (Department of Health, 2002) four types of assessment are specified to be included in the overall process: contact (including the collection of basic personal information), overview, specialist (such as that relating to particular medical conditions) and comprehensive assessment. The specific tools to be used and the way co-ordination is to be achieved between the different stages and settings of assessment are being left to local negotiation and agreement. However, individual Trusts (with the aid of local geriatricians and psychiatrists for the older age group) will be required to ensure that all health care settings in their province are aligned to the single assessment process within their locality, so that consistency of assessment is achieved across all their services (Department of Health, 2002). Alongside this, however, renal units themselves need to ensure that systems are in place to deliver a comprehensive and integrated team assessment. To this aim, it would seem important that the following issues are addressed.

Firstly, that there is a systematic approach to assessment in place to ensure that health and social circumstances in the broadest sense are explored as early as possible prior to the commencement of dialysis. This should occur even where patients already have frequent contact with health or social services, since it has still been found in such cases that physical, social and psychological problems are missed or may go unreported (Department of Health, 2001). Secondly, that family or other key carers are included in the assessment process, so that all relevant issues (such as realistic functional abilities or problems at home) are accounted for (Health Advisory Service, 1998) and carers' own needs acknowledged (Department of Health, 2002). Finally, that good coordination is achieved throughout the assessment process between members of the multidisciplinary renal team. The SNMAC report (2001) states that all too often, older people are assessed separately by different disciplines within a team, and uni-disciplinary plans devised for care from each staff group. To enhance this process, therefore, and avoid duplication or fragmentation of effort, staff should integrate documentation and make it centrally and readily available to the whole team (Department of Health, 2001).

Further to the single assessment process, once dialysis treatment has commenced there is an additional need to ensure that these chronically ill older patients receive regular reviews of their holistic needs as they age. Best practice would seem to indicate regular home visits for older dialysis patients, since once patients leave hospital, staff may be unaware of changing home circumstances, social needs, motivation and the ability to carry out or comply with treatment (Steinman, 1999). However, resource limitations may prevent this ideal being fulfilled in many units. At the very least, therefore, the NSF for Older People (2001) recommends that every time an older person is admitted to hospital, staff should be aware that they may have needs beyond the reason for their attendance and should explore these issues.

### Ensure service provision for older renal patients is based on a multidisciplinary and preventative approach to care

Good multidisciplinary working is essential for the effective care of older renal patients, because of the need to co-ordinate a range of care interventions to meet the ongoing and often complex needs of this group (Levin et al., 1997; Oreopoulos, 1997; Winchester and Rakowski, 1998; Hazzard, 1999; Stack and Messana, 2000). However, it has been found that, even where there might be a good mix of relevant disciplines within a renal unit team, systems in place may hinder team working. In the study by Meyer and Bentley (2002), for example, the number of settings within the renal unit (such as peritoneal and haemodialysis areas, in-patient wards and specialist clinics) were found to pose great challenges for communication even amongst single disciplines. Increased provision of satellite dialysis units and outreach clinics in local district general hospitals further added to problems. To counter such issues, renal services may need to consider a range of initiatives to enhance communication between staff groups and settings. For example, the development of common records and the introduction of link personnel between dialysis areas and in-patient wards are two ideas being introduced at the unit studied.

However, not only does older people's care need to be based on good multidisciplinary working, it also needs to be preventative in approach, so that emerging problems are identified ahead of crisis and effective responses made to reduce long-term dependency (Department of Health, 2001). One difficulty facing renal staff, however, is that the culture of care may tend towards addressing immediate renal issues or acute complaints, rather than addressing management of co-morbidities, for example. This may result in the systems underlying services working against efforts to promote preventative health care.

As an example, although a number of multidisciplinary team meetings were held during each week in the renal unit studied by Meyer and Bentley (2002), these meetings tended to only review in-patients of the unit, or patients in the community with acute problems. There was, therefore, no formal multidisciplinary forum where information obtained through telephone, home visit or informal contact with older patients or carers could be shared that related to more chronic problems, or to early indications of decline. As a result, social workers and occupational therapists in particular felt that many opportunities to intervene early were missed, because there was no opportunity for the team as a whole to review concerns from different professional perspectives. Staff were also often left feeling isolated regarding concerns they might have, which led to reluctance to explore wider issues with older patients. Instead, matters were left until the situation became more acute. It may be necessary, therefore, for renal services to review the role and scope of current multidisciplinary meetings and to raise awareness amongst staff of the particular importance for older patients of adopting a more preventative and rehabilitative approach to care.

## Ensure renal units have access to the right mix of specialists and resources to address the holistic needs of older renal patients

It has been recommended that all renal patients should have access to dieticians, social workers, pharmacists and other specialist roles alongside medical and nursing care, because of the need to co-ordinate a range of care interventions to meet the ongoing, often complex needs of this group (Kidney Alliance, 2001). However, further emphasis is also given in the literature to the need for renal staff to work more closely with other specialists and health care providers outside renal services, in order to meet the specific needs of the older age group. Particular mention is given to the involvement of geriatricians and GPs in care planning and resource provision (Oreopoulos, 1997; Hazzard, 1999). This stems from a need for care to combine clinical expertise in dialysis treatment with specialist knowledge of the changing physiology of age.

Renal physicians face the challenge of identifying and modifying factors contributing to debility in older renal patients before they become too advanced (Latos, 1996). Provision of support from specialists in older people's health care is seen as one means of improving knowledge and awareness amongst renal staff and is a key recommendation of the NSF for Older People (Department of Health, 2001).

However, a particular problem for both older patients and staff would seem to be that of balancing the management of renal-related conditions with those of other illnesses or age-related problems. Patients in frequent contact with renal units may naturally look to their nephrologist to fulfil a primary care role (Bender and Holley, 1996). Nevertheless, these doctors may not have the necessary knowledge, time or ready access to resources necessary for the most effective management of older patients' care.

At the same time, however, GPs may have insufficient renal expertise and therefore be uncertain of how to manage treatment of other conditions themselves alongside patients' regular renal therapy. As a result, despite the difficulties posed by distance over large catchment areas, it would seem important for renal staff to improve clarification over areas of responsibility in care and to strive for good levels of communication with GPs and others (Kidney Alliance, 2001). Furthermore, renal staff should take responsibility for providing clearer signposting for older patients regarding how to use health and social care systems, since it has been found that older people themselves are often confused as to who they should approach for help and advice. As a result, some older people may 'fall through the net' in terms of obtaining appropriate and timely intervention with emerging difficulties (Meyer and Bentley, 2002).

All these areas are highlighted as being crucial to the improvement of standards of older peoples' care across the health service in the NSF for Older People (Department of Health, 2001). Specific further recommended action to address the issues again include improving holistic assessment, improving the sharing of assessment findings across health and social services, increasing investment in rehabilitation services and adaptation equipment, and greater involvement of elderly care, rehabilitation and mental health specialists in specialist health settings, especially for those with complex co-morbidities or mental health problems.

Nevertheless, tertiary services such as renal care face particular problems in accessing services and equipment and working with specialist teams, because their patient populations tend to cover such wide geographical areas. Great differences may exist across boroughs within catchment areas in terms of provision and availability of equipment and support services for older people. This may lead to delays in discharge from hospital, problems with equity of access to care and ongoing difficulties for older people and carers trying to maintain independence at home (Meyer and Bentley, 2002). It would therefore seem a priority for greater recognition to be given nationally for the need to properly resource the community interface with specialist services like renal care, if real improvements are to be made in this area.

### Promote better awareness of the particular needs of this age group and ensure staff have the appropriate skills and resources to meet these needs

With the removal of overt age-based selection criteria, older patients are now increasingly forming the majority of acute and specialist service populations (Department of Health, 2000b). Nevertheless, negative attitudes are known to persist within the health service towards the care of this group (SNMAC, 2001). As a result, older people may be regarded as inappropriate users of acute resources by staff, or as 'bed blockers' when discharge from hospital is slower than that of other age groups. As nursing and other roles have become more specialised, meeting the physical needs of this group in particular has been increasingly delegated away from the core trained nursing group: either to health care assistants or to specialists post holders, such as continence advisors.

As a result, it has been found that nurses may not always have the adequate knowledge, skills and awareness to meet the needs of older people in many acute and specialised settings (Health Advisory Service, 1998; Davies et al., 1999; Meyer and Bentley, 2002). The Department of Health's Standing Nursing and Midwifery Advisory Committee (SNMAC) also suggests that too much focus has been given to educating nurses in specialised technical skills for the care of younger adults with single conditions, whereas, in reality, the majority of adults making use of acute health services are older people likely to have multiple co-morbidities who require knowledge of quality care to meet basic needs. As a consequence, the Committee recommended that core skills for nurses in the adult branch of training nationally need to be re-examined to address this issue.

Whilst such recommended changes to nurse education may help improve care of older renal patients in the long term, it would also seem necessary for work to be conducted with existing nursing (and other professional) staff at renal units now, to ensure staff have the necessary knowledge and skills to provide a high standard of care for their older age group. Senior managers of renal services may, however, need to devise a more cohesive and directive policy to address this matter, since, when given the choice, staff may choose courses seen as more directly relating to renal care over those focused on the care of older people per se (Meyer and Bentley, 2002).

Better liaison between renal services, elderly care specialists and other relevant post holders (such as continence specialists) might also be of benefit for renal staff as a means of accessing up-to-date advice on more specific areas of care. Trusts are being encouraged in the NSF for Older People (Department of Health, 2001) to provide specialist old-age multidisciplinary teams to help manage those with complex co-morbidities across acute settings generally. This might be a further way for renal staff to access advice in meeting older peoples' needs alongside renal priorities.

### Encourage greater openness and reflection amongst staff to address ageist attitudes towards older dialysis patients

Although older people are now the majority of users across the spectrum of services within the NHS (Department of Health, 2000a), the SNMAC report (2001) recommends that a cultural change in attitudes needs to occur across the NHS in recognition of this fact. In other words, older patients now need to be seen as an ongoing and key focus for services, rather than regarded as peripheral to the 'normal' patient population. Previous investigation of staff attitudes to older people has often revealed that stereotypical and negative views of attributes are held in relation to this patient group. These will need to be challenged if care is to be improved. Some staff interviewed by Meyer and Bentley (2002), for instance, expressed a number of assumptions about older renal patients that were in marked contrast to the experiences voiced by older patients in the study. These included views that older people would be less distressed by the impact of their diagnosis and treatment than younger patients, were less capable of understanding and retaining information, and were more likely to see treatment as a positive social experience because otherwise they tended to have inactive and socially empty lifestyles.

Such attitudes have been found to be relatively common amongst NHS staff generally (SNMAC, 2001). Some of the impacts on care suggested to be associated with such negative attitudes include reduced equity of access to services (Department of Health, 2001) and reduced expectations in patients' abilities to rehabilitate or recover (Health Advisory Service, 1998). Along with other areas within the NHS, therefore, it would appear that managers within renal services need to encourage a greater openness and reflection of these issues amongst staff, and consider ways of reducing the impact of any negative attitudes on the care of older dialysis patients.

Nevertheless, whilst addressing ageist attitudes amongst individual staff may play a part in improving standards of care for older patients, additional recognition needs to be given to other pressures placed on staff and resources by the increased numbers of older people making use of services. The SNMAC report (2001) also highlights the role that insufficient resources, poor skill mix and poor physical environment of care may play in promoting negative attitudes to older patients amongst staff. Findings by Meyer and Bentley (2002) would further support this. Here, staff related that they felt frustration in having to provide care for growing numbers of older patients because they perceived that they could not provide good care for this group, owing to a lack of time, or to not being able to access necessary equipment or help for patients. This situation appeared to be exacerbated by a number of factors, including a lack of appropriately trained staff, a failure to account for the increased time needed by older people, a failure to match increases in numbers or dependency of patients using the service with increases in staff deployment and a lack of community provision of relevant equipment and services.

It would seem necessary in future, therefore, that renal services review such issues within their service configuration and raise any identified community deficits with service commissioners, as a further means of improving staff attitudes to the increasing numbers of older people requiring care.

## Summary

Older people now form a significant part of the renal population, both nationally and internationally. Whilst much in the care of this age group will be in common with younger renal patients, nevertheless, specific factors associated with ageing may further complicate renal disease and the treatment process in the older age group. Until now, it would appear that there has been little reflection, on the part of either care providers or researchers, as to whether services adequately support those older patients receiving renal replacement therapy.

Current recognition of the need to improve standards of older peoples' care generally throughout the National Health Service (Department of Health, 2001) would, therefore, seem to make more work in this area essential. However, some emerging findings from the renal field (as well as from other health care settings) already indicate a number of key areas where care of this group can be improved. These include the need for renal practitioners to adopt a more preventive and holistic mode of care for older dialysis patients (such as by improving pre-dialysis care and assessment) and to promote better co-ordinated multidisciplinary team working.

Staff also need to be provided with ongoing training and education to help them improve their levels of understanding of older patients' potential needs and to guarantee the possession of suitable and up-to-date skills for care delivery. Of key additional importance, however, is the need for greater recognition to be given to increased funding of renal services in the light of the growing numbers of older renal patients. The potential complexity of needs and likely greater dependency of many older dialysis patients demand that units be better resourced in terms of staff numbers, relevant specialist support and equipment if the standard of care for older renal patients is truly to be improved.

# References

Bender, F.H. and Holley, J.L. (1996) Most nephrologists are primary care providers for chronic dialysis patients: results of a national survey. *American Journal of Kidney Diseases* **28** (1), 67–71.

Bhatnagar, V. (1998) Ethical issues involved in dialysis for the elderly. *Geriatric Nephrology and Urology* **8** (2), 111–14.

Davies, S., Laker, S. and Ellis, L. (1999) *Dignity on the Ward: Promoting Excellence in Care. Good Practice in Acute Hospital Care for Older People.* Help the Aged, London.

Department of Health (2000a) *The National Plan for the NHS.* Stationery Office, London.

Department of Health (2000b) *Shaping the Future NHS: Long Term Planning for Hospitals and Related Services.* Consultation document on the findings of the National Beds Inquiry. Stationery Office, London.

Department of Health (2001) *National Service Framework for Older People.* Department of Health, London, www.doh.gov.uk/nsf/olderpeople.htm.

Department of Health (2002) *Single Assessment Process: Key Implications, Guidance for Local Implementation and Annexes to the Guidance.* Department of Health, London, www.doh.gov.uk/scg/sap/index.htm.

Grapsa, I. and Oreopoulos, D.G. (1996) Practical ethical issues of dialysis in the elderly. *Seminars in Nephrology* **16** (4), 339–52.

Harries, F. (1996) Psychosocial care in end-stage renal failure. *Professional Nurse* **12** (2), 124–6.

Hazzard, W.R. (1999) Ageing kidneys in an ageing population: how does this impact nephrology and nephrologists? *Geriatric Nephrology and Urology* **9** (3), 177–82.

Health Advisory Service (1998) *'Not Because They Are Old'.* HAS, London.

Hines, S., Babrow, A.S., Badzek, L. and Moss, A. (1997) Communication and problematic integration in end-of-life decisions: dialysis decisions among the elderly. *Health Communication* **9**, 199–217.

Ifudu, O., Dawood, M., Iofel, Y., Valcourt, J. and Friedman, E. (1999) Delayed referral of Black, Hispanic and older patients with chronic renal failure. *American Journal of Kidney Diseases* **33** (4), 728–33.

Jungers, P. (2002) Late referral: loss of chance for the patient, loss of money for society. *Nephrology Dialysis Transplantation* **17** (3), 371–5.

Khan, I.H., Catto, G.R., Edward, N. and MacLeod, A.M. (1994) Chronic renal failure: factors influencing nephrology referral. *Quarterly Journal of Medicine* **87** (9), 559–64.

Kidney Alliance (2001) *End Stage Renal Failure – A Framework for Planning and Service Delivery.* www.kidneyalliance.org.uk.

Kutner, N.G. (1996) Rehabilitation of the elderly patient on dialysis. *Geriatric Nephrology and Urology* **6**, 81–8.

Latos, D.L. (1996) Chronic dialysis in patients over age 65. *Journal of the American Society of Nephrology* **7** (5), 637–46.

Levin, A., Lewis, M., Mortiboy, P., et al. (1997) Multidisciplinary pre-dialysis programmes: quantification and limitations of their impact on patient outcomes in two Canadian settings. *American Journal of Kidney Diseases* **29**, 533.

Meyer, J. and Bentley, J. (2002) *The Experience of Care of Older End-Stage Renal Patients in Receipt of Long-term Dialysis.* City University, London.

Meyer, J., Bridges, J. and Spilsbury, K. (1999) Caring for older people in acute settings: lessons learned from an action research study in accident and emergency. *NT Research* **4** (5), 327–39.

Oreopoulos, D.G. (1997) Should geriatric ethics differ from general medical ethics when considering the elderly for dialysis? *Contemporary Dialysis and Nephrology* **18** (7), 22–4, 30.

Royal College of Physicians (2000) *Management of the Older Medical Patient: Teamwork in the Journey of Care.* Working Party Report. RCP, London.

Schrag, W.F., Campbell, M., Ewert, J., et al. (1999) Multidisciplinary team renal rehabilitation: interventions and outcomes. *Advances in Renal Replacement Therapy* **6** (3), 282–8.

Stack, A.G. and Messana, J.M. (2000) Renal replacement therapy in the elderly: medical, ethical, and psychosocial considerations. *Advances in Renal Replacement Therapy* **7** (1), 52–62.

Standing Nursing and Advisory Committee (SNMAC) (2001) *Caring for Older People: A Nursing Priority. Integrating Knowledge, Practice and Values.* Department of Health, London.

Steinman, T.I. (1999) The challenges of geriatric nephrology managed care/disease management. *Geriatric Nephrology and Urology* **9** (2), 115–21.

UK Renal Registry (2000) *Third Annual Report.* December. Southmead Hospital, Bristol.

Winchester, J.F. and Rakowski, T.A. (1998) End-stage renal disease and its management in older adults. *Clinics in Geriatric Medicine* **14** (2), 255–65.

# Chapter 8
# Diabetes and Renal Failure

*Sara Youngman*

## Introduction

Diabetes remains one of the largest causes of established renal failure (ERF) in the UK (Renal Registry, 2002). The management of these two chronic illnesses presents specific challenges for the multidisciplinary team, not least because of the significant number who are referred to the renal specialist with late-stage renal insufficiency and a concomitant increased level of co-morbidity. This chapter aims to review the care for this group of patients, but also to highlight the management of prevention and detection of diabetes in those patients predisposed to the disease. Nephropathy complicates diabetes and vice versa; however, it is evident that much can be done to improve outcomes for these patients in both their quality and quantity of life.

## Renal failure and diabetes

The incidence of both renal failure and diabetes represents a worldwide epidemic. It is predicted that the requirement for renal replacement therapy will grow by 7–10% per annum, despite UK take-on rates for renal replacement therapy still lagging behind other developed countries such as Japan, the USA and Canada (Maynard and Cordonnier, 2001).

There will be a substantial increase in the incidence and prevalence of type II diabetes over the coming decades owing to an increase in age, obesity and ethnic diversity, with the predominate increase being in the Asian and African-Caribbean population (Harvey et al., 2001). However, how far numbers of patients with diabetes and established renal failure will increase is still unclear. It is hoped that with good nursing and medical management in primary care the transition to ERF can be prevented or reduced.

# Detection of renal failure in patients with diabetes

Healthy kidneys excrete less than 30 mg albumin in 24 hours. Microalbuminuria (MA) (excretion of 30–300 mg protein/24 hours) can be used as an early marker of renal damage. Testing can be carried out on an early-morning urine sample (EMU), where the albumin–creatinine ratio is measured. False positives can occur with infection, strenuous exercise or menstrual contamination. A positive MA screen is defined as an albumin:creatinine ratio of more than 2 mg/mmol in at least two out of three collections (Mogensen et al., 1995).

However, debate continues around the long-term cost–benefits of testing. Tabaei et al. (2001) found that MA testing may not be as sensitive and specific a predictor of nephropathy as previously suggested, as in their study of over 200 subjects, the predictive value positive of MA as a marker of risk for DN was 43%, and the predictive value negative was 77%. However, the incidence and progression of MA were significantly associated with poor glycaemic control and duration of diabetes between 10 and 14 years. It appears that the predictive marker of MA is still in doubt.

It may be prudent to test those with type I diabetes for MA after 5 years following diagnosis of diabetes, as carried out in some diabetes centres, although some centres screen annually for MA (Kirby, 2002). The National Service Framework (NSF) for Diabetes gives clear guidance, and recommends that all those with type II diabetes who are not already receiving treatment with an angiotensin-converting enzyme (ACE) inhibitor should receive annual surveillance for MA.

Studies advocate the use of ACE inhibitors (ACE Inhibitors in Diabetic Nephropathy Trialist Group, 2001) to protect against progression of diabetic nephropathy, with pre- and 2 weeks post-medication measurements of serum urea and creatinine to detect renal insufficiency and renal artery stenosis. More recently, angiotensin 2 receptor blockers (Tarnow et al., 1999) and calcium channel blockers studies have implied equal success.

Table 8.1 reviews the care and management of patients once MA has been confirmed.

**Table 8.1**  Care and management of patients with positive microalbuminuria (MA). (Adapted from NICE Guideline, 2002.)

- Repeat screen for MA every 2 months.
- Optimise glycaemic control (HbA1c below 6.5–7.5%, *see below*).
- Maintain blood pressure below 135/75 mm Hg.
- Treat hypertension with angiotensin-converting enzyme (ACE) inhibitor.
- Measure, assess and manage cardiovascular risk factors aggressively and educate about smoking cessation.
- Monitor renal function (24-hour urine testing for creatinine clearance, serum urea and electrolytes at each visit).

# Referral to the renal unit

A later marker of renal disease is proteinuria. Once detected (usually more than 0.5 g protein/24 hours or serum creatinine of more than 125 µmol/l) the patient needs to be referred to a nephrologist. However, it is important to recognise that detection of MA and proteinuria may be as a result of other glomerular disease (e.g. membranous nephropathy, minimal change disease, IgA nephropathy, Henoch–Schonlein purpura). Other key indicators include a proteinuria within 5 years of diagnosis of diabetes, or, as diabetic nephropathy is a chronic manifestation, an acute onset of renal disease. In those patients routinely screened, overt proteinuria will need further immunological screening and a diagnostic renal biopsy to confirm the underlying cause.

In any event, the Renal Association (2002) recommends that all those with progressive renal insufficiency and a plasma creatinine above 150 µmol/l and/or a rapidly rising plasma creatinine should be referred to a specialist nephrology service for assessment and follow-up.

It is preferable that preparation for dialysis commences as soon as possible and patients should have input from the whole multiprofessional team, including physicians, pre-dialysis nurses, anaemia co-ordinators, dietitians and counsellors.

# Diabetes and renal disease

There are many ways to manage diabetes and methods vary only slightly within the context of renal disease. Because the kidney excretes insulin, any endogenous or exogenous insulin (regardless of whether this is administered orally or by injection) will have a longer half-life, and the extent of this increased activity will in turn depend upon the degree of renal impairment. Prior to a diagnosis of renal disease, patients may therefore present with either perfect glucose control or unexplained hypoglycaemic episodes without a recent change to their routine.

Those with type II diabetes continue to produce endogenous insulin, but the quantity is insufficient to meet either their dietary intake or their body mass. Following dietary education, an oral hypoglycaemic agent (OHA) may be indicated. Sulphonyureas are excreted by the liver, which explains the renal preference for this class of OHA. Other OHAs such as biguanides (e.g. metformin, which is usually the first line of treatment for patients who are overweight) will have limited use for those with renal disease. These are only prescribed for those who have received a renal transplant, and who have near-normal renal function.

Those with type II diabetes who have reached the maximum dose of OHA or those with type I diabetes (who do not produce any endogenous insulin) will require subcutaneous insulin. The regimen prescribed may take many forms, from once, twice or four times per day, to continuous insulin infusion pumps or intraperitoneal insulin regimes. The aim of any prescribed pattern of medication is to maintain blood glucose within normal range to prevent further micro- or macro-vascular complications. The normal range is 4–7 mmol/l before meals (pre-prandial) and no higher than 10 mmol/l 2 hours after meals (post-prandial).

One consistent measure of glycaemic control is HbA1c (normal range 5–7%, but different laboratories may have different normal values). The HbA1c test measures the effect of glucose on haemoglobin A. As red blood cells have a life span of 90–120 days, during this time glucose in the blood attaches itself to the haemoglobin, changing parts of the red blood cells. These parts can be separated out from the red blood cells in the laboratory to give an indication of the average blood glucose level during the lifetime of a red blood cell.

HbA1c is a preferable long-term marker of glycaemic control, compared with self-administered blood glucose monitoring. In renal disease where haemoglobin is fragile, consideration needs to be given to recent blood transfusion, and haematinics such as percentage hypochromasia. Thus any marker reflecting glucose control should not be viewed in isolation but should be interpreted within a wider context.

# Haemodialysis

Although haemodialysis (HD) may not be the first therapy of choice for those with diabetes because of difficulties with vascular access and ability to tolerate fluid shifts, many patients may do well particularly if they have good support and on-going education (McMurray et al., 2002). However, many challenges remain and this section will review the main difficulties facing those with diabetes on dialysis.

## Hypoglycaemia

For those with diabetes who opt for HD, hypoglycaemia may be a common symptom. However, there are simple remedies for this including:

- A reduction in OHA or subcutaneous injection pre-HD. Insulin should never be omitted entirely for those who have type I diabetes because of the risk of ketoacidosis.
- A carbohydrate load pre-HD may be sufficient to maintain the blood glucose level throughout the dialysis session; however, any pre-existing gastroparesis with delayed stomach emptying must be taken into consideration. Such conditions cause diversion of blood supply for a longer period and may cause the patient to become nauseous and hypotensive during dialysis.
- More commonly used is a glucose-containing dialysate – as little as 1% will often maintain the blood glucose throughout dialysis.

## Vascular access

Access for HD is often the Achilles' heel of diabetes care. Early venogram and referral to a vascular surgeon will result in a pre-emptive functioning fistula thereby avoiding the need for temporary dialysis catheters and their associated risks. Blood vessels are, however, often less suitable for fistulae and complications such as 'steal syndrome' remain real possibilities. For these patients vascular access is achieved through semi-permanent catheters and graft access, and good planning and follow-up may improve fistula survival (Ravani et al., 2002). Peritoneal dialysis (PD) is a viable alternative treatment option and many of those with diabetes (and their clinicians) may choose this form of renal replacement therapy in the first instance.

## Blood pressure control

Initial therapy will consist of non-pharmacological interventions, e.g. lifestyle changes, sodium restriction, weight loss, exercise programmes, cessation of smoking and reduction of alcohol intake (Kaplin and Gifford, 1996). For those with diabetes, hyperinsulinaemia and extracellular fluid excess will contribute to hypertension as insulin can increase sympathetic activity and promote sodium retention (Renderee et al., 1992). A target blood pressure within 5 mmHg of 120/70 mmHg is desirable (Hanson Zanchetti and Carruthers, 1998; Adler et al., 2000).

Occasionally hypertension during HD may be as a result of acute actuation of the rennin–angiotensin system by reduction in the intravascular volume, induced by intradialytic ultrafiltration. Adding a small dose of ACE inhibitor at the start of dialysis may ameliorate this phenomenon.

A common presentation in the hypertensive patient is left ventricular hypertrophy, and is associated with an enhanced incidence of heart failure, ventricular arrhythmias and sudden cardiac death (Lovell et al., 2000). The Kaplin–Meier survival curve for 3755 patients enrolled on the Heart Outcomes Prevention Evaluation (HOPE) trial (HOPE Study Investigators, 2002) confirmed a significant reduction in the relative risk of cardiovascular and cerebral vascular events, demonstrating a vasculoprotective and renoprotective effect on patients with diabetes.

Organisations such as the World Health Organization (1999), British Hypertension Society (Ramsey et al., 1999) and the USA Joint National Committee (1997) advocate pharmacological intervention in a patient with an average 24-hour blood pressure above 130/85 mmHg. Loop diuretics such as thiazides will have a limited effect in renal disease once the glomerular filtration rate (GFR) falls below 20 ml/min. Secondary hyperparathyroidism can raise intracellular calcium, which can lead to vasoconstriction and consequently hypertension.

Twenty-four-hour blood pressure monitoring will also identify those patients who do not demonstrate the normal nocturnal decline in blood pressure, increasing the risks attached to hypertension.

An inability to shift fluid between vascular compartments due to autonomic neuropathy or hypoalbuminaemia resulting from nephrotic syndrome or malnutrition will result in the low colloid oncotic pressure and reduced plasma-filling rate, and can cause the patient to become hypotensive.

During HD, techniques to ensure the patient's comfort will vary and may include the following:

- Blood volume monitoring and sodium profiling will allow careful and appropriate fluid removal (see Chapter 4).
- Sequential ultrafiltration.
- Priming the circuit with a colloid solution.
- Omitting or decreasing anti-hypertensive medication pre-HD.
- Maintaining hematocrit on HD with 2–4 l of oxygen.
- Not taking meals before and during HD to prevent diversion of circulating blood volume to the stomach often prolonged with gastroparesis.
- Exercise on HD to aid venous return.
- Maintaining haemoglobin (see Chapter 3) as anaemia reduces the viscosity and peripheral vascular resistance, thereby impairing the ability to maintain blood volume during ultrafiltration.

Increased thirst secondary to hyperglycaemia is one of the main causes of fluid overload, often accompanied by hyperkalaemia. Once glucose is restored to normal, the patient will be able to comfortably cope with his/her fluid allowance. This list is by no means exhaustive and a combination of interventions may be required.

## Peritoneal dialysis

In contrast to HD, PD provides a near-euvoleamic state maintained by the almost continuous ultrafiltration and sodium removal during dialysis. A patient's preference for a particular dialysis modality may be influenced by his or her co-morbid conditions. PD is often a challenge for the patient with pre-existing retinopathy and autonomic neuropathy affecting manual dexterity. In addition, social circumstances, level of independence and degree of motivation are of equal importance.

Maintaining blood glucose within the normal range is desirable so that the potential osmotic gradient between dialysate and plasma promotes optimal ultrafiltration (and, to a lesser extent, solute clearance). Treating elevated blood glucose resulting from the use of hypertonic dialysate solutions can be remedied in several ways. Increases in OHA or commencing subcutaneous insulin are obvious strategies. Less common strategies include the use of intraperitoneal (IP) insulin protocols (administration of a short-acting insulin added to the dialysate: dosage will depend on the glucose content of the fluid, e.g. 2–4 i.u./l of 1.36% glucose dialysate, or the use of a non-glucose-based PD solution (see Chapter 5)).

Hyperglycaemia will not only decrease dialysis efficiency by reducing the potential to ultrafiltrate, but also may cause the patient to drink excessively. If fluid overload and unmanageable oedema results, intermittent ultrafiltration on HD may be required.

## Transplantation

Another treatment option for those with diabetes is one of transplantation, either kidney-alone or combined kidney–pancreas transplant.

The main consideration pre-transplantation is close examination of blood vessels, including femoral and carotid Doppler studies, exercise tolerance test, echo cardiogram and coronary angiogram, repeated every 2 years to ensure graft and patient survival post-operatively. Many units will opt for revascularisation (Andrews and Brecker, 2002), which will decrease cardiac morbidity and mortality, as there is an obligation not only to the recipient but also to the donor to ensure best possible outcome.

Simultaneous combined kidney–pancreas (SPK) transplants may be selected for those with type I diabetes, the rationale being that not only will normoglycaemia improve quality of life, but also the vessels will be preserved and the graft maintained (Reddy et al., 2003). Transplant surgical time is doubled, and complications from either bladder or bowel anastomoses give rise to post-operative complications and a prolonged post-operative hospitalisation. Urinary amylase is a marker of rejection, and as the amylase level falls, it predicts pancreas graft rejection. An elevated random blood glucose is a sign of graft failure, but then it is often too late for intervention. The combined SPK has demonstrated improvement in pre-existing neuropathies, but this may take several years to manifest (Navorro et al., 1997).

## Diabetes post-renal transplantation

Patients may develop diabetes post-transplantation, either through excessive weight gain due to medication, or due to feelings of well-being resulting in excessive eating and lack of exercise. The latter can be more easily remedied. Immunosuppressive agents such as corticosteroids, cyclosporine and tacrolimus have diabetogenic qualities. For those patients who develop diabetes post-transplant, there are many possible scenarios; either the diabetes disappears as the drugs are reduced and the patient continues on his/her healthy eating programme, or the patient may need to commence an OHA or insulin therapy. The education and co-operation of these patients remains paramount in the management of diabetes, as the raised glucose will promote vessel damage with subsequent loss of graft and inability to have further transplants (see Chapter 6).

## Nutrition

Healthy eating is the cornerstone to diabetes management; and a healthy eating plan has to be achievable and realistic (see Chapter 12). It is well recognised that patients often experience a loss of appetite or reduced dietary intake as a consequence of their renal disease. While renal replacement therapy may ameliorate many of the elements promoting anorexia, other contributing factors give rise to the aetiology of protein-calorie malnutrition. These include proteinuria resulting from the underlying kidney disease, intraperitoneal loss of proteins and amino acids (these losses increase significantly during peritonitis episodes), and, as described earlier in the chapter, the gastroparesis that many patients with diabetes may experience. Inadequate dialysis (of either modality) puts these patients at high risk of malnutrition.

The relationship developed between the dietician and the patient cannot be overemphasised and is key to the patient's well-being. Correction of anaemia and effective pre-dialysis education will provide solid foundations for dialysis. Those with diabetic nephropathy who have established renal failure (ESF) may have had a lifetime of dietary restrictions, and the renal dietician has a difficult task in providing the balance and maintaining adequate nutrition. Recent education programmes (DAFNE Study Group, 2002) are progressively empowering patients to understand and adapt to their disease, producing encouraging results and interest in the diabetes world.

## National Service Framework (NSF) for Diabetes

Diabetes was the fourth NSF to be published (Department of Health, 2003). It sets out a national programme to improve health care for people with diabetes, and the first of the two-part document identifies 12 key standards. These standards embody the holistic approach detailed in the Expert Patient (Department of Health, 2002). Each of the standards has been stratified to levels 1–4 according to the amount of supporting evidence available. Their emphasis is upon the development of a systematic approach to care, working closely with the Primary Care groups, and they advocate a patient-centred approach to management of diabetes detailing key interventions and implications for service planning (Chaplin, 2003). Table 8.2 shows the 12 standards of the Diabetes NSF.

These standards alongside the recent National Institute of Clinical Excellence (NICE) (2002) guidelines, focusing on blood glucose, hypertension, retinopathy and early renal failure management, should ensure that the number of patients reaching established renal failure is kept to the minimum.

**Table 8.2**  The 12 standards of the NSF for Diabetes.

| |
|---|
| (1)  Prevention of diabetes – details prevalence of type II diabetes. |
| (2)  Identification of people with diabetes – aimed at early detection of diabetes. |
| (3)  Empowering people with diabetes – encourages partnership in the decision-making process. |
| (4)  Clinical care of adults with diabetes – aimed at the reduction of risks associated with diabetes. |
| (5)  Clinical care of children and young people with diabetes – acknowledges that this clinical care requires an individualised patient approach which is linked to adult services. |
| (6)  Management of diabetic emergencies – provides guidance on managing changes in blood glucose. |
| (7)  Care of people with diabetes during admission to hospital – aimed at consistency of care during hospital admissions. |
| (8)  Diabetes and pregnancy – seeks to empower and support women in pregnancy. |
| (9)  Detection and management of long-term complication – this final section covers three standards involving: |
| (10) Surveillance |
| (11) Guidelines |
| (12) Integrated health and social care. |

# Dyslipidemia in diabetes

Accurate lipid measurement can only be achieved in the absence of excessive glucose and nephrotic syndrome. Dietary advice, such as eating of oily fish Omega 3 to lower triglycerides, is not appropriate for patients on dialysis due to their reduced phosphate allowance. The rationale for reducing lipids is well documented (Haffner et al., 1999), and treatment goals remain the same as for those without diabetes: a total cholesterol level of less than 5.2 mmol/l, and for those with ischaemic heart disease one of less than 4.8 mmol/l.

# Routine screening

## *Eyes*

Direct ophthalmology by well-trained personnel remains the most cost-effective method of screening. In line with recent NICE (2002) guidelines, thorough routine eye screening consists of retinal screening at time of diagnosis and biannually thereafter, together with prompt referral to the ophthalmologist if abnormalities are detected. Screening and maintenance of normoglycaemia and normotension will preserve the retina.

## *Feet*

Hill et al. (1996) found that the prevalence of foot problems (foot problems are defined here as ulcers, infections, gangrene or amputation of toes, feet or lower or upper leg) was significantly greater in a group of patients with end-stage renal disease (ESRD) (25%) compared with a group without ESRD (10%).

Annual foot screening for all those with diabetes is recommended by the Diabetes NSF, but particularly for patients who attend for haemodialysis in hospital, foot care is not always optimum. For those patients in renal failure, screening should be undertaken alongside their routine renal appointments or when on haemodialysis. The assessment for peripheral vascular disease will include:

- Examination of the leg, general appearance, colour, fluid status, any signs of ulceration, recent scarring or infection.
- Pedal pulses and comparison with previous readings.
- Skin temperature.
- Skin thickness, texture, cracking, dryness.
- Hair growth in the lower extremities starting with the toes, absence indicating loss of circulation.
- Pedobarography plantar pressures can be monitored effectively. Intervention is achieved with the use of orthotic devices or specialised footwear to allow redistribution of pressure and avoidance of ulceration.

Some complications are more easily remedied than others and careful monitoring will pre-empt further complications and will protect the patient from pain and amputation. Particular attention needs to be made to those with permanent femoral graft formation, as without doubt this will divert the circulation further. Knowles (1998) provides further reading.

## Summary

Diabetes and renal disease combined present a great challenge for the multidisciplinary team, and the importance of prevention cannot be underestimated (Locatelli et al., 2003). It may appear that often the patient chooses to ignore the multitude of information given, but it must be recognised that the nature of these two chronic illnesses combined is at times overwhelming.

Medical professionals, who attempt to assimilate proven anatomical and physiological responses, recent clinical research and current practice guidelines to provide consistent information and care, also expect patients to both understand and appreciate the complexities of the two disease processes. It is to be hoped that this chapter has emphasised that this will only ever be achieved through working in partnership with patients and their carers.

## References

ACE Inhibitors in Diabetic Nephropathy Trialist Group (2001) Should all patients with type 1 diabetes mellitus and microalbuminuria receive angiotensin-converting enzyme inhibitors? A meta analysis of individual patient data. *Annals of Internal Medicine* **134**, 370–379.

Adler, A.L., Stratton, I.M., Neil, H.A., et al. (2000) Association of systolic blood pressure with macrovascular and microvascular complications of type 2 diabetes (UKPDS 36): a prospective observational study. *British Medical Journal* **321**, 412.

Andrews, P.A. and Brecker, S.J. (2002) Premature arteriosclerosis associated with diabetic renal disease. *British Journal of Diabetes and Vascular Disease* **2** (2), 128–9.

Chaplin, S. (2003) Key messages of the National Service Framework for Diabetes: delivery strategy. *Practical Diabetes International* **20** (1).

DAFNE Study Group (2002) Training in flexible, intensive insulin management to enable dietary freedom in people with type 1 diabetes: dose adjustment for normal eating (DAFNE) randomised control trial. *British Medical Journal* **325**, 746.

Department of Health (2002) *The Expert Patient. A New Approach to Chronic Disease Management for 21st Century.* Department of Health, London.

Department of Health (2003) *National Service Framework for Diabetes: Delivery Strategy.* www.doh.gov.uk/nsf/diabetes.

Haffner, S.M., Alexander, C.M., Cook, T.J., et al. (1999) Reduced coronary events in simvastatin-treated patients with coronary heart disease and diabetes or impaired fasting glucose level: subgroup analysis in the Scandinavian Simvastatin Survival Study. *Archives of International Medicine* **159** (22), 2661–7.

Hanson Zanchetti, A. and Carruthers, S.G. (1998) Effects of the intensive blood-pressure lowering and low-dose aspirin in patients with hypertension: principal results of the Hypertension Optimal Treatment (HOT) randomised trial. *Lancet* **351**, 1755.

Harvey, J.N., Rizvi, K., Craney, L., Messenger, J., Shah, R. and Meadows, P.A. (2001) Population based survey and analysis of trends in the prevalence of diabetic nephropathy in type 1 diabetes. *Diabetes Medicine* **18** (12), 998–1002.

Heart Outcomes Prevention Evaluation (HOPE) Study Investigators (2002) The effects of ramipril on cardiovascular and microvascular outcomes in people with diabetes mellitus. Results of the HOPE and MICRO HOPE substudy. *Lancet* **355** (9200), 253–9.

Hill, M.N., Feldman, H.I., Hilton, S.C., Holechek, M.J., Ylitalo, M. and Benedict, G.W. (1996) Risk of foot complications in long-term diabetic patients with and without ESRD: a preliminary study. *ANNA Journal* **23** (4), 381–6.

Joint National Committee (1997) The sixth report on the Joint National Committee in detection, evaluation and treatment of high blood pressure. *Archives of International Medicine* **157**, 2413.

Kaplin, N.M. and Gifford, R.W. (1996) Choice of initial therapy for hypertension. *JAMA* **275** (20), 1577–80.

Kirby, M. (2002) Screening for microalbuminuria. *British Journal of Diabetes and Vascular Disease* **2** (2), 106–109.

Knowles, A. (1998) Care of the diabetic foot. *Journal of Wound Care* **6** (5), 227–30.

Locatelli, F., Canaud, B., Eckardt, K.U., Stenvinkel, P., Wanner, C. and Zoccali, C. (2003) The importance of diabetic nephropathy in current nephrological practice. *Nephrology Dialysis Transplantation* **18** (9), 1716–25.

Lovell, B.H., Blasé, A., Beverley, H. and Carabello, B.A. (2000) Left ventricular hypertrophy pathogenesis, detection and prognosis. *Circulation* **4**, 102–470.

McMurray, S.D., Johnson, G., Davis, S. and McDougall, K. (2002) Diabetes education and care management significantly improve patient outcomes in the dialysis unit. *American Journal of Kidney Diseases* **40** (3), 566–75.

Maynard, C. and Cordonnier, D. (2001) The late referral of diabetic patients with renal insufficiency to nephrologist has a high human and financial cost. *Diabetes Metabolism* **27**, 517–21.

Mogensen, C.E., Keane, W.F., Bennett, P.H., Jerums, G., Parving, H.H., Passa, P., Steffes, M.W., Striker, G.E. and Viberti, G.C. (1995) Prevention of diabetic renal disease with special reference to microalbuminuria. *Lancet* **346** (8982), 1080–84.
NICE Guideline (2002) *Management of Type 2 Diabetes – Renal Disease, Prevention and Early Management.* www.nice.org.uk.
Navorro, X., Sutherland, D.E. and Kennedy, W.R. (1997) Long term effects of pancreatic transplantation on diabetic nephropathy. *Annals of Neurology* **42** (5), 727–36.
Ramsey, L.E., Williams, B. and Johnston, G.D. (1999) British Hypertension Society guide-lines for hypertension management. *British Medical Journal* **319**, 630.
Ravani, P., Marcelli, D. and Malberti, F. (2002) Vascular access surgery managed by renal physicians: the choice of native arteriovenous fistulas for hemodialysis. *American Journal of Kidney Diseases* **40** (6), 1264–76.
Reddy, K.S., Stablein, D., Taranto, S., Stratta, R.J., Johnston, T.D., Waid, T.H., McKeown, J.W., Lucas, B.A. and Ranjan, D. (2003) Long-term survival following simultaneous kidney–pancreas transplantation versus kidney transplantation alone in patients with type 1 diabetes mellitus and renal failure. *American Journal of Kidney Diseases* **41** (2), 464–70.
Renderee, H.A., Omar, H.A., Motala, A.A. and Seedat, M.A. (1992) Effect of insulin therapy on blood pressure in NIDDM patients with secondary failure. *Diabetes Care* **15**, 1258.
Renal Registry (2002) *The Fifth Annual Renal Registry Report.* www.renalreg.com.
Tabaei, B.P., Al-Kassab, A.S., Ilag, L.L., Zawacki, C.M. and Herman, W.H. (2001) Does microalbuminuria predict diabetic nephropathy? *Diabetes Care* **24** (9), 1560–66.
Tarnow, L., Rossing, P., Jenson, C. and Parving, H.H. (1999) The long term effect of nisoldipine and lisinipril in type 1 diabetic patients with diabetic nephropathy. *Diabetes Care* **23** (12), 1723–4.
World Health Organization (1999) International Society of Hypertension guidelines for the management of hypertension. *Journal of Hypertension* **17** (20), 151–83.

# Further reading

DCCT Research Group (1992) Lipid and lipoprotein levels in patients with IDDM: diabetes control and complications trial experience. *Diabetes Care* **15**, 886.
DCCT Research Group (1993) Treatment of diabetes in the development and progres-sion of long term complication in insulin-dependent diabetes. *New England Journal of Medicine* **329**, 977–86.
DCCT Research Group (1995) The effect of Intensive therapy on the development and progression of diabetic nephropathy in the Diabetes and Complications Trial. *Kidney International* **47** (6), 1703–1720.
Lameire, N. (2000) Pathogenesis and treatment of diabetic nephropathy. *EDTNA/ERCA Journal* **26** (2), 8–10.
UK Prospective Diabetes Study Group (1998) Tight blood pressure control and the risk of macrovascular and microvascular complications in type 2 diabetes. UKPDS 38. *British Medical Journal* **317**, 703–713.

# Chapter 9
# Infection Control in Renal Care

*Judith Hurst*

## Introduction

Despite the many advances in the care and treatment of those with renal insufficiency and established renal failure (ERF), infection is the second highest cause of death, after cardiovascular causes, and 71.6% of mortality from infection is caused by septicaemia (United States Renal Data System, 1999). In the renal population, mortality associated with sepsis is 50 times that seen in the general population and accounts for around 30% of all hospital admissions (Sarnak and Jaber, 2000).

Additionally, in the haemodialysis population between 25 and 50% of infections are associated with vascular access, most notably central venous catheters (CVCs), causing major morbidity rates for these patients (Rickard, 2001). Those undergoing haemodialysis have severe alterations in cell-mediated immunity, and thereby increase their risk of contracting infections and reducing their protective responses to vaccination. The renal community must place the utmost importance on prevention and management of potential infectious incidences.

## Historical perspective and types of organism

Whilst there may be issues related to how a person may be exposed to infection control during care and treatment, control of infections that may already be present in patients prior to renal replacement therapy (RRT) should be considered, such as hepatitis, human immunodeficiency virus (HIV) and methicillin-resistant *Staphylococcus aureus* (MRSA). In this section the prevention of the spread of infection and the control of infections that are already present will be considered. It is important that these issues in all areas of renal care (and not just haemodialysis) are evaluated in order to ensure a healthy environment for staff, patients and carers alike.

## Rosenheim Report and universal precautions

In response to a number of viral hepatitis outbreaks in renal units in the UK in the late 1960s, the Rosenheim Report (Department of Health and Social Security, 1972) set out guidelines for the prevention and control of infections. These included barrier methods for staff to use when caring for those infected with a virus, the screening of blood products for transfusion and the segregation of those patients identified as being infected with the virus.

Whilst these guidelines did much to reduce the incidence of hepatitis in renal units, the guidelines have not been updated regularly to include a number of other sources of infection. Indeed, it was only in 2002 that the Department of Health published the long-awaited update. Some speculate that in the meantime practice may have been relaxed in light of technological advances in RRT and our understanding of the treatment of infections when they do occur (Zuckerman, 2002).

Of course there are many reasons why infections occur in renal units, and one of the compounding factors in modern times is that renal units now accept patients of all ages with a much wider range of underlying renal diseases at an annual rate of around 96 new patients per million population. Transplantation rates are currently around 30 per million population per year. As renal professionals we see patients in an ever-expanding renal population who are increasingly frail, and therefore more vulnerable when exposed to infections, and are likely to have poorer outcomes.

## Types of organisms, aetiology and spread vectors

The parenteral routes of transmission of blood-borne viruses (BBV) are well known, but several studies more recently have indicated that exogenous routes perhaps play a pertinent role in the spread of infection. For example, Corcoran et al. (1994) and Sanchez-Tapias (1999) demonstrated nosocomial spread when patients dialysed next to each other and this was a significant risk factor in the infection of hepatitis C virus (HCV). The patients were infected with the same genotype of BBV that could not be traced in their haemodialysis equipment, from transfusions or other physical contact usually associated with transmission. Hence nosocomial spread in the dialysis environment was the likely route.

It has been noted that the longer the time on dialysis, and the older the patient, the greater the risk for infection with a BBV. What is not clear is whether this infection is due to risk factors associated with RRT, or something related to the renal disease process itself. Generally though, incidence of outbreaks has demonstrated breaches in safety precautions and lack of dialysis machine sterilisation (Balshaw and Casey, 2000).

The EDTA report in 1995 (Valderrabano et al., 1995) revealed an average prevalence of HCV of 18% among haemodialysis patients, although there is a wide variation among the different countries: 1% in Finland to 44% in Egypt (Valderrabano et al., 1995). Hepatitis G (HGV) has more recently been identified and prevalence in the European haemodialysis population is estimated at between 3.1 and 57.5% (Cocco et al., 1998). Whilst these figures do not demonstrate a large challenge in the UK, incidence across Europe and in some parts of the world, where patients travel to visit family or on holiday, is far greater, and rather different approaches to infection control procedures are adopted.

HIV has not been demonstrated to be transmitted frequently in dialysis units. The only cases where this has been the case is where inadequate cleaning or reuse of equipment have occurred, or when equipment designed for single use was reused (Velandia et al., 1995).

# Infection and renal replacement therapy

## Haemodialysis

Stevenson (2002) states that epidemiological data clearly establish that a major risk for vascular access infections is the type of access used for haemodialysis, with temporary catheters demonstrating the greatest risk and native arterio-venous fistulae (AVF) the least risk.

Staff-patient ratios have been demonstrated to play an important contribution to infection rates in dialysis units. Petrosillo et al. (2001) demonstrated how understaffing situations increased the risk of HCV infection occurrences through nosocomial transmission, and higher rates of infection generally occur when new or inexperienced staff manipulate vascular access. Taylor et al.'s study in 1998 reviewed an increasing haemodialysis bacteraemia, concluding that this was associated with reliance on CVCs for vascular access during a period of health care restructuring.

The European Best Practice Guidelines for Haemodialysis (European Renal Association, 2002) state that:

'. . . staff training for fistula cannulation is mandatory to avoid poor needle insertion' and that 'catheter connection, disconnection and interventions should be performed under aseptic conditions by trained dialysis staff with the patient and the nurse wearing a surgical mask.'

These guidelines are based on research that indicates that excessive manipulation of catheters and the use of barrier methods reduce contamination of catheters (Marr et al., 1998).

Many investigators have evaluated cleaning and sterilising methods used in the maintenance of haemodialysis machines. However, studies more recently have been concerned with the potential impact of contamination of the dialysate solution. Considering that patients come into contact with around 400 l of water per week, the contamination of this fluid will cause acute reactions, or chronic damage and cytokine reaction (Pansini et al., 2001).

Pansini's study measured levels of colony forming units (CFUs) and endo-toxin units (EUs) from dialysate solution that was made from sterile concentrate and non-sterile concentrate. Not surprisingly the dialysate from the sterile sources produced the lowest levels of EUs and CFUs, but even the other recording revealed contamination levels below that of the European recommended guideline values for safe dialysate. This highlights the need for guidelines to be continually updated, and for the whole dialysis equipment to be kept clean and disinfected appropriately. See Chapter 14 for further discussion on water quality.

Various cleaning solutions for access have been recommended. Whilst the National Kidney Foundation Kidney Disease Outcomes Quality Initiative (NKF-K/DOQI) guidelines (National Kidney Foundation, 2000) recommend an AVF is cleaned with soap, followed by 70% alcohol and/or 10% povidone-iodine, Dickenson (1997) argues that chlorhexidine is superior to the use of alcohol and povidone-iodine in the prevention of central catheter infections. Indeed, some manufacturers state that some of the catheter materials may actually be adversely affected by the iodine-based solutions.

The NKF-K/DOQI guidelines recommend that both patients and staff should wear a mask for all haemodialysis catheter procedures that remove caps and access the patient's blood stream, and for all catheter-dressing changes. Additionally, it is suggested that povidone-iodine and mupirocin ointment at the catheter site can reduce the incidence of catheter infections. However, Schneeberger et al. (1998) highlight that operating dialysis machines with gloves may be a potential source for nosocomial infection and complacency amongst staff. Hands still need to be washed after the gloves have been removed, as breaks in the gloves can cause the hands to be contaminated during a procedure.

Each patient should be assigned all his or her own equipment needed for the dialysis procedure. This should include his/her own supply tray, clamps, medications and if possible blood pressure cuff. All should be cleaned after use.

---

**Discussion point**

An EDTNA/ERCA survey (referenced in Elseviers and Van Waeleghem, 2003) on vascular access showed that across renal units in Europe:

- 32–83% of units used sterile gloves
- 28–63% of units used masks
- 6–63% used eye protection
- 0–100% used aprons

When the results were collated and comparisons made of the hygienic scores, Belgium had the highest score of 2.25 out of a maximum score of 3, and the UK had a score of 0.9.

Can you suggest how this information may be used to develop practice?

What compounding factors could be identified that may prevent renal units complying with infection control guidelines?

## *Peritoneal dialysis*

Whilst body fluids are not accessed for dialysis in the same way for peritoneal dialysis (PD), infective incidences have been reported concerning the disposal of PD waste. Further discussion on infection in PD can be found in Chapter 5.

## *Transplantation*

Much is known about the risk factors associated with immunosuppressive therapy, but what of those patients known to be infected with a BBV wishing to be considered for a transplant? Whilst in the shorter term no differences are observed in graft and patient survival rates for those with a BBV compared with those without, liver lesions seem to be more apparent in those infected by HCV for more than 10 years, especially when co-infected with HBV (Lezaic et al., 2003). Further discussion on infection and transplantation can be found in Chapter 6.

# Prevention

Hand washing is still one of the most effective methods of infection control. However, the solutions used to clean hands have come in for some scrutiny. Pittet (2002) demonstrated that the disinfectant gels commonly used to clean hands between patients are less effective than both disinfectant rinses and soap and water. The gel needs more than 30 seconds to achieve effective decontamination, whereas the other mediums are effective within the average application time of 8–15 seconds. Hence, review of the efficacy of the hand washing process is in itself necessary for the on-going monitoring of infection control in the clinical environment.

The Department of Health and the Renal Association have recommended immunisation of patients for HBV since 1994, but surveys have shown that in 1995 49% of renal units were not offering this immunisation to any group with chronic renal failure. Ray et al.'s study (2002) demonstrates that although rates of immunisation have improved in recent years (29% not immunising any patient group), most renal units still fail to follow current guidance. It appears that partial coverage for immunisation of the renal population is the norm, in terms of both incomplete vaccination schedules and the numbers of patients who are offered immunisation.

Collaborative and shared care management with those involved in the care and treatment of those with renal insufficiency has not been developed in any meaningful way. This model of care is not new, as the management of erythropoeitin has already been developed, enhancing collaboration between renal units and general practitioners. Whilst some could argue that the response rate, and thereby effective immunisation, in the renal population does not necessarily justify the cost, it is noted and recommended that immunisation should begin in the pre-end-stage period when response rates are more favourable and remain so once RRT has commenced. Indeed, other reasons why a non-response is seen should be considered, as malnutrition has been identified as negatively influencing the response to vaccination.

Different doses of the vaccine have been studied and higher doses have been noted to be more successful in achieving an effective immunisation status. Other vaccination strategies can be of benefit to the vulnerable renal population. Each patient should be individually assessed and considered for yearly influenza vaccination, and kept up to date with tetanus and diphtheria toxoids (European Renal Association, 2002).

## Best practice guidelines

It is recommended that staff should wear gowns or scrub suits in the renal areas, and wear gloves for any patient contact, including taking blood pressure. However, Belkin (1997) noted that there is no evidence to suggest that clean standard-issue uniforms play a part in the spread of infection in the hospital environment, although it is necessary when caring for patients with known BBV as part of isolation barrier procedures.

How may patients view these precautions, and what impact may it have on their experience of the renal care and treatment they receive? It has been suggested that clinical staff gowned, gloved and wearing a mask and approaching a patient may create more psychological barriers for the patient concerning his/her worth and personal identity (Gaskill et al., 1997). However, it should be noted that some patients have reported that being cared for in isolation has a positive impact on their care delivery. Each member of the care team delivers their care at one time and not as a series of task-orientated visits. To be left in peace for periods of time was considered beneficial to their overall treatment and recovery (Lendemeijer, 1997).

It could be questioned whether isolation procedures are strictly necessary. Several of the guidelines considered already state that those patients infected should be cared for in isolation. However, some authors question this, stating that if universal precautions are applied correctly then the need for isolation is superfluous (Cerrai et al., 1998; Jimenez et al., 1999). So it could be argued by what criteria patients should be isolated. If it is known that transmission can occur through endogenous and exogenous routes, and renal unit staff comply with controlling the exogenous factors, will all future transmission be eliminated? Indeed not.

So who should be isolated, and what proportion of the renal unit's resources should be utilised in isolation versus the educative and preventative measures to reduce the incidence of infections in the first place? The Renal Association (2002) recommends that carriers of hepatitis B should be dialysed in separate rooms on dedicated machines. Those patients with hepatitis C should be dialysed on separate shifts and units should move towards providing separate rooms for such patients. Those patients with HIV should be considered for segregation, but this is based on local risk assessment, and their machines treated as for patients with hepatitis C; the machine can be used by other patients provided that the dialysis circuit has been adequately decontaminated and the external surface cleaned with suitable disinfectant between use (Renal Association, 2002, p. 118).

# Future developments

Already renal units are utilising policy documents and risk assessment exercises in order to plan the management and prevention of infections. However, to rely on national or international guidelines only to inform care would seem to ignore the very individual needs of those who we are seeking to protect – the staff and patients. It is suggested that an individual approach to the needs and challenges of individual renal units uses the broader guidelines to develop the unit's own protocol and audit measures in the prevention and control of the particular dynamics of its renal environment.

A shared governance approach is needed to improve infection control and access care. Table 9.1 shows a summary of good practice in the prevention of infection in renal units.

**Table 9.1**   Summary of good practice in the prevention of infection in renal units.

General universal precautions should be observed, including the following:

- Patients awaiting the start of RRT should be immunised against HBV as soon as possible while their plasma creatinine level remains relatively low.
- All long-term dialysis patients should be immunised against HBV.
- Testing for HBV and HCV should take place every 3 months, and for HIV annually, once the patient's consent has been obtained.
- Only staff demonstrating their own HBV immunity should care for HBV-positive patients. Indeed, wherever possible staff should only care for those infected with BBVs during one shift.
- Patients positive to HBV and HCV should be dialysed in separate rooms, and those with HIV should be considered for segregation.
- All units should have a documented infection control policy which should include nasal screening for *Staphylococcus aureus* (SA).
- Patients using a temporary CVC should have 2% mupirocin ointment or povidone-iodine ointment applied at the end of each dialysis session.
- PD patients positive to SA should have mupirocin cream applied to their exit site, or receive eradication therapy.
- Concentrates and water used for dialysis should meet the standards set out in the European Best Practice Guidelines (2002).

# References

Balshaw, A. and Casey, J. (2000) One haemodialysis unit's experience of hepatitis B. *EDTNA/ERCA Journal* **26** (1), 17–19.

Belkin, N.L. (1997) Use of scrubs and related apparel in health care facilities. *American Journal of Infection Control* **25** (5), 401–404.

Cerrai, T., Michelassi, S., Ierpi, C., Toti, G., Zignego, A.L. and Lombardi, M. (1998) Universal precautions and dedicated machines as cheap and effective measures to control HCV spread. *EDTNA/ERCA Journal* **24** (2), 43–8.

Cocco, M., Amoruso, M., Lavanna, S., Mariotti, D., Bertoni, G., Sinelli, N. and Brizzolara, R. (1998) Is hepatitis G virus a real risk for haemodialysis patients? *EDTNA/ERCA Journal* **24** (3), 36–7.

Corcoran, G.D., Brink, N.S., Millar, C.G., et al. (1994) Hepatitis C infection in haemodialysis patients: study of risk factors. *Journal of Infection* **28**, 279–85.

Department of Health and Social Security (1972) *Report of the Rosenheim Advisory Group – Hepatitis and the Treatment of Chronic Renal Failure*. DHSS, London.

Dickenson, L. (1997) Central venous catheter site care: chlorhexidine versus povodine-iodine. *American Nephrology Nursing Association Journal* **24** (3), 349–58. Elseviers, M.M. and Van Waeleghem, J.P. (2003) European Dialysis and Transplant Nurses Association/European Renal Care Association. Related articles, links complications of vascular access: results of a European multi centre study of the EDTNA/ERCA Research Board. *EDTNA ERCA Journal* **29** (3), 163–7.

European Renal Association (2002) European Best Practice Guidelines Expert Group on Hemodialysis. Section 6. Haemodialysis-associated infection. *Nephrology Dialysis Transplantation* **17** (Suppl 7), 72–87.

Gaskill, D., Henderson, A. and Fraser, M. (1997) Exploring the everyday world of the patient in isolation. *Oncology Nursing Forum* **24** (4), 695–700.

Jimenez, D.A., Gonsalez, C., Rivera, F. and Enriquez, R. (1999) Isolation of HVC patient is sufficient in reducing the annual incidence of HCV infection, but is it really necessary? *Nephrology Dialysis Transplantation* **14**, 1337–9.

Lendemeijer, B. (1997) The use of isolation in psychiatry – a literature study (in Dutch). *Verpleegkunde* **12** (1), 15–26.

Lezaic, V., Djukanovic, L.J., Blagojevic, R. and Radivojevic, D. (2003) Long-term outcome of kidney transplantation in patients with hepatitis B or C positive. *Clinical Transplantation* **17** (1), 75–6.

Marr, K.A., Long, L. and Fowler, V.G. (1998) Incidence and outcome of *Staphylococcus aureus* bacteraemia in haemodialysis patients. *Kidney International* **54**, 1684–9.

National Kidney Foundation (2000) *NKF-K/DOQI Guidelines for Vascular Access. Prevention of Complications: Infection*. www.kidney.org/professionals.

Pansini, S., Degaetano, R., Boccassini, D. and Turi, E. (2001) Microbiological survey of dialysate: advantage of use of sterile bag concentrate. *EDTNA/ERCA Journal* **27** (3), 132–3.

Petrosillo, N., Gilli, P., Serraino, D., Dentico, P., Mele, A., Ragni, P., Puro, V., Casalino, C. and Ippolitto, G. (2001) Prevalence of infected patients and understaffing have a role in hepatitis C virus transmission in dialysis. *American Journal of Kidney Diseases* **37** (5), 1004–1010.

Pittet, D. (2002) Promotion of hand hygiene: magic, hype, or scientific challenge? *Infection Control in Hospital Epidemiology* **23** (3), 118–19.

Ray, S., Samuel, T., Hawker, J. and Smith, S. (2002) Hepatitis B immunization in renal units in the United Kingdom: questionnaire study. *British Medical Journal* **324** (7342), 877–8.

Renal Association (2002) *Treatment of Adults and Children with Renal Failure. Standards and Audit Measures*, 3rd edn. Royal College of Physicians, London.

Rickard, N.A. (2001) Central venous catheters: infection and patient susceptibility. *British Journal of Nursing* **10** (16), 1044, 1046, 1048, 1050, 1052, 1056.

Sanchez-Tapias, J.M. (1999) Nosocomial transmission of hepatitis C virus. *Journal of Hepatology* **31** (Suppl 1), 107–112.

Sarnak, M.J. and Jaber, B.L. (2000) Mortality caused by sepsis in patients with end-stage renal disease compared to the general population. *Kidney International* **58**, 1758–64.

Schneeberger, P.M., Toonen, N., Keur, I. and van Hamersvelt, H.W. (1998) Infection control of hepatitis C in Dutch dialysis centres. *Nephrology Dialysis Transplantation* **13** (12), 3037–40.

Stevenson, K.B., Hana, E.L., Lowder, C.A., Adcox, M.J., Davidson, R.L., Mal, N.C., Narasimhan, N. and Wagnild, J.P. (2002) Epidemiology of hemodialysis vascular infections from longitudinal infection surveillance data: predicting the impact of NKF-DOQI clinical practice guidelines for vascular access. *American Journal of Kidney Diseases* **39** (3), 549–55.

Taylor, G.D., McKnezie, M., Buchanan-Chell, M., Caballo, L., Chui, L. and Kowalewska-Grochowska, K. (1998) Central venous catheters as a source of haemodialysis related bacteraemia. *Infection Control in Hospital Epidemiology* **19** (9), 643–6.

United States Renal Data System (1999) Annual data report. Causes of death. *American Journal of Kidney Diseases* **43** (Suppl 1), s87–94.

Valderrabano, F., Jones, E.H. and Mallick, N.P. (1995) Report on management of renal failure in Europe, XXIV 1993. *Nephrology Dialysis Transplantation* **10** (Suppl 5), 1–25.

Velandia, M., Fridkin, S.K. and Cardenas, V. (1995) Transmission of HIV in dialysis centre. *Lancet* **345**, 1417–22.

Zuckerman, M. (2002) Surveillance and control of blood-borne virus infections in haemodialysis units. *Journal of Hospital Infection* **50** (1), 1–5.

# Further reading

Advisory Committee on Immunization Practices (1993) Recommendations of the Advisory Committee on Immunization Practices (ACIP) use of vaccines and immunoglobulins in persons with altered immunocompetence. *Mortality and Morbidity Weekly Report* **42** (RR-4), 1–18.

Ansell, D. and Feest, T. (2002) *The Fifth Annual Report of the UK Renal Registry.* www.renalreg.com.

Centers for Disease Control and Prevention (1995) HIV transmission in a dialysis centre – Columbia, 1991–1993. *Morbidity and Mortality Weekly Report* **44**, 404–402.

Department of Health (2002) *Good Practice Guidelines for Renal Dialysis/Transplantation units. Prevention and Control of Blood-Borne Virus Infection.* Department of Health, London.

Chapter 10
# Sexual Dysfunction and Renal Disease
*Martin Steggall and Sandra Gann*

## Introduction

Sexual function is not merely the simple matter of integrating desire, blood supply and nerve supply, but a complex process that demands many physical and psychological conditions to be right for the individual concerned.

This section will introduce the concept of sexuality, and specific physical issues facing those with established renal failure will be discussed. Assessment and treatment options will be reviewed, alongside general guidelines for setting up a sexual dysfunction clinic or referring patients to specialist services.

## Sexuality and sexual dysfunction

Sexual dysfunction is common in patients with renal disease (Palmer, 1999). Traditionally sexual dysfunction has been divided into organic (physical) causes and psychogenic (psychological) causes, and these are often treated separately. However, such an approach fails to acknowledge the complex nature of sexuality and, furthermore, whether the sexual dysfunction is purely organic or psychogenic in origin is of little importance to the individual coping with it. Treating just the organic or psychogenic cause often results in the failure of any treatment programme (Steggall and Gann, 2002).

It is important to address issues relating to sexuality in patients with long-term chronic illness. Sexuality is a basic human instinct and like other human instincts it does not necessarily have to be gratified, but it does need to be acknowledged. If ignored it can be destructive and the source of much discontent and misery, leading to social isolation and even suicide.

Each individual is unique and the time to think about sexual issues will be unique to each individual (Hawton, 1985). It is important for patients to know that sexual issues are not taboo and can be discussed appropriately whenever it is important for the patient to do so. It is the health professional's responsibility to put sexuality on the agenda rather than leave it to the patient to raise.

One of the misconceptions about sexuality is that most people are enjoying regular and good-quality sexual relationships, and that men in particular can have erections whenever they want. Crowe (2002) reported that erectile disorders affect approximately 10% of all men, with incidence increasing with age. Premature ejaculation is complained of in up to 30% of men, delayed ejaculation by 8% and loss of libido or sexual interest in 16%. Sexual dysfunction in women tends to be less well publicised, but includes vaginismus, decreased libido, vulvodymia (persistent pain in the vulva) and inability to orgasm (Palmer, 1999).

Whilst erectile disorders affect approximately 10% of the sexually active population, arousal dysfunction may be more prevalent, affecting more than 40% of sexually active pre-menopausal women, with a higher incidence in post-menopausal women reported (Riley, 2000). However, Laumann et al. (1999) noted that women rarely present with loss of arousal but instead loss of desire or a specific physical symptom such as dyspareunia (pain on intercourse) or anorgasmia (no orgasm).

Normal sexual arousal in women requires intact sensory nerves of the vulva and pelvic floor muscles, an adequate blood supply to the genitalia to allow increased flow to the labia and clitoris, and vaginal lubrication (Riley, 2000). The effects of long-term medical problems and chronic disease that change these processes are as significant to women as men.

It can be seen therefore that sexual dysfunction is common in the 'general' population and will be exacerbated by established renal failure (ERF). Pain, discomfort and poor body image all contribute to sexual dysfunction and, consequently, loss of sexual desire (Williams, 1989).

However, even when well, no individual should expect to be able to be sexually responsive if his or her basic underlying needs are not met. They should not be tired or worried about interruptions; they should not be feeling upset or angry with their partner. Sometimes a patient presenting with erectile dysfunction may describe a situation where he is feeling 'impotent' in a work or social situation. This can be a common contribution to sexual difficulties.

As men have their sexual organs outside their body, it is obvious if and when they have a problem. However, women too experience difficulties sexually for all the same reasons yet it is less likely to be acknowledged or addressed even by themselves. An ongoing successful relationship usually requires a capacity for commitment and intimacy as well as the physiological changes that accompany arousal, i.e. increased blood flow and neurological interpretation.

Patients with ERF may have some or all of these problems to contend with, as a chronic medical condition often leads to poor body image and low self-esteem. It can affect the way the individual sees him- or herself being able to fulfil the 'normal' role of husband/mother, breadwinner, etc. If you have lived with a body that produces only pain, fear and discomfort, it is difficult to be confident in the possibility that you can also experience pleasure and intimacy.

It is also important to understand how patients have previously expressed their sexuality within or outside the relationship, to ascertain what is normal to them and what they hope to achieve. However, for young patients with ERF who have had life-long problems, they have not had the chance to mature and become sexual in the way their peers have. The case example below outlines the complexity of the problems faced by young people with chronic disease.

## Case example

Tom[1] required dialysis from the age of 12. At 21 years of age he had a successful renal transplant and it was thought he had been given the opportunity to lead a 'normal' life. However, once his physical problems were removed he reported anger that his sexual issues had not been addressed. He felt that neither family nor medical colleagues had given him the opportunity to discuss his feelings at being unable to express his sexual needs during adolescence. He also felt that his medical condition and his body image prevented him from forming satisfactory relationships, and at the age of 35, when he presented to the clinic, he had not had the opportunities of other people his age to meet a partner. This left him feeling very alone and apart from others in society. He had been treated for depression in the past and had received psychological counselling, but the sexual issues had not been addressed. Tom was initially provided with a 'medical' treatment plan that failed, and required joint psychosexual counselling and further medical management for resolution of his sexual dysfunction.

There are often different anxieties or fears depending on the age and marital status of the patient. Mature patients sometimes worry about their partner's sexual needs and what the implications are for the relationship long term; sometimes it is the partner who feels guilty that they no longer feel desire for someone they have nursed and attended to personal bodily functions. Clearly sexuality, and its expression, has many facets that need to be considered in caring for such patients.

## The sexual cycle

Any sexual relationship has both physical and psychological components. It is important to be able to break down the sexual cycle into the three main stages of excitement or desire, arousal or orgasm, and resolution (Masters and Johnson, 1966) in order to identify exactly where any sexual dysfunction lies (Crowe, 2002).

---

[1] Name of patient has been changed to preserve confidentiality.

The first stage of the sexual cycle is desire or libido. The myth is that men have a constant desire for sex, whilst it is acknowledged that women's desire can vary at different times of the month. Often a woman's desire lies just under her consciousness, but she can be aroused once being caressed. For men and women desire is dependent on feeling that another desires them. A change in body image that can accompany ERF can dramatically affect self-esteem and libido.

The second stage is arousal, when each person is aware that they are feeling sexual and wanting to be sexual. This is usually a response to some stimulant, whether alone and enjoying pictures or stories, or with another and responding to thoughts and sensations. Arousal will often lead to orgasm, but does not have to. Either partner can enjoy excitement levels of arousal, which die down rather than finish with orgasm and/or ejaculation. Some women enjoy orgasms by manual stimulation rather than by penetration during sexual intercourse. Likewise, some men find it more difficult to ejaculate inside their partner than alone. What is important is that each person enjoys the experience and does not try to achieve unrealistic 'goals' (Stanway, 2001).

The final phase of the sexual cycle is the resolution period. This is essential for the man. At 18 years of age the refractory requirement, i.e. the time taken for the body to 'recover' from ejaculation, is very short, but over the lifespan the man requires a longer recovery time – from a few hours to a few days depending on each individual. The female arousal phase usually takes longer than the man's, but once at their peak it is biologically possible for women to have more than one orgasm in any 'encounter'. For men and women the urgency of lovemaking changes over the years, but the ability to express oneself sexually remains one of choice for each person (Stanway, 2001).

The first step to achieving a mutually satisfying sexual relationship is to feel comfortable about expressing feelings of wanting to be close to your partner. It may be important to change the 'goals' – not to attempt sexual intercourse all the time but find other ways of expressing sexual feelings with each other.

Permission giving is an important task to acknowledge and sometimes permission not to have a penetrative sexual relationship is important. It may well be that positions that have not previously been tried are more comfortable and less tiring. The answers of course are not in a textbook but with each individual.

The key to the sexual cycle is communication, and communication is sometimes harder than actions (Crowe, 2002). Individuals need to be able to communicate their physical and emotional needs to their partners. Fear or embarrassment can often lead to isolation; individuals can cope without sexual intercourse but cannot cope without intimacy or 'closeness' in a relationship. Sometimes individuals like to have the opportunity to talk these issues through in clinic either with their partner or alone, so it is essential that health professionals be at ease with their own communications skills.

Individuals with established renal failure may have to contend with the psychological effects of chronic illness *and* disordered physiology, most commonly uraemia, which can cause sexual dysfunction.

**Table 10.1**  Effects of uraemia. (Adapted from Lue, 2002.)

- Arterial (atherosclerosis).
- Neurologic (peripheral neuropathy).
- Psychologic (added stress and depression).
- Medication (hypertension).
- Endocrine (hyperprolactinaemia, hypogonadism, hyperparathyroidism).

## Effects of uraemia

Uraemia may result in endocrine dysfunction with lowered testosterone and elevated luteinising hormone (LH), follicle stimulating hormone (FSH) and prolactin. Decreased testosterone production and possible uraemic toxins on the testes have been implicated in erectile dysfunction (ED) (Carson and Patel, 1999). Hyperprolactinaemia caused by an increased production or a reduced metabolism of prolactin, or induced by drugs, is common and is also implicated in erection failure.

Uraemia affects all body systems and the common effects are shown in Table 10.1. Excess prolactin may be produced which can affect potency and libido in men and women. After successful renal transplant, erections/libido may improve from an organic perspective, but many psychogenic issues may remain; therefore sexual dysfunction can still occur in this group of patients.

Elevated uric acid or uraemia is common in renal disease; proteinuria is found which can result in loss of antithrombin III, causing a predisposition to thromboembolic complications; and hypertension is common, accelerating loss of renal function. Antihypertensive medication is well documented in the genesis of sexual dysfunction, especially in the male (Fogari and Zoppi, 2002). Women with renal failure may have amenorrhoea or other menstrual abnormalities, inhibition of arousal and loss of libido, whereas men may have erectile dysfunction and loss of libido (Palmer, 1999).

Erythropoietin may affect the hypothalamic-pituitary axis, responsible for normal sexual and reproductive functions (Tokgoz et al., 2002). The hypothalamus releases gonadotropic releasing hormone (GnRH) which is transferred to the adenohypophysis (anterior pituitary), where the gonadotropic hormones LH and FSH are released. Medication that affects dopamine, serotonin or noradrenaline has been implicated in affecting release of the hormones, resulting in decreased sexual function.

## Physiology of the male sexual response

Visual or tactile stimulation results in nerve impulses transmitted to the penis which stimulate the release of neurotransmitters. The release of nitric oxide and prostaglandins results in activation of guanylate and adenylate cyclase, increasing local concentrations of cGMP and cAMP (Brewster et al., 2001).

**Table 10.2**  Effects of medication. (Adapted from Lue, 2002.)

| Antihypertensives: Betablockers, calcium antagonists, ACE inhibitors | Induces sexual dysfunction by actions at the central or peripheral level, e.g. $\alpha$-adrenergic receptor agonists, methyldopa acts by depleting neurotransmitters, by direct actions at the corporal level or by dropping systemic blood pressure on which the patient has relied to maintain an intracorporal pressure sufficient for development of penile rigidity. |
|---|---|
| Diuretics: Thiazide diuretics | Usually causes sexual dysfunction when used in combination with anti-hypertensives, but spironolactone blocks testosterone synthesis and competitively binds to androgen receptors. Thiazide is a common cause of impotence; some diuretics may also cause decreased libido. |
| Cardiovascular drugs: Lipid-lowering, digoxin | Digoxin can cause sexual dysfunction because it blocks the Na-K-ATPase pump, resulting in a net increase intracellular calcium and subsequent increased tone in the corporal smooth muscle.<br>Lipid-lowering medication enhances metabolism of androgens. Betablockers may impair libido. |
| Anti-androgens: Oestrogens, LHRH analogues and testosterone | Block androgen synthesis; examples include spironolactone, oestrogen and ketoconazole which lower serum testosterone. |

These chemicals cause relaxation of the smooth muscle and the cavernosal arteries dilate, increasing blood flow into the cavernosal sinuses. As they fill, the sinuses compress the blood vessels that allow blood to exit the penis, resulting in reduced venous outflow from the corpus cavernosa. The corpora become engorged, increasing their length and girth and becoming rigid, so causing an erection. Reduction in the release of chemicals coupled with the metabolism of cGMP and cAMP by phosphodiesterases reduces inflow, increases outflow and detumescence occurs (Brewster et al., 2001).

Any condition that interferes with this system will cause erection failure, and a prime causal factor is that of anti-hypertensive medication and calcium-channel blockers. All anti-hypertensive medications have the potential to cause erection failure since they prevent the endothelium from contracting (Fogari and Zoppi, 2002). In addition, there are profound changes to body image and energy levels in chronic illness. This combination therefore renders individuals with renal diseases a high chance of sexual dysfunction. The effects of medication are shown in Table 10.2.

## Physiology of the female sexual response

The female sexual response is similar to the male in that it is dependent on tactile and psychogenic stimulation. The tactile stimulation provides a neural input with attendant release of chemicals. The vascular response results in engorgement of the corpora of the clitoris and clitoral erection, although the degree of clitoral involvement varies considerably. Vaginal lubrication occurs by transudation of fluid through the vaginal wall, which vasocongests and becomes a purplish colour (Johnson and Everitt, 1995). The vagina expands and the labia majora engorges with blood. Any medical condition or medication that interferes with normal blood flow can affect females in a similar way to that seen in males. The psychogenic effects are the same as in males, although, as previously stated, female sexual responses are generally slower to start than the male.

## Specific male sexual dysfunction: erectile dysfunction

Erectile dysfunction is defined as the inability of a man to gain an erection of sufficient quality for intercourse (Kirby and Eardley, 1991). Diagnostic tools can help identify the severity of erection failure, for example the International Index of Erectile Function (IIEF); however, the usefulness of such an index is debatable since the clinician looks to assist the patient in resolving sexual dysfunction, which does not necessarily mean improving the quality of the erection, given the sexual cycle described.

The incidence of erectile dysfunction is thought to be approximately 2.6% in the general population of men aged 40–69 years (Meuleman, 2002). However, the incidence appears to be higher in individuals with renal problems. Castro et al. (2001) noted that up to one half of patients with established renal failure have erectile dysfunction. Approximately three-quarters of this group, however, regain function after renal transplant, but erectile dysfunction may occur in one third with a bilateral transplant with vascular anastomosis to the hypogastric artery. (This would be a logical finding as the arterial blood supply to the penis is from a branch of the hypogastric artery.)

A common finding is that patients with renal disease, who therefore have a known organic cause of their erectile dysfunction, also had significant psychogenic factors that influenced the condition and its treatment.

## Assessment

Despite media images, our sexuality is usually a private subject and not one that a patient or a professional will feel at ease in addressing. There are difficulties in knowing what words to use and whether you can understand exactly the problem the patient is experiencing. It can be difficult to listen to a patient if the health professional is worrying about how he/she should respond.

The key to treating sexual dysfunction is identification. A simple assessment could include questions such as 'I notice that you are taking XYZ drug. Some individuals can have difficulty with sex drive or erections following taking this medicine. Have you had any trouble?'. A detailed assessment would not be required; the patient could be asked if he or she would like referral to a nurse specialist in sexual dysfunction, and further advice and information sought.

For many cultures, discussion about sex or sexual dysfunction may be forbidden or taboo, which presents a dichotomy to the nurse caring for these patients. Does the nurse broach this potentially difficult subject or not? The position adopted locally, where there is a high proportion of Muslims, is that of information giving; if the patient knows that there is help available, it is up to the patient to decide if he or she wants to access it. It is important to appreciate the need to broach sexual issues sensitively and to respect both cultural and religious norms that make discussion of sex more limited or difficult for practitioners, patients and partners. Often the consequence of denying sexual function, in terms of intercourse and intimacy associated with sexual contact, is relationship distress and breakdown.

## Investigations

Prior to referral for specialist advice, urea and electrolytes and a hormone profile should be completed. These tests include luteinising hormone (LH), follicle stimulating hormone (FSH), testosterone (for men), sex hormone binding globulin (SHBG), prolactin, and an electrolyte assessment. Although the hormone profile is invariably within normal ranges, there may be an undiagnosed hormonal imbalance that will require endocrinological investigation.

Referral for specialist advice is relatively simple provided a sexual dysfunction clinic has been established locally. Often all that are required are a letter of introduction and a copy of the hormone profile results. A full assessment will be completed in the clinic (see Table 10.3).

## Treatment options (male)

Irrespective of the cause of sexual dysfunction, only seven treatments are available to men, which are:

- Psychosexual counselling.
- Apomorphine hydrochloride (Uprima®).
- Phosphodiesterase type V inhibitors, e.g. sildenafil citrate (Viagra®), tadalafil (Cialis®) and vardenafil (Levitra®).
- Medicated Urethral System for Erections (MUSE®) – intra-urethral alprostadil pellet.
- Intracavernosal injection of prostaglandin $E_1$ – Caverject Dual Chamber® or Viridal Duo®.
- Vacuum devices.
- Surgery – prosthesis.

**Table 10.3**  Sexual dysfunction assessment. Reproduced from Steggall and Gann (2002) with kind permission of EMAP Healthcare.

| Assessment | Rationale | Implication for treatment |
|---|---|---|
| Surgical history | Assess whether there has been surgical damage to the hypogastric artery, through, for example, renal transplant | May need to offer more aggressive management in terms of intracavernosal injection or vacuum device, to encourage blood flow in men |
| Medical history | Assess the level of renal function, type and frequency of dialysis | Important when considering the metabolism of the medications available |
| Current medication | Assess risk of potential drug interactions, for example, antibiotics enhance plasma levels of Sildenafil | Check for contra-indications to medication that can improve localised blood flow |
| Allergies | Interaction with treatment | Interaction with treatment |
| Tobacco | Assess vascular damage | Give lifestyle advice |
| Alcohol | Desensitises the individual to stimulation | Potential to effect success of treatment |
| **Specific history** | | |
| Description of the problem | Erection failure, loss of desire, or rapid ejaculation, duration of problem, anorgasmia, vaginismus, etc. | Guides management |
| Gradual or sudden onset | Organic or psychogenic causes? | Gradual onset suggests an organic cause whereas sudden onset suggests a psychogenic cause |
| Early morning tumescence (applies to males only) | Is the blood supply intact? | May need locally acting medication if blood flow is poor |
| Libido | Assess desire and the impact of performance anxiety | Often absent in long-term sexual dysfunction; possible compensatory mechanism or a form of communication |
| Is penetration possible? | Assess strength of erection/lubrication | Assess blood flow; may indicate 'strength' of medication required |
| Current sexual relationship | Need to know if there is some sexual activity | Absence of intimacy is important – for the medication to work some type of sexual stimulation is required |
| Psychological factors: social problems (particularly prior to onset of problem) | Anxieties inhibit function | Feelings of 'impotence' in other areas will be reflected in sexuality – need to resolve underlying problem |
| Performance anxiety | Maintains problem | Break cycle of failure/restore confidence |
| Does the partner know of the patient's visit? | Status of relationship | Address unresolved issues with both partners |

**Table 10.4** Summary of treatments for erection failure. Reproduced from Steggall and Gann (2002) with kind permission of EMAP Healthcare.

| Treatment | Dosage guide | Mode of action |
|---|---|---|
| Uprima® (apomorphine hydrochloride) | 3 mg sub-lingual (need at least 6 doses before excluding) | Dopaminergic receptors, increase blood flow to the penis |
| Phosphodiesterase type V inhibitors | Viagra®: 25–100 mg (recommend start dose of 50 mg, increasing to 100 mg) Cialis®: 10–20 mg (recommend 10 mg start dose) Levitra®: 5–20 mg (start at 5 mg); should be tried on eight occasions | Phosphodiesterase type V inhibitor, increases blood flow to the penis |
| Medical Urethral System for Erections, MUSE® (alprostadil pellet) | 250–1000 μg (depends on whether the patient can pass urine) | Increases blood flow to the penis through the action of prostaglandin E$_1$; however, it is important to be able to urinate in case of the side effect of urethral burning |
| Intracavernosal alprostadil injections (Caverject Dual Chamber® and Viridal Duo®) | 2.5–60 μg | Increased blood flow by the same action as MUSE although the delivery of the medication is direct into the corpus cavernosa; thus absorption in the urethra is not required |
| Vacuum pumps | These devices draw blood into the corpus cavernosa under pressure. A constriction band will help to keep the blood in place but must be removed after 30 minutes | Non-pharmacological; draws blood into the corpus cavernosum under pressure. This option is useful in patients with multiple pathologies where drug interaction is a problem. The major advantage is that there are no potential side effects, other than leaving the constriction band in place |
| Surgery (prostheses) | — | Prosthesis – artificial implants replace the corpus cavernosum – erection gained 'on demand'. May be unsuitable for immunocompromised patients or others at high risk during surgery |
| Psychosexual therapy (behavioural programme with counselling of underlying issues) | Weekly or regular attendance with 'exercises to do at home' | Breaks pattern of failure, removes anxiety and restores confidence |

Such options tend to focus on 'medication' solutions for males. The relative merits of each option are shown in Table 10.4; however, it is essential that an assessment of renal function is made, taking into consideration additional information such as manual dexterity and co-existing pathologies.

Sildenafil is thought to be as effective in patients with renal disease as it is in the general population of patients with erectile dysfunction (Juergense et al., 2001), and there are no differences in side effects in those with renal failure (Chen et al., 2001).

The efficacy of these treatments can be variable and dependent on patient motivation. It is essential to take time to assess and teach patients about the various treatment options; this can markedly improve patient acceptability and efficacy. Clearly, if there are unresolved psychosexual issues, then there is a powerful barrier to block the efficacy of the medication. In some circumstances, the medication may provide an erection, but the patient may still complain of sexual dysfunction because of unresolved fears of intimacy. It is also important to take the partner's views/desires into consideration, as a negative response from a partner will maintain an individual's sexual dysfunction.

## Future treatment options

Tadalafil (Cialis®) and vardenafil were released in early 2003. Vardenafil appears to be similar in action and side effects to Sildenafil, and well tolerated (Porst et al., 2001). The mode of action of Tadalafil is also similar to that of Sildenafil, but the half-life is much longer, which may have the benefit of helping the patient to regain some degree of spontaneity. The side-effect profile is also similar, so it must be used with caution in renal failure. Dosages of 10 mg have been given to patients with renal insufficiency, but there is little clinical data at this stage to evaluate the effects; therefore an individual risk evaluation needs to be undertaken when prescribing (Brock et al., 2002, Lilly ICOS, 2002).

## Specific concerns in management

The Department of Health guidelines (Health Service Circular, 1999) for the prescription of these medications includes research from Johnson et al. (1994), who report that the average number of times that the 40- to 60-year-old male age group have intercourse is once a week, and therefore suggest that GPs prescribe to reflect this. A feature of chronic illness is long-term sexual dysfunction. This means that any treatment is unlikely to be successful on the first few attempts, which will result in performance anxiety where patients are under such pressure to perform that the pressure itself causes erection failure. Clearly, such guidelines fail to recognise the effect that delayed treatment and performance anxiety have on patients, especially with chronic illnesses.

Rigid adherence to the prescribing guidelines will have implications on successful and rapid outcome, by exacerbating fear of failure and performance anxiety. Patients could be recommended to take the medication more frequently than once per week, using the rationale that this will lower anxiety levels related to the expected outcome of the medication. Once a successful treatment regime has been established, the patient could then decrease his treatment demand to once a week.

**Table 10.5**  Some treatment options for female sexual dysfunction.

| | |
|---|---|
| Psychosexual therapy (behavioural therapy): self-focus and sensate focus | These are programmes practised over several weeks combining relaxation techniques and exercises with opportunity to explore underlying issues |
| Lubricants – KY or 'Senselle' | Solutions or lubricants such as KY-Gel or 'Senselle' gel may assist where there is vaginal dryness |
| Hormone replacement therapy (HRT) | For some menopausal women, HRT has been found to assist in arousal |
| Sildenafil | Assists in engorgement of blood to the female genital tract |

## Treatment options (female)

Both men and women can suffer sexual anxieties and specific dysfunction. It is interesting to note that female sexual dysfunction has a much lower profile than male sexual dysfunction within the medical profession, although arousal dysfunction may affect more than two in every five sexually active pre-menopausal women, with a higher incidence than this in post-menopausal women not receiving oestrogen replacement (Riley, 2000).

Often, arousal dysfunction reflects a sexual drive or desire disorder. Women with arousal or desire difficulties may also present with other sexual dysfunctions such as dyspareunia or anorgasmia. Methods of recording genital sexual arousal and genital blood flow are now being used in research and in the future could be useful in providing information to the patient and clinician about where the problem is in the sexual cycle.

Currently, psychosexual therapy and/or oestrogen replacement is effective in overcoming arousal problems and other dysfunctions for many women for whom organic causes have been excluded. Sildenafil has been found to be of benefit in female patients by changing vaginal lubrication and clitoral sensitivity, although the precise role of Sildenafil in this group of patients has yet to be fully researched and evaluated in the UK before it can be registered for treatment purposes (Kaplan et al., 1999). The treatment options for females are shown in Table 10.5.

## Referrals and clinics

Advice has been given on how to assess patients and the options for treatment/management programme have been identified. Many departments provide a sexual health service, including Urology, Genito-Urinary Medicine, Psychological Medicine and other specialist clinics. In the absence of specialist services, patients could be referred to national organisations such as Family Planning or Relate or to private clinics for further advice.

It may be possible to set up a sexual dysfunction clinic. A core speciality team would need to include medical, nursing and a psychosexual therapist or clinical psychologist. The patient would need a joint medical and psychological assessment, as described, before treatment is offered. Specialist training in erectile dysfunction is available in many centres, such as Urology, Genito-Urinary Medicine and other specialist clinics. Given the effects of uraemia discussed, patients would require a hormone profile and correction of any uraemia before referral.

The key elements to any sexual dysfunction clinic are:

- Time.
- A safe environment.
- Training to undertake management of these patients.

The fundamental principle in assisting patients with sexual dysfunction is that of offering an opportunity for discussion. Discrete advertising in the clinical area empowers patients to decide for themselves whether they want to seek treatment.

## Summary

Sexual dysfunction is a common finding in both men and women with established renal failure. Disturbances include erectile dysfunction in men, decreased blood flow to the female genitalia affecting sensation or lubrication, menstrual abnormalities in women, and decreased libido and fertility in both sexes. Although such problems are organic in origin, and related to uraemia and other pathologies, there is often a significant element of psychogenic dysfunction, whether through decreased libido, fatigue or performance anxiety.

A key feature of successful management of sexual dysfunction is that of identification. Clearly one of the main goals of treatment for ERF is the resolution of electrolyte imbalance and blood pressure control, but once achieved the emphasis should be on returning the individual to a 'normal' lifestyle, and sexuality forms a part of this.

## Useful contact

Sexual Dysfunction Association
Helpline: 0870 774 3571
www.sda.uk.net

## References

Brock, G.B., McMahon, C.G., Chen, K.K., Costigan, T., Shen, W., Watkins, V., Anglin, G. and Whitaker, S. (2002) Efficacy and safety of Tadalafil for the treatment of erectile dysfunction: results of integrated analyses. *Journal of Urology* **168**, 1332–6.

Brewster, C., Cranston, D., Noble, J. and Reynard, J. (2001) Urological oncology. In: *Urology: A Handbook for Medical Students* (Brewster, C., Cranston, D., Noble, J. and Reynard, J., eds). Bios Scientific Publishers, Oxford.

Carson, C.C. and Patel, M.P. (1999) The epidemiology, anatomy, physiology, and treatment of erectile dysfunction in chronic renal failure patients. *Advances in Renal Replacement Therapy* **6**, 296.

Castro Prieto, R.M., Anglanda Curado, F.J., Regueiro Lopez, J.C., Leva Vallejo, M.E., Molina Sanchez, J., Saceda Lopez, J.L. and Requena Tapia, M.J. (2001) Treatment with Sildenafil citrate in renal transplant patients with erectile dysfunction. *British Journal of Urology International* **88**, 241–3.

Chen, J., Mabjeesh, N.J., Greenstein, A., Nadu, A. and Matzkin, H. (2001) Clinical efficacy of Sildenafil in patients on chronic dialysis. *Journal of Urology* **165**, 819–21.

Crowe, M.J. (2002) Sexual dysfunction and sexual therapy. *Psychiatry* **1**, 60–63.

Fogari, R. and Zoppi, A. (2002) Effects of antihypertensive therapy on sexual activity in hypertensive men. *Current Hypertension Reports* **4** (3), 202–210.

Hawton, K. (1985) *Sex Therapy – A Practical Guide*. Oxford University Press, Oxford, pp. 56–94.

Health Service Circular (1999) *HSC 1999/148. Treatment for Impotence.* Department of Health, London, www.doh.gov.uk – link to HSC for full guidelines.

Johnson, A., Wadsworth, J., et al. (1994) Sexual attitudes and lifestyles survey, UK 1990–1991. In: Health Service Circular *HSC 1999/148 Treatment for impotence.* Department of Health, London, www.doh.gov.uk – link to HSC for full guidelines.

Johnson, M.H. and Everitt, B.J. (1995) Coitus and fertilization. Chapter 8. In: *Essential Reproduction* (Johnson, M.H., Martin, H. and Everitt, B.J., eds), 4th edn. Blackwell Science, Oxford.

Juergense, P.H., Botey, R., Wureth, D., Finkelstein, S.H., Smith, J.D. and Finkelstein, F.O. (2001) Erectile dysfunction in chronic peritoneal dialysis patients: incidence and treatment with Sildenafil. *Peritoneal Dialysis International* **21** (4), 355–9.

Kaplan, S.A., Reis, R.B., Kohn, I.J., Ikeguchi, E.F., Laor, E., Te, A.E. and Martins, A.C. (1999) Safety and efficacy of Sildenafil in postmenopausal women with sexual dysfunction. *Urology* **53** (3), 481–6.

Kirby, R.S. and Eardley, I. (1991) Initial assessment of patients with erectile dysfunction. Chapter 6. In: Kirby, R.S., Carson, C.C. and Webster, G.D. (1991) *Impotence: Diagnosis and Management of Male Erectile Dysfunction.* Butterworth Heinemann, Oxford.

Laumann, E.O., Paik, A. and Rosen, R.C. (1999) Sexual dysfunction in the United States: prevalence and predictions. *Journal of the American Medical Association* **281**, 537–44.

Lilly ICOS (2002) *Cialis: Summary of Product Characteristics.* Lilly ICOS, Indianapolis.

Lue, T.F. (ed.) (2002) *Atlas of Impotence*, 2nd edn. Current Medicine, Philadelphia.

Masters, W.H. and Johnson, V.E. (1966) *Human Sexual Response.* Little Brown & Co., Boston.

Meuleman, E.J. (2002) Prevalence of erectile dysfunction: need for treatment? *International Journal of Impotence Research* **14** (Suppl 1), S22–8.

Palmer, B.F. (1999) Sexual dysfunction in uremia. *Journal of the American Society of Nephrology* **10** (6), 1381–8.

Porst, H., Rosen, R., Padma-Nathan, H., Goldstein, I., Giuliano, F., Ulbrich, E. and the Vardenafil Study Group (2001) The efficacy and tolerability of Vardenafil, a new, oral, selective phosphodiesterase type 5 inhibitor, in patients with erectile dysfunction: the first at-home clinical trial. *International Journal of Impotence Research* **13**, 192–9.

Riley, A. (2000) Do all women need sex? In: *Proc British Society of Sexual and Impotence Research (BSSIR)/Impotence Association Conference 2000*, Spring Meeting. British Society for Sexual Medicine, www.bssm.org.uk.

Stanway, A. (2001) *Sexuality and Cancer. A Guide for People with Cancer and their Partners.* CancerBacup, London.

Steggall, M.J. and Gann, S.Y. (2002) Assessing patients with actual or potential erectile dysfunction. *Professional Nurse* **18**, (3), 155–9.

Tokgoz, B., Utas, C., Dogukan, A., Oymak, O. and Kelestimur, F. (2002) Influence of long term erythropoietin therapy on the hypothalamic–pituitary–thyroid axis in patients undergoing CAPD. *Renal Failure* **24** (3), 315–23.

Williams, W. (1989) *It's Up to You: Overcoming Erection Problems.* Harper Collins, London.

# Chapter 11
# Issues in Nephrology, Dialysis and Transplantation for Minority Ethnic Groups

*Gurch Randhawa*

## Introduction

The Department of Health's (DoH's) Tackling Health Inequalities 2002 Cross-Cutting Review identified that not only do health gaps still exist in the UK but also, in some cases, they are growing ever wider.

> 'There are wide geographical variations in health status, reflecting the multiple problems of material disadvantage facing some communities. These differences begin at conception and continue throughout life. Babies born to poorer families are more likely to be born prematurely, are at greater risk of infant mortality and have a greater likelihood of poverty, impaired development and chronic disease in later life. This sets up an inter-generational cycle of health inequalities.' (DoH, 2002a)

This statement reflects the shift in focus of policy during the last 20 years in which there has been a growing interest in the health of minority ethnic populations in the UK.

Throughout this period, the provision of renal services for minority ethnic groups has become a particularly important area of debate. This is in part due to the observation of high rates of established renal failure (ERF) (as a result of diabetic nephropathy) among South Asian and African-Caribbean populations in the UK and the disproportionately higher numbers of South Asians and African-Caribbeans represented on transplant waiting lists.

Throughout this chapter 'South Asians' and 'African Caribbeans' are used to describe the minority ethnic groups in the UK. There is a lack of available data for other minority ethnic groups.

# Background

South Asians (those originating from the Indian subcontinent) and African-Caribbean communities have a high prevalence of type 2 diabetes: recent studies indicate a prevalence rate four times greater than white people. It has been reported that 20% of South Asians aged 40–49 have type 2 diabetes, and by the age of 65 the proportion rises to a third (Raleigh, 1997).

A further complication is that diabetic nephropathy is the major cause of ERF in South Asian and African-Caribbean patients receiving renal replacement therapy (RRT), either by dialysis or transplantation. Nationally, this higher relative risk, when corrected for age and gender, has been calculated in England as 4.2 for the South Asian community and 3.7 for those with an African-Caribbean background (Roderick et al., 1996). Data from Leicester show that South Asians with diabetes are at 13 times the risk of developing ERF compared to 'white' Caucasians (Burden et al., 1992). Thus, not only are South Asians and African-Caribbeans more prone to diabetes than white people, but also they are more likely to develop ERF as a consequence.

Importantly, the South Asian and African-Caribbean populations in the UK are relatively young compared to the white population. Since the prevalence of ERF increases with age, this has major implications for the future need for RRT and highlights the urgent need for preventive measures (Randhawa, 1998a). The incidence of ERF has significant consequences for both local and national NHS resources. The National Renal Review (DoH, 1994; National Health Service Executive, 1996) estimated an increase over the next decade of 80% in the 20 000 or so patients receiving RRT and a doubling of the current cost, about £600 million a year, of providing renal services (Raleigh, 1997).

Kidney transplantation is the preferred mode of RRT for patients with end-stage renal failure. There are currently over 5500 people on the transplant waiting list in the UK – the majority waiting for kidney transplants, but substantial numbers also waiting for heart, lung and liver transplants. However, a closer examination of the national waiting list reveals that some minority ethnic groups are greater represented than others.

The situation is clear: there is an urgent need to address the number of African-Caribbean and South Asian patients requiring a kidney transplant, otherwise the human and economic costs will be very severe. In the short term there needs to be a greater number of donors coming forward from these communities to increase the pool of suitable organs (Exley et al., 1996a; Randhawa, 1998a). In the long term, there needs to be greater attention paid to preventive strategies to reduce the number of African-Caribbeans and South Asians requiring RRT. The latter can only be achieved if we begin to address the problem of poor access to services for minority ethnic groups (Randhawa, 2003).

## Improving access to services

The National Service Framework (NSF) for Diabetes highlights the importance of access to services, in particular to meet the needs of minority ethnic groups (DoH, 2002b). The working draft of the NSF for Renal Services is also focusing on 'renal disease complicating diabetes' and emphasises inequalities experienced by minority ethnic groups (DoH, 2002c). However, there is evidence that knowledge of diabetes and its complications is poor among South Asians and African-Caribbeans (Nazroo, 1997; Johnson et al., 2000). Preliminary evidence also suggests that quality of health care for South Asians and African-Caribbeans is inadequate and compliance poor (Raleigh, 1997; Johnson et al., 2000). There is also a low-uptake of hospital-based diabetes services, with growing evidence that South Asians are subsequently referred later for renal care, and are more likely to be lost to follow-up (Jeffrey et al., 2002). Late referral may reduce opportunities to implement measures to slow progression of renal failure, or to prepare adequately for RRT, adding to morbidity and mortality.

The World Health Organization (WHO) Study Group on diabetes (1994) notes that resources should be directed to improving the quality of preventive care in primary care settings and to public health interventions for controlling diabetes. Education, early diagnosis and effective management of diabetes are important for safeguarding the health of susceptible populations and for long-term savings for the NHS (Raleigh, 1997). Most encouragingly, recent studies from the US and Finland have demonstrated that modest lifestyle changes can reduce the risk of developing overt type 2 diabetes by more than 58% in susceptible groups (Tuomilehto et al., 2001; Diabetes Prevention Program Research Group, 2002). Furthermore, various interventions, such as tight blood pressure control, effective use of angiotensin converting enzyme (ACE) inhibitors or angiotensin receptor (ATR) blockers, and tight blood sugar control can significantly delay the progression of diabetic nephropathy (UK Prospective Diabetes Study Group, 1998; Feest et al., 1999; Brenner et al., 2001; Cinotti and Zucchelli, 2001; Lewis et al., 2001; Lightstone, 2001).

## Improving transplantation rates

Unfortunately, the transplant option may be medically and economically favourable but in reality is not as forthcoming due to constraints concerning the severe lack of donors from the African-Caribbean and South Asian populations. This could be attributed to two main reasons – a lack of awareness concerning organ donation and transplantation and low referral rates to the Intensive Care Unit (Exley et al., 1996a; Darr and Randhawa, 1999). It must be stressed that these factors are not unique to the African-Caribbean and South Asian population and have relevance to other members of the UK's public. Furthermore, it is extremely important to recognise that the African-Caribbean and South Asian communities in the UK are heterogenous and thus it is important to familiarise oneself with the demographics of the local population (Khan and Randhawa, 1999).

## *Increasing awareness of the need for organ donors among the African-Caribbean and South Asian communities*

Unfortunately, very little research has been devoted to this area. The relatively few studies that have been carried out consistently show that South Asians are supportive of organ donation and transplantation, but are simply not aware of the specific needs for organs from their community (Exley et al., 1996a; Darr and Randhawa, 1999).

A growing amount of literature has shown that the role of religion has been known to play an important part in the decision to donate organs (Randhawa, 1998b). The religious beliefs of the major faiths of the UK's African-Caribbeans and South Asians, namely Islam, Hinduism, Sikhism, Buddhism and Christianity, have been scrutinised in the literature. None of the religions objects to organ donation in principle, although in some there are varying schools of thought. What is interesting, however, is that the position of one's religion is used by many people in informing their decision as to whether to donate or not (Randhawa, 1998b). This has been highlighted in several studies conducted abroad (Callender, 1989; Kyriakides et al., 1993; Spina et al., 1993). Unfortunately, this issue has not been prominent in research carried out in the UK, but the findings of a pilot study to examine the attitudes towards organ donation and transplantation among a cross section of the UK's South Asian population have shed some light on the matter (Randhawa, 1998b). It was found that far from being a barrier to organ donation, the respondents were more supportive of donation, and transplantation in general, when they were aware of the position of their religion with regards to these issues. This highlights the importance of education and raising awareness among the South Asian public (Exley et al., 1996a; Darr and Randhawa, 1999).

The Department of Health has produced a range of educational material (including leaflets, posters and videos) in the main South Asian languages to increase awareness of transplant-related issues. However, current evidence shows that further thought is required regarding the dissemination of this literature among African-Caribbean and South Asian populations (Exley et al., 1996a; Randhawa, 1998b; Darr and Randhawa, 1999). Care needs to be taken in specifying the target population, selecting the persons who will communicate the campaign appeal, designating the methodology of appeal delivery and deciding upon the content of the appeal. There are indications from pilot work in the UK and research overseas involving minority ethnic groups that appeals for African-Caribbean and South Asian donors may be more effectively communicated by employing a grassroots, community networking approach (Exley et al., 1996a; Darr and Randhawa, 1999; Khan and Randhawa, 1999). Figure 11.1 sets out how this community-based approach may be operationalised in practice.

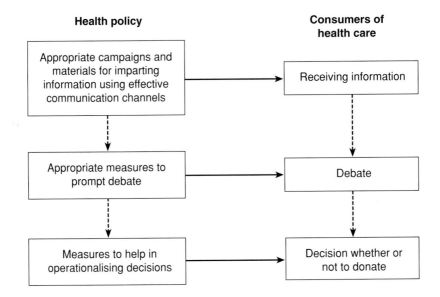

**Figure 11.1**  Stages for consideration in the development of a comprehensive approach to organ procurement (Reproduced from Darr and Randhawa, 1999 with kind permission of the Institute of Health Promotion and Education).

## Low referral rates to the intensive care unit

The vast majority of organs are procured from ventilated patients in the Intensive Care Unit (ICU) who have suffered some form of cerebrovascular accident (Gore et al., 1992; Randhawa, 1997). Thus, an important point to consider is whether African-Caribbean and South Asian patients are reaching the ICU so that they may be considered to be potential donors. It may be that the African-Caribbean and South Asian population are simply not dying of the relevant cause or are not being referred to the ICU, rather than an unwillingness to become donors (Exley et al., 1996b).

Again, there is very little research in this area. Gore et al. (1992) carried out a comprehensive audit of all ICU deaths in the UK and the suitability to become organ donors. However, the main drawback to this study was that the ethnic group of patients was not recorded. A pilot study in Coventry was carried out which sought to determine admission rates of South Asian and non-South Asian patients to ICUs (Exley et al., 1996b). The results indicate that South Asians were less than half as likely to be admitted to an ICU than non-South Asians. These findings have serious implications, as they indicate that there are fewer instances where the health professional has an opportunity for making a request for organs from South Asian families.

Another important finding of this study was that the rates of referral from the ICU to the transplant unit were the same for South Asians and non-South Asians, as were subsequent donation rates (Exley et al., 1996b) Thus, the results of this preliminary study suggest that lower rates of organ donation among the South Asian population are related to the initial low admission rates to the ICU. Related to this, there is preliminary evidence emerging to suggest that the number of brain-stem deaths is lower among minority ethnic groups.

## Looking to the future

It is clear that minority ethnic groups are disproportionately affected by renal health problems both in terms of access to appropriate services and the higher prevalence of renal complications.

A major undertaking for researchers and clinicians in the UK will be to explore *access* to and the progression through the diabetes and 'renal disease complicating diabetes' care pathways, and to identify health beliefs and experiences associated with diabetes and diabetic renal complications among African-Caribbean and South Asian groups. A systematic exploration of these subjects would provide a valuable resource for health professionals working with these groups and allow for the development of a culturally competent diabetes and renal care service which is sensitive to the needs of minority ethnic groups (Randhawa, 2000). Specifically, there are gaps in:

- Identification of cultural beliefs and practices relevant to diabetes and diabetic renal disease self-management. These include attitudes to medication and attendance at family doctor appointments, and at diabetes and nephrology services for routine monitoring.
- Examination of referral patterns to hospital-based diabetic services, and subsequent attendance.
- Exploration of referral patterns to nephrology services.
- Exploration of the relevance of current renal complications education programmes for minority ethnic groups.

The National Kidney Research Fund launched the ABLE (A Better Life through Empowerment) campaign in 2002, which aims to redress some of the above issues by education and raising personal awareness of kidney health issues among minority ethnic groups.

Concomitantly, there needs to be an increase in the supply of organs from the African-Caribbean and South Asian population to alleviate the burden on current waiting lists and for those patients on dialysis. This process can only begin if the public are in an informed position to consider and debate the issues surrounding organ donation and transplantation. Central to attaining this goal is increased levels of health education and awareness of the specific problems within the African-Caribbean and South Asian population. It has been suggested previously by commentators that religion acts as a prohibitor to organ donation among the South Asian population, but empirical research seems to suggest otherwise.

The position of one's religion towards donation is used by individuals as a helpful guide in reaching their decision as to whether to donate or not (Randhawa, 1998b). The introduction of community-based information programmes needs to be evaluated to assess whether this impacts upon the number of African-Caribbeans and South Asians on the Organ Donor Register.

Attention also needs to be given to the number of South Asian patients who are eligible to become organ donors in the ICU. The limited research conducted so far suggests that low rates of organ donation by South Asian people may be related to factors pertaining to the low admission to ICUs rather than to those relating to the donation of organs (Exley et al., 1996b). There is a clear need for extensive research in this area. Preliminary evidence also suggests that the number of brain-stem deaths is lower among minority ethnic groups. An audit of potential donors identifying ethnicity is urgently required to substantiate this. Within the ICU also, there need to be clear guidelines on how to approach the family when making a request for their loved one's organs, with specific training and counselling in a multicultural environment (Randhawa, 1997). Alongside these initiatives, efforts to promote living-related kidney donation among Asian families need to be implemented, especially in the light of low admission rates to ICUs and the subsequent low cadaveric donation rates.

It is only when these issues are addressed adequately that we will begin to see renal services that truly meet the needs of a multi-ethnic and multi-faith population within the UK.

# References

Brenner, B.M., et al. (2001) Effects of losartan on renal and cardiovascular outcomes in patients with type 2 diabetes and nephropathy. *New England Journal of Medicine* **345**, 861–9.

Burden, A.C., McNally, P.G., Feehally, J. and Walls, J. (1992) Increased incidence of end-stage renal failure secondary to diabetes mellitus in Asian ethnic groups in the United Kingdom. *Diabetic Medicine* **9**, 641–5.

Callender, C.O. (1989) The results of transplantation in Blacks: just the tip of the iceberg. *Transplantation Proceedings* **21**, 3407–3410.

Cinotti, G.A. and Zucchelli, P.C. (2001) Effect of lisinopril on the progression of renal insufficiency in mild proteinuric non-diabetic nephropathies. *Nephrology Dialysis Transplantation* **16**, 961–6.

Darr, A. and Randhawa, G. (1999) Public opinion and perception of organ donation and transplantation among Asian communities: an exploratory study in Luton, UK. *International Journal of Health Promotion and Education* **37**, 68–74.

Department of Health (1994) *Health Care Strategy Unit. Review of Renal Services*. Department of Health, London.

Department of Health (2002a) *Tackling Health Inequalities 2002 Cross-Cutting Review*. Department of Health, London.

Department of Health (2002b) *National Service Framework for Diabetes: Standards*. Department of Health, London.

Department of Health (2002c) *National Service Framework for Renal Services.* www.doh.gov.uk/nsf/.

Diabetes Prevention Program Research Group (2002) Reduction in the incidence of type 2 diabetes with lifestyle intervention or metformin. *New England Journal of Medicine* **346**, 393–403.

Exley, C., Sim, J., Reid, N.G., Jackson, S. and West, N. (1996a) Attitudes and beliefs within the Sikh community regarding organ donation: a pilot study. *Social Science and Medicine* **43**, 23–8.

Exley, C., Sim, J., Reid, N.G., Booth, L., Jackson, S. and West, N. (1996b) The admission of Asian patients to intensive therapy units and its implications for kidney donation: a preliminary report from Coventry, UK. *Journal of Epidemiology and Community Health* **50**, 447–50.

Feest, T.G., Dunn, E.J. and Burton, C.J. (1999) Can intensive treatment alter the progress of established diabetic nephropathy to end-stage renal failure? *Quarterly Journal of Medicine* **92**, 275–82.

Gore, S.M., Cable, D.J. and Holland, A.J. (1992) Organ donation from intensive care units in England and Wales: two year confidential audit of deaths in intensive care. *British Medical Journal* **304**, 349–55.

Jeffrey, R.F., Woodrow, G., Mahler, J., Johnson, R. and Newstead, C.G. (2002) Indo-Asian experience of renal transplantation in Yorkshire: results of a 10 year survey. *Transplantation* **73**, 1652–7.

Johnson, M., Owen, D. and Blackburn, C. (2000) *Black and Minority Ethnic Groups in England: The Second Health and Lifestyles Survey.* Health Education Authority, London.

Khan, Z. and Randhawa, G. (1999) Informing the UK's South Asian communities on organ donation and transplantation. *EDTNA/ERCA Journal* **25**, 12–14.

Kyriakides, G., Hadjigavriel, P., Hadjicostas, A., et al. (1993) Public awareness and attitudes toward transplantation in Cyprus. *Transplantation Proceedings* **25**, 2279.

Lewis, E.J., et al. (2001) Renoprotective effect of the angiotensin-receptor antagonist irbesartan in patients with nephropathy due to type 2 diabetes. *New England Journal of Medicine* **345**, 851–60.

Lightstone, L. (2001) *Preventing Kidney Disease: The Ethnic Challenge.* National Kidney Research Fund, Peterborough.

National Health Service Executive (1996) *Renal Purchasing Guidelines: Good Practice.* NHS Executive, Leeds.

National Kidney Research Fund (2002) *ABLE (A Better Life Through Empowerment) Campaign.* www.nkrf.org.uk/pages/research/.

Nazroo, J.Y. (1997) *The Health of Britain's Ethnic Minorities.* Policy Studies Institute, London.

Raleigh, V.S. (1997) Diabetes and hypertension in Britain's ethnic minorities: implications for the future of renal services. *British Medical Journal* **314**, 209–212.

Randhawa, G. (1997) Enhancing the health professional's role in requesting transplant organs. *British Journal of Nursing* **6**, 429–34.

Randhawa, G. (1998a) The impending kidney transplant crisis for the Asian population in the UK. *Public Health* **112**, 265–8.

Randhawa, G. (1998b) An exploratory study examining the influence of religion on attitudes towards organ donation among the Asian population in Luton, UK. *Nephrology Dialysis Transplantation* **13**, 1949–54.

Randhawa, G. (2000) Increasing the donor supply from the UK's Asian population: the need for further research. *Transplantation Proceedings* **32**, 1561–62.

Randhawa, G. (2003) Developing culturally competent renal services in the United Kingdom: tackling inequalities in health. *Transplantation Proceedings* **35**, 21–3.

Roderick, P.J., Raleigh, V.S., Hallam, L. and Mallick, N.P. (1996) The need and demand for renal replacement therapy amongst ethnic minorities in England. *Journal of Epidemiology and Community Health* **50**, 334–9.

Spina, F., Sedda, L., Pizzi, R., et al. (1993) Donor families' attitudes toward organ donation. *Transplantation Proceedings* **25**, 1699–701.

Tuomilehto, J., et al. (2001) Prevention of type 2 diabetes mellitus by changes in lifestyle among subjects with impaired glucose tolerance. *New England Journal of Medicine* **344**, 1343–50.

UK Prospective Diabetes Study Group (1998) Intensive blood-glucose control with sulphonylureas or insulin compared with conventional treatment and risk of complications in patients with type 2 diabetes (UKPDS 33). *Lancet* **352**, 837–53.

WHO Study Group (1994) *Prevention of Diabetes Mellitus*. World Health Organization, Geneva.

# Chapter 12

# Renal Nutrition

*Debbie Sutton*

## Introduction

This section seeks to reflect issues of current interest in renal dietetics, and to highlight areas of controversy. Where there is evidence on which to base guidelines, references are given, but much dietetic advice and nutritional support described here is based on best practice.

Basic information regarding renal diets is kept to a minimum in this chapter as it can readily be found elsewhere (e.g. Vennegoor, 2002). More emphasis is given here to stimulating thought as to what governs eating behaviour and what models may be used to bring about change. It is not desirable to be too prescriptive when teaching renal nutrition to patients. Although many patients, and some renal clinicians, find it convenient to have lists of 'Foods to Avoid' and 'Foods to Eat', when long-term dietary habits are at stake, it is preferable to encourage informed choice and selection of foods.

The renal population has changed in recent years and now includes a significant proportion of older patients and patients with co-morbidity. The watchword for these groups is malnutrition and emphasis is placed on encouraging patients to eat. It is important that this emphasis should not give the impression that the content of the diet does not matter. There are plenty of nourishing foods that those with renal failure can safely eat, but the person giving the dietary advice must have a thorough understanding and knowledge of the nutritional principles involved.

The essential skill in tackling renal diets is being able to transform a 'prescription' for nutrients (protein, phosphate, potassium, etc.) into a tasty selection of foods, suited to each patient's individual preferences, tastes, finances, cooking ability and social circumstances.

## Conservative management

Conservative management looks set to become high profile as a positive treatment option, rather than a euphemism for 'no treatment'. Forty years ago, conservative management was the only option for most people with established renal disease, but it fell out of favour as dialysis became more widely available. It is now likely to be introduced as a therapy option along with haemodialysis, peritoneal dialysis and transplantation.

The Renal National Service Framework (NSF) (Department of Health, 2004) has designated one of its modules 'End of Life Care', reflecting the growing recognition by health care professionals that dialysis is not necessarily a life-enhancing procedure, and may not even be a life-prolonging one. As more patients grow old on dialysis, and more older people have established renal failure (ERF), it is important to recognise the importance of individual choice of suitable therapy. Preliminary work by Chandna et al. (1999) has suggested that it is possible to identify and predict those patients for whom dialysis is unlikely to be a success. Significant co-morbidity, often but not always with advanced age, can make dialysis an unhappy, distressing and ultimately unsuccessful experience for some patients.

Dietary management has always played a significant role in the non-dialytic treatment of chronic renal failure. Before the availability of dialysis, it would have been almost all there was on offer. The main aim was to reduce protein intake to a level that provided minimum requirements alongside essential amino-acids, whilst maintaining adequate energy from fat and carbohydrate. Control of protein also restricts phosphate. With the help of specially manu-factured low protein products such as flour, bread and pasta, a low-protein, high-energy diet could be achieved and uraemic symptoms controlled.

The provision of energy from non-protein sources is very important (Rigalleau et al., 1997), not just to maintain a healthy body weight, but to try to prevent the conversion of protein to glucose via gluconeogenesis, since one of the by-products of this pathway is urea. This leads to a rise in serum urea and its associated symptoms just the same as if excessive dietary protein had been eaten, thus negating the hoped-for benefits of reducing protein intake.

Even if dietary protein intake is reduced, it should be provided at a level that maintains body protein stores. World Heath Organisation (WHO) recom-mendations for this are 0.6 g/kg body weight (WHO, 1985). Calories needed for metabolism and activity should come from fat and carbohydrate. Euro-pean guidelines (EDTNA/ERCA, 2001) suggest 0.8–1.0 g protein and 30–35 calories/kg ideal body weight, depending on age and activity levels.

Dietary assessment may well reveal that protein intake has spontaneously reduced to this level already. Studies have shown that as glomerular filtration rate (GFR) declines, so does protein intake quite independently of any dietary advice, usually due to loss of appetite and decreased enjoyment of eating (Passey et al., 2001).

Assessment must examine body weight and energy intake. Many patients with ERF will have been losing weight, often for months. If they are over-weight, this may have passed unnoticed, unremarked or even may have been a cause for congratulation. Certainly it seems illogical to prescribe extra calories for someone who already has a generous store. However, it is important to assess whether they are losing fat or muscle. Weight loss of more than 1 kg per week probably means some loss of lean body mass. Feeling unwell and lethargic probably means that usual activity levels are reduced, with resulting reduction in muscle mass. Bio-impedance measures or skin-fold callipers, properly used, can monitor body composition (Heyward, 1998).

Lean body weight *must* be maintained in order to prevent muscle wasting. Under starvation conditions, metabolic changes take place that aim to preserve body mass by reducing activity and providing energy requirements from muscle breakdown. Not only does this lead to loss of lean body mass, reduced basal metabolic rate (BMR) and malnutrition, but also it results in the production of urea. Glucose generated from muscle protein goes through the same biochemical pathways as dietary protein.

The debate over the use of low-protein diets continues to cause controversy. Apart from relieving symptoms, much work has gone into investigating whether these diets actually slow the rate of deterioration of renal function. Experimental work on partially nephrectomised rats indicated that there was an effect (Brenner et al., 1982), but attempts with human subjects have proved inconclusive, not least because of the difficulties associated with encouraging patients to follow a fairly complicated and restrictive diet. Two major multicentre prospective randomised trials were carried out in the 1990s to try to reach a final conclusion to the controversy: the Northern Italian Co-operative Study (1991) and the Modification of Diet in Renal Disease (MDRD) Study (1998) from the USA. Neither study was able to show a conclusive result. The difference in protein intake between control and intervention groups was not, in practice, sufficiently great to be able to detect changes. The 'normal' protein groups tended to under-consume and the 'low' protein groups to over-consume.

A major concern over the use of any reduced protein diet is that it may lead to malnutrition. Properly monitored, this need not be the case, as a patient who is offered no dietary advice at all is more likely to become malnourished than one who is being regularly monitored in a low clearance clinic (Passey et al., 2001).

Traditionally, animal protein has provided 70% of the estimated protein requirements for a patient on a low-protein/high-energy diet, in the belief that the nearer the amino-acid pattern of the dietary proteins is to that of human protein, the more efficiently the protein will be used. Empirical observation on the urea levels and phosphate levels achieved by vegetarians on low-protein diets led to work studying the utilisation of amino-acids from vegetarian diets in terms of protein turnover and re-use of amino-acids from the amino-acid pool (Passey et al., 2001). The conclusion is that all amino-acids are adequately provided from a diet made up of 70% vegetable protein.

There is no doubt that urea levels can be well controlled with dietary manipulation. Other electrolytes, in particular potassium and phosphate, can also be controlled. There is a need for careful explanation and a thorough understanding of the biochemistry behind the advice, as well as an unending supply

**Table 12.1**  Practical advice for conservative management.

- Increase dietary energy by fortifying normal food
- Add spreading fat to potatoes and vegetables
- Use oil-based salad dressings
- Fry (in suitable oil) instead of grilling
- Use glucose instead of sugar – it is less sweet than sugar but has the same calorie value weight for weight so more is needed to achieve the desired taste
- Use full cream milk

of recipes, menus, encouragement and monitoring by the renal team. Considerable commitment and motivation on the part of the patient is also needed, and the family/carer also needs to be involved. The positive point is that patients do feel better. The nausea, tiredness and distorted taste sensation can be improved, which makes it worth persevering. Table 12.1 identifies some practical advice for conservative management.

# Haemodialysis (HD)

Fluid and potassium have always been the key issues for patients on HD. However, in recent years thrice-weekly dialysis, improved dialysis technology and more older people on dialysis have caused the emphasis to shift. Dietary potassium seldom needs the restrictive approach that many experienced renal workers were taught. The reduced length of time between sessions means there is less time for potassium levels to build up in the bloodstream. The habitual diet of many older people and their eating patterns means that they may not include many high-potassium foods in their diet. They are less likely to eat fast foods or to snack between meals. The size of their appetite makes it likely that their portion sizes will be low, and there is little need to make many alterations.

So avoidance of malnutrition is the priority. Bringing about changes in eating habits that can be maintained long term is important, especially since the shortage of donor organs means that patients may face a long time on dialysis waiting for a transplant. Transplant outcome may be at risk if patients have become malnourished whilst on dialysis (Chertow et al., 1996). Regular review and assessment with suitable dietary advice and intervention is important. This is an area where a Dietetic Assistant (DA) may have a role. An assessment by a dietitian and the development of an action plan where needed can be followed up by a DA. One UK unit has ceased to use Intra Dialytic Parenteral Nutrition (IDPN) since employing a DA, who has been able to encourage patients to take a high-calorie drink instead (personal communication).

Work carried out on measuring the success of HD patients at making dietary changes indicates that for the first 3 months they do not achieve much, in spite of advice to increase their protein intake and maintain a good energy intake (Pollock et al., 1997). It is to be hoped that appropriate monitoring of patients in nephrology or low clearance clinics will mean that dialysis is commenced before patients have become seriously unwell and undernourished.

Commencing dialysis, either HD or peritoneal dialysis (PD), is clearly going to have a profound effect on patients and their families. They will be given a great deal of new information, there may be setbacks and complications as dialysis is established and the complete upheaval of their lifestyles can hardly be imagined. This is not likely to be an auspicious time to offer advice about protein exchanges, fruit and vegetable allowances and complicated instructions about double boiling potatoes. Neither will it help to inform them that from now on chips, chocolate and crisps are forbidden foods.

European Guidelines (EDTNA/ERCA, 2001) state that an HD diet should aim to provide 1.0–1.2 g/kg protein per kg ideal body weight and 30–35 calories/kg depending on age, activity levels and body weight. Potassium levels should be 1.0 mmol/kg, but it is very important to review each individual's biochemistry. Many factors influence serum potassium. If pre-dialysis levels are consistently less than 6.0 mmol/l, there is no need to alter dietary potassium. If they are consistently more than 6.0 mmol/l then dietary potassium should be reduced, if necessary to less than 1.0 mmol/kg. Phosphate intake may need to be reduced. Many good sources of protein are also high in phosphate, which can make achieving the required protein intake difficult within the recommended 30 mmol phosphate per day. Phosphate binders are often used and it is important to emphasise the need to take phosphate binders with every meal and snack.

In the late 1990s it was thought that high phosphate levels could be treated leniently if it appeared that an adequate dietary intake was being achieved. In terms of setting priorities, a balanced dietary intake may in some cases be more beneficial than good phosphate control. It is now felt that issues surrounding long waits for transplants, increased risk of heart disease and longer times on dialysis make this attitude unacceptable. Many renal units are exploring ways of improving phosphate control, often by training dietitians to manipulate phosphate binder dosage in conjunction with education concerning high-phosphate foods. Encouraging results have been achieved by developing protocols that adopt a co-ordinated approach to patient education, dialysate calcium concentration and the timing and use of phosphate binders. Table 12.2 summarises the European nutrition guidelines for HD (EDTNA/ERCA, 2001).

**Table 12.2** Summary of European dietary guidelines for haemodialysis (EDTNA/ERCA, 2001).

| | |
|---|---|
| Energy | Less than 60 years: 35 kcal/kg IBW/day |
| | More than 60 years: 30–35 kcal/kg IBW/day |
| Protein | 1–1.2 g/kg IBW/day |
| Fluid | 500 ml/day plus equivalent of daily urine output |
| Potassium | 1 mmol/kg IBW/day or 50–65 mmol/day |
| Sodium | No added salt, i.e. 80–110 mmol/day |
| Phosphate | 32–45 mmol/day |

# Peritoneal dialysis (PD)

The established dietary advice for PD patients is high protein, low energy. High protein is necessary because protein lost mainly as albumin into the dialysate fluid must be replaced by eating protein. Low energy is required because a significant number of calories are absorbed from the glucose in the dialysis fluid. Metabolic balance studies carried out in the early days of PD are widely cited as the evidence base for this advice (Blumenkrantz et al., 1982).

The 1982 study was carried out on eight men undergoing PD. They were fed high-energy diets providing either 0.98 or 1.44 g/kg protein per day. Mean nitrogen balance was neutral with the lower protein intake group and strongly positive with the high protein intake group. The conclusions drawn were that PD patients required at least 1.1 g/kg protein/day, and that to allow for variability 1.2–1.3 g/kg was 'probably preferable'. The high-energy intake would have ensured that protein was not used as an energy source. As a result of this one study, dietary recommendations have been set at 1.2 g protein/kg lean body weight and 25 kcal/kg, with an expectation that there will be energy available from glucose in the PD fluid. Individual variation is considerable, but between 300 and 1000 kcal/day may be expected to be absorbed by this route.

As long ago as 1996, papers were being published that suggested that PD patients did not achieve the recommended protein intake, but that many seemed to do well on this therapy, despite intakes of around 0.8 g/kg protein (Bergstrom and Lindholm, 1994). Not many studies describe measures of dietary energy intake, but those that do indicate that it is often low (Sutton et al., 2001).

In spite of this, many PD patients become overweight, so it is important to carefully examine the distribution of body fat. There may be significant central adiposity, although legs, arms and across the shoulders may be quite wasted. An assessment of dietary intake and a measure of nutritional status is often helpful. It is not necessarily the case that dietary restriction is the answer. The dietary intake must be designed to provide appropriate minerals and vitamins. Too restrictive a calorie allowance may jeopardise levels of these micronutrients.

## *Body weight and body composition*

Many PD patients have a body mass index (BMI) higher than 25, suggesting they are overweight. BMI is a useful measure, but it cannot differentiate between muscle and fat. In the normal population, a BMI between 20 and 25 is considered to cover the ideal body weight range. Below 20 suggests undernutrition and above 25, overweight or obesity.

When calculating protein and energy requirements, ideal body weight (IBW) should be used, that is, the weight that would give a BMI of between 20 and 25. If a more precise figure is needed, that which gives a BMI of 23 is commonly used. It is important that the IBW that has been used to base calculations is known, so that precise comparisons can be made between outcomes.

## Assessment

Assessment is discussed within the PD section because of the confusion that can arise around body weight issues; however, many of the points in this section may be applied to all those with renal disease.

The lack of clear nutritional markers and the difficulties and inaccuracies inherent in collecting accurate dietary information make it hard to choose outcomes that truly reflect nutritional status. A number of parameters can be measured. They can be considered within the following groups: dietary assessment, anthropometry and biochemistry.

Dietary information may be collected from interviews, food records, recall, frequency questionnaires or food diaries. Anthropometry includes weight, BMI, skinfold measurements, bio-electrical impedence, dual-energy X-ray absorptiometry (DEXA) scanning, handgrip dynomometry and exercise tests such as a sit-to-stand test and a walk/stairs test. Such tests will give an indication of body composition and muscle strength and can monitor change over time. Subjective global assessment (SGA) is a helpful tool that includes a range of parameters that may influence dietary intake, availability of nutrients and energy expenditure. A score is allocated which classifies each subject as well nourished, mildly malnourished or at risk (Kalantar-Zadeh et al., 1999). Table 12.3 shows ways in which nutritional status of those on PD may be assessed.

**Table 12.3**  Assessment of nutritional status in PD.

| Body weight | Dietary intake | Subjective global assessment (SGA) |
|---|---|---|
| How does it compare with IBW? | Try a 24-hour recall | Find out what other influences there are on intake and energy expenditure. |
| Calculate BMI: $\frac{\text{Weight in kg}}{(\text{Height in m})^2}$ | Start with the meal most recently eaten and work backwards. | Recent weight change? |
| Use a BMI chart to calculate the patient's BMI in the normal range | Ask about portion sizes – slices, spoonfuls, bowlfuls, packets used. | Anorexia, nausea, vomiting? |
|  | Use a portion handbook to make an estimate of protein and energy intake. | Functional ability and activity levels – is your patient really using 35 kcal/kg or is he/she sitting in front of a TV all day? |
|  | Compare intake with requirements. | Do they have any co-morbid conditions that might affect requirements and activity levels, e.g. arthritis, pulmonary disease. |

It is reasonable to base recommendations on IBW since fat is largely inert and does not metabolise in the way that lean tissue does. Significant overestimates may be likely if based on actual body weight, as the following example demonstrates.

*Example*

A 59-year-old lady, weighing 78 kg and who is 165 cm tall.
Current BMI = $78/1.65^2$ = 28.6.
This puts her in the 'overweight' range.
Dietary requirements based on this weight would be:

   Protein = 94 g ($78 \times 1.2$)                     Calories = 2730 ($78 \times 35$)

Taking ideal body weight to be the weight at which BMI = 23, i.e. the middle of the 'healthy' range, the calculation looks rather different:

   IBW = 63 kg.   Protein = $63 \times 1.2$ = 76 g.   Calories = $63 \times 35$ = 2205

Remembering that the energy recommendations include glucose from the dialysate, this lady probably needs to eat around 1800 kcal/day to maintain her weight.

The BMI calculation can also be used to suggest a healthy weight range; a weight within the 20–25 'healthy' section. Continuing with the above example, this would be 55–68 kg.

Be prepared to revise recommendations if previously ill and underweight patients regain flesh weight. It may be helpful to encourage exercise at appropriate level. For example: using stairs instead of a lift, getting on or off the bus at the next stop along the route, cycling to the local shops. Regained weight should be muscle as well as fat.

Guard against restricting calories to a level that will endanger intakes of vitamins and minerals. A minimum calorie level of 1400 kcal/day should be enough to sustain micronutrient intake at recommended levels, which are the same for people with renal failure as the normal age and sex matched population. Patients using high glucose bags, or who are high transporters, may benefit from changing to a non-glucose fluid in order to control weight. Their calorie intake may well be appropriate. Discourage use of high glucose concentration bags as a means of controlling fluid balance. These bags mean more dialysate calories, which leads to weight gain. If the patient is not clear about the difference between fluid and flesh weight gains, he or she may continue with an inappropriate use of these bags, ending up both dehydrated and heavier before the misunderstanding is identified.

It is worth noting that no correlation has been found between serum albumin and nutritional status or nutritional intake, yet low serum albumin is still widely used as a referral criterion for dietary advice (CANADA–USA (CANUSA) Peritoneal Dialysis Group, 1996). There is no single marker of nutritional status in PD or any other patients. Serum albumin is undoubtedly below normal in many PD patients, for reasons that are not entirely clear. Losses into the dialysate may be significant, but if this was the only reason, then all patients might be expected to show low levels. Raised C-reactive protein (CRP) appears to correlate with low serum albumin, implying that inflammation and an acute

**Table 12.4**  Summary of European dietary guidelines for peritoneal
dialysis (EDTNA/ERCA, 2001).

| | |
|---|---|
| Energy | < 60 years: 35 kcal/kg IBW/day<br>> 60 years: 30 kcal/kg IBW/day<br>including calories from peritoneal absorption of glucose |
| Protein | 1.0–1.2 g/kg IBW/day for active non-catabolic patients<br>1.5 g/kg IBW/day if the patient has peritonitis |
| Fluid | 800 ml/day plus equivalent of daily urine output |
| Potassium | 50–65 mmol/day and modify according to serum levels<br>Aim for serum potassium of 3.5–5.5 mmol/l |
| Sodium | No added salt: 80–110 mmol/day |
| Phosphate | 32–45 mmol/day |

phase response may be implicated (Han et al., 1996). Table 12.4 summarises
the European nutrition guidelines for PD.

# Behavioural changes

One model that may be usefully adapted to help patients make dietary changes
is that of Prochaska and Diclemente (1986). Originally developed to show
the process through which patients change addictive behaviour, it may also
be applied to the changing of risky behaviour. An example of behaviour
that dialysis patients may need to address is that of controlling potassium
and fluid.

A clear and balanced explanation of fluid balance and the metabolic role of
potassium is a good starting point. Education is critical to understanding the
consequences of continuing the risky behaviour and accepting the need to
change. Until the benefits of change outweigh the costs, action is unlikely. A
patient who each lunchtime has a pint of beer with his friends will need more
than persuasion and threats to make him see the need to change. Rather than
labelling such a patient as non-compliant it would be more useful to spend
time helping that patient articulate the difficulties he perceives in making a
change, offer him alternatives (e.g. whisky) and offer support. Talking to other
patients who have made similar changes may be useful.

When making change, a clear goal, a realistic plan and plenty of support
and rewards will help progress. This is the time to offer information about
nutrients – good sources of protein, high-energy foods, potassium content
of fruit and vegetables, high phosphate foods, portion sizes and quantities.
Maintaining change is almost certain to involve the occasional relapse. It is
important to teach patients that this does not mean that they have failed
– provide strategies for damage limitation and tips on how to get back on
course.

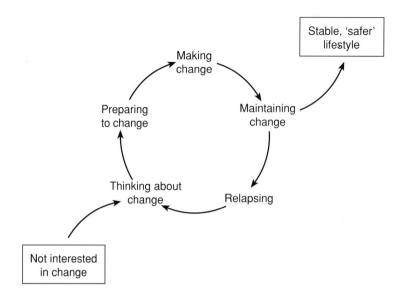

**Figure 12.1**   The process of change. (Adapted from Prochaska and Diclemente, 1986.)

There should be no need to use words such as 'avoid', 'cut out' or 'do not eat'. On any renal diet it should be possible to incorporate all kinds of foods provided the relative quantities are understood.

Figure 12.1 shows a change model that may be useful in helping patients adapt to a new diet.


## Practical tips for all patients on dialysis

Some renal units, for example satellite units, may not have a specialist renal dietitian available to give advice. The following suggestions may be helpful:

- Always check biochemistry before giving any dietary advice.
- Always take a dietary history so you can use your patient's usual eating pattern, likes and dislikes to inform your advice.
- Increase protein intake by fortifying normal foods. Aim to keep portions small, but more concentrated.
- Add grated cheese to mashed potato (check phosphate levels).
- Add dried skimmed milk powder to ordinary milk, then use in drinks, on cereal, for custard and sauces (check potassium levels).
- Encourage a meal pattern of small, tasty meals with regular snacks.
- Bread-based products are generally low in fat, low in potassium, high in energy and contain useful quantities of protein, e.g. bread, rolls, bagels, crumpets, muffins, iced buns.

- Work with your renal dietitian to develop a summary chart of commonly eaten high phosphate foods.
- Work with your renal dietitian to develop a summary chart of commonly eaten high potassium foods too.
- Develop a resource folder or scrapbook from food labels to give ideas for low potassium, low phosphate meals, e.g. pizzas, ready meals, biscuits, pies, buffet snacks.

## Transplantation

The main concern of most patients following successful transplant is the freedom to eat and drink whatever they want, whenever they want it. The main concern of the clinical team following successful transplant should be to encourage a pattern of eating and behaviour that will do everything possible to prevent coronary heart disease (CHD), as 40% of transplanted patients die with functioning grafts from CHD or related disorders (Kasiske et al., 1996).

It is important to maintain contact in the weeks following successful transplant. Weight may well go up and diet may be inappropriate, but in the long term both can be controlled. Repressive and discouraging advice too early may cause patients to avoid situations where unsought dietary advice may be offered.

### *Safe eating*

'Safe' eating information offers a neutral approach and may be offered prior to discharge. Transplant patients, in common with other immunosuppressed patients, are genuinely at risk from infections, including food poisoning. Information about correct storage and cooking, looking at sell-by dates and taking care to follow reheating and microwave instructions is very important. Patients should be sure to choose cheeses made from pasteurised milk and avoid egg products using raw egg or egg white.

### *Normal eating and how to achieve it*

Patients who may have started dialysis as children when all their meals were provided from home may have a very hazy idea as to what 'normal' eating actually is. Following transplantation they may need help with food choices and portion sizes. There are several models of a balanced diet, but Table 12.5 may be a useful starting point as a daily guide.

Eating this combination ensures an adequate intake of protein, iron, calcium and vitamins. Fatty or sugary foods may be incorporated according to appetite and appropriate body weight. Most foods in this category have very little in the way of nutrients, only calories. These foods include crisps, sweets, chocolate, cakes, biscuits and puddings, but there need be no mention of 'good' food and 'bad' food!

**Table 12.5** The 5-2-2-5 plan for a healthy eating diet.
(Adapted from *The Balance of Good Health*, Health
Education Authority, 1996.)

| |
|---|
| 5 – portions of starchy carbohydrate-rich foods<br>2 – portions of protein foods, e.g. meat, fish, eggs, beans<br>2 – portions of dairy foods, e.g. milk, yoghurt, cheese<br>5 – portions of fruit and vegetables. |

Portion size should be based on appetite and desirable body weight. For an older lady, five portions of starchy food could be a slice of toast, two Rich Tea biscuits, a small potato and a round of sandwiches for tea. For a younger, active man, it would be two or three Weetabix, two digestive biscuits, two rounds of sandwiches, a dish of pasta and some toast at bedtime. What is important is maintaining the relative proportions of the different food groups. Depicted as a plate model, one third of the plate should be starchy foods, one-third fruit and vegetables and the last third divided between protein and dairy with a little slice of fatty/sugary extras. Healthy eating is straightforward!

### Steroid-induced diabetes

Patients who develop diabetes as a result of steroid therapy will need sensitive handling, since the perception of diabetic diets may be that they will be restrictive. However, a 'diabetes diet' actually correlates very well with the type of diet currently recommended to the population as a whole and dovetails easily with the heart-protecting balanced diet described above (Scottish Intercollegiate Guidelines Network, 1999). Education about regular carbohydrate (CHO) intake and increased CHO required during exercise may also be relevant (Diabetes UK, 2003).

## Acutely ill/acute renal failure

Acutely ill patients with renal impairment present a challenge. For those clearly unable to eat normally, parenteral nutrition or tube feeding will be required. Unlike most patients, many standard-feeding regimes will not be suitable. Fluid and electrolyte balance are the main concerns, and may need to be altered on a daily basis.

A particularly challenging group to care for are those patients with acute renal failure who are not particularly traumatised. It can be incredibly difficult to persuade them, their relatives and even some staff that they need to eat. Their appetite is often poor, they probably have a reduced fluid allowance and the task of persuading without resorting to threats and bullying requires considerable patience and perseverance. Shifts in body fluid often disguise and confuse actual body weight, so even simple weighing may not be useful.

Food charts can be helpful, if carefully filled in. Success or failure in achieving an agreed regime may be greatly helped by having a ward housekeeper, dietetic helper or nutrition assistant who takes on the role of maintaining records, offering snacks and supplements at regular intervals and helping with menu choices.

Acutely ill patients suffering significant fluid losses or with greatly increased requirements, for example those with burns, cannot hope to meet nutritional requirements during this acute phase. They are likely to be in negative nitrogen balance, with amino-acids being taken from the breakdown of skeletal muscle. Whatever the estimate of nitrogen losses, only levels of 0.2g N/kg can be effectively utilised, regardless of adequate provision of energy from fat and carbohydrate.

Requirements for protein and energy may be assessed using recognised equations such as Schofield et al., (1985) and Elia (1990). Recommendations for vitamins and minerals are not well documented, but may safely be considered to be the same as for healthy people (Department of Health, 1991). Excessive doses of vitamin C should be avoided as oxalate deposition has been reported (Friedman et al., 1983). The following guide shown in Figure 12.2 may be useful in caring for those who are acutely ill.

As the patient improves, monitor and evaluate the above stages. If tube fed, feed overnight and introduce at least two meals before withdrawing

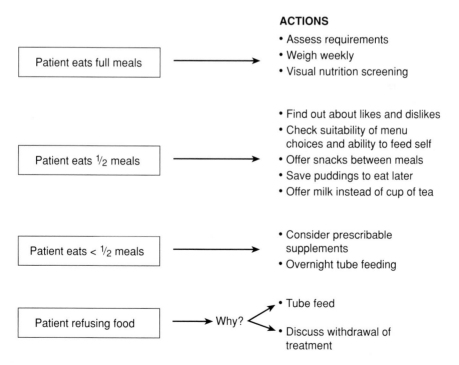

**Figure 12.2**    A suggested guide for nutritional intervention.

feed. If the patient is receiving supplements, reduce by one a day as food increases.

# Role of renal dietitian

The following summary taken from a Renal Nutrition Group (RNG) poster outlines what renal dietitians can offer. Availability varies and, at least in the UK, most renal dietitians are based in regional renal centres.

## Who are we?

- State-registered dietitians with a degree qualification.
- A specialist interest and nutritional expertise in all aspects of renal disease.

## What do we do?

- We take responsibility for the nutritional care of renal patients at all stages of renal disease.

## How do we do this?

- We advise patients on how to change their diets to meet individual needs for nutrients such as protein, phosphate, potassium and salt.
- We review patients regularly and monitor nutritional status using several recognised methods, e.g. dietary intake assessment, nutrition risk tools, anthropometric measurements.
- We advise on nutrition support methods if indicated.
- We teach patients how to adapt recipes and make sensible choices when eating out, in order that they can continue to enjoy food and eating.
- We regularly audit our work.

## How do we learn and develop skills?

- Renal dietitians have access to many groups and associations for training and support, such as the Renal Nutrition Group (RNG), National Kidney Federation (NKF) and EDTNA/ERCA.

## What next?

- Renal dietitians are increasingly leading research, audit projects and are involved in the long-term planning for UK renal services.
- National and European standards and nutritional guidelines have been developed and audited to ensure best practice.

# Summary

Maintaining a good nutritional status for those with renal disease is challenging. The strict diets prescribed for the control of uraemic symptoms and fluid balance have moderated in recent years, in recognition of the changing renal population. The approach to dietary management should be individualised to each patient and his/her usual appetite, food intake and biochemistry, and should be as flexible as possible. This means that it is essential for the practitioner to have an in-depth knowledge of the principles of renal diets, and an ability to apply these principles in practical ways.

It must be recognised that other factors affect nutritional status, such as inflammation, the patient's inability to exercise and the psycho-social aspects of renal disease. There will always be a need to explain why specific elements in food are so important in established renal failure, so good patient education must be at the forefront of a renal dietician's expertise. A flexible, individualised approach enables patients to make informed choices and results in good nutritional outcomes.

# References

Bergstrom, J. and Lindholm, B. (1994) Nutritional assessment and therapeutic outcome in CAPD patients. *EDTNA-ERCA Journal* **20**, 11–19.

Blumenkrantz, M.J., Kopple, J.D., Moran, J.K. and Coburn, J.W. (1982) Metabolic balance studies and dietary protein requirements in patients undergoing CAPD. *Kidney International* **21**, 849–61.

Brenner, B., Meyer, T.W. and Hostetter, T.H. (1982) Dietary protein intake and the progressive nature of kidney disease. *New England Journal of Medicine* **307** (11), 652–9.

CANADA–USA (CANUSA) Peritoneal Dialysis Group (1996) Adequacy of dialysis and nutrition in CAPD: association with clinical outcomes. *Journal of the American Society of Nephrology* **7**, 198–207.

Chandna, S., Schultz, J., Lawrence, C., Greenwood, R. and Farrington, K. (1999) Is there a rationale for rationing chronic dialysis? A hospital based cohort study of factors affecting survival and morbidity. *British Medical Journal* **318**, 217–23.

Chertow, G.M., Lazarus, J.M. and Milford, E.L. (1996) Quetelet's index predicts outcome in cadaveric kidney transplantation. *Journal of Renal Nutrition* **6**, 134–40.

Department of Health (1991) *Dietary Reference Values for Food Energy and Nutrients for the UK. Report on Health and Social Subjects*, no. 41. DoH, London.

Department of Health (2004) *National Service Framework for Renal Services. Part One: Dialysis and Transplantation.* www.doh.gov.uk/nsf/renal.

Diabetes UK (2003) *Patient education materials.* www.diabetes.org.uk.

EDTNA/ERCA (2001) *European Guidelines for the Nutritional Care of Adult Renal Patients.* www.edtna-erca.org.

Elia, M. (1990) Artificial nutritional support. *Medicine International* **82**, 3392–6.

Friedman, A.L., et al. (1983) Secondary oxalosis as a complication of parenteral alimentation in acute renal failure. *American Journal of Nephrology* **3**, 248.

Han, D.S., Lee, S.W., Kang, S.W., et al. (1996) Factors affecting low values of serum albumin in CAPD patients. *Advances in Peritoneal Dialysis* **12**, 288–92.

Health Education Authority (1996) *The Balance of Good Health.* Ministry of Agriculture, Fisheries and Food, London.

Heyward, V.H. (1998) Practical body composition assessment for children, adults and older adults. *International Journal of Sport Nutrition* **8**, 285–307.

Kalantar-Zadeh, K., Kleiner, M., Dunne, E., et al. (1999) A modified quantitative subjective global assessment of nutrition for dialysis patients. *Nephrology Dialysis Transplantation* **14**, 1732–8.

Kasiske, B.L., Guijano, C., Massey, S.A., et al. (1996) Cardiovascular disease after renal transplantation. *Journal of the American Society of Nephrology* **7**, 158–65.

Modification of Diet in Renal Disease Study Group (1998) Effect of dietary protein restriction on nutritional status in the MDRD study. *Kidney International* **52**, 778–91.

Northern Italian Cooperative Study Group (1991) Prospective, randomised, multicentre trial of effect of protein restriction on progression of chronic renal insufficiency. *Lancet* **337**, 1299–304.

Passey, C., Bunker, V., Higgins, B., et al. (2001) The scientific value and acceptance by pre-dialysis patients of low protein diets consisting of animal versus vegetable protein. In: *Proc 11th International Conference on Nutrition and Metabolism in Renal Disease*, Japan, Abstract.

Pollock, C.A., Lloyd, S., Ibels, F.-Y., et al. (1997) Protein intake in renal disease. *Journal of the American Society of Nephrology* **8**, 777–83.

Prochaska, J.O. and Diclemente, C.C. (1986) Towards a comprehensive model of change. In: Miller, W.R. and Heather, N. (eds) *Treating Addictive Behaviors: Processes of Change.* Plenum, New York.

Rigalleau, V., Combe, C., Blanchetier, V., et al. (1997) Low protein diet in uraemia: effects on glucose metabolism and energy production rate. *Kidney International* **51**, 1222–7.

Schofield, W.N., Schofield, C. and James, W.P.T. (1985) Basal metabolic rate – review and prediction. *Human Nutrition: Clinical Nutrition* **39**, 1–96.

Scottish Intercollegiate Guidelines Network (SIGN) (1999) *Lipids and the Primary Prevention of Coronary Heart Disease; a National Clinical Guideline.* Publication no. 40. SIGN, Edinburgh.

Sutton, D., Talbot, T. and Stevens, J.M. (2001) Is there a relationship between diet and nutritional status in CAPD patients? *Peritonitis Dialysis International* **21** (Suppl 3).

Vennegoor, M. (2002) Renal Nutrition. In: Thomas, N. (ed.) (2002) *Renal Nursing.* Baillière Tindall, Edinburgh.

World Health Organization (1985) *Energy and Protein Requirements.* Technical Report Series no. 724. WHO, Geneva.

# Further reading

ERA/EDTA (2002) Nutritional status in dialysis patients: a European consensus. *Nephrology Dialysis Transplantation* **17**, 563–72.

K/DOQ1 (2000) Clinical practice guidelines for nutrition and CRF. *American Journal of Kidney Diseases* **6** (Suppl 1), 140.

Mitch, W.E. and Saulo, K. (1998) *Handbook of Nutrition and the Kidney*, 3rd edn. Lippincott-Raven, Philadelphia.

Renal Association (2002) *Guidelines for the Treatment of Adult Renal Patients,* 3rd edn. Royal College of Physicians, London.

Renal Nutrition Group/British Dietetic Association (1998) *Setting Standards and Achieving Optimal Nutritional Status.* www.bda.uk.com.

Thomas, B. (2001) *Manual of Dietetic Practice*, 3rd edn. Blackwell Science, Oxford.

# Chapter 13
# Psychological Care

*Mike Kelly, Cathal Gallagher and Celia Eggeling*

## Introduction

The movement of life is a constant tension between chaos and order. In infancy, within the security and the enfolding, protective and stimulating love of a family, the infant develops from the chaos of emotions and feelings towards a child who learns to live with a certain level of separateness, independence and autonomy. However, once a certain order has been achieved adolescence arrives with its new tide of impulses and drives to be confronted and assimilated, bringing once again the chaos that pushes the teenager to learn to relate in a new way, to develop a growing independence and to move towards young adulthood where responsibilities can be assumed. It appears that there is an ongoing cycle of chaos challenging us to develop an order in our lives that can again disintegrate and needs to be re-ordered.

Throughout life there is the disorder created by sickness, accidents, loss of work and loss of friends – all the crises that destroy carefully laid plans and security. These crises, and especially chronic illness, can sometimes bring with them a loss of reference points and a crumbling of the structured existence that has given life a certain security. They can reawaken unresolved development issues that need to be confronted in order to live a more integrated life. Renal disease can be such a trauma, with the result that many aspects of a patient's and family's life can be thrown into turmoil.

## Brief history of psychological care

The treatment of those with renal disease has advanced considerably over the past 40 years. The 1960s saw the development of a network of hospital dialysis units and the development of home haemodialysis (Stevens, 2002). The first nephrologist in the UK was appointed during this time. By the mid 1970s 68% of haemodialysis patients were dialysing at home. As the service expanded the realisation grew that the provision of haemodialysis places was never going to grow fast enough to accommodate the number of patients requiring treatment. The 1980s saw the expansion into satellite units. By 1986, with the development of peritoneal dialysis, 42% of patients dialysed by this method. The number of satellite units continued to grow and by 1998 73 were operating in the UK. With the development of satellite units and the expansion of hospital-based haemodialysis places the numbers of home haemodialysis patients dropped significantly. Today only 2% of haemodialysis patients dialyse at home (Ansell and Feest, 2001).

From the early days it was recognised that a chronic illness like renal failure had psychological consequences. This is attested to, for example, in Kaplan-de-Nour's study carried out in the late 1960s (Kaplan-de-Nour and Czackes, 1968). Dr Murray Parkes reminded us to keep in mind the link between the physical illness and the psychological consequences of such an illness. He wrote, 'we need to cultivate a sensitivity to the possible psychological influences of the physical illnesses that come our way' (Murray Parkes, 1998). Doctors, nurses, social workers, chaplains, psychologists and latterly counsellors are testament to the recognition of the link between the physical and psychological. However, historically it would be fair to say that developing a service to provide psychological and emotional support to patients was patchy rather than uniform.

The reasons why this is so are complex and many. A major reason is that initiatives taken were locally driven rather than nationally planned. For example, some psychology departments made links with renal units to facilitate the needs of their students. Or a particular member of staff saw a need and responded to it informally. This resulted in some renal units developing psychological and emotional support for patients, and in some cases families, while others provided minimal support.

## Through loss, shock, denial and dependency towards hope

Advances in medical technology have transformed the way many operations are carried out and the way treatment is administered. This has led to an increased sense of hope and optimism among professionals and patients (Nichols, 1989). Yet there is a growing body of evidence (Buchanan and Abram, 1989; Fallowfield, 1990; Radley, 1994) that shows that a diagnosis of any chronic illness, like renal failure, provokes a range of emotional responses which evoke feelings about loss. That loss could be loss of employment, reduced functioning of the kidney or the inability to complete familiar tasks. In other words, diagnosis of a chronic illness, such as renal failure, provokes psychological distress.

This is reflected in the figures from a study carried out in 24 dialysis units in 1995 by Gudex (Gudex, 1995). The results confirm the level of psychological distress; with 68% of patients acknowledging that their social and personal relationships were seriously affected by renal disease. Almost 30% admitted to being unable or less able to perform usual activities. Nichols (1984) also concluded that 'the vast body of the literature on renal failure echoes a recurring theme – life in renal failure is hugely stress laden for the majority of those involved'.

When a person receives the news that he or she has renal failure and that dialysis, in its various forms, will be the mode of treatment, reactions vary. One of the most common immediate reactions is psychic numbing, in other words, denial. A common response to the recommendation that soon an individual will have to commence dialysis is 'Don't worry, I will continue taking the pills and I will be fine'. To a patient this may seem a reasonable response, yet many readers will recognise that these patients are in denial. Denial may manifest itself as not adhering to diet or medication, drinking over the fluid allowance, failure to attend appointments and possibly more frequent admissions to hospital.

The most common word patients use to describe the moment they are told they have renal failure is 'shock'. Patients recall this time as a time of uncertainty, confusion and incomprehension. Questions flood the mind; how did this happen? Did I do something to cause this illness? Am I going to die? Up to this point life had its own rhythm. The ordinary stresses and strains of daily life could be coped with. Life functioned, despite all its 'ups and downs'. Life had its equilibrium. With the diagnosis of renal failure, this equilibrium shifts. The outcome can be significant psychological stress. The familiar coping mechanisms no longer function or function inadequately.

Holkamp (2002) speaks about the psychological distress of making a decision about donating an organ from a recently deceased loved one. The psychological distress she described is similar in those facing renal failure. She writes, 'a stressful life event is one that is not fully in accord with an individual's usual working models. It contains unfamiliar material that threatens the individual's equilibrium and destroys the expectation that things will remain the same'. The fact that life has drastically changed and will never be the same again is one of the primary causes of the psychological distress felt by those with renal disease. A book read by many renal patients puts it as 'kidney failure has a massive impact on the whole of a person's life' (Stein and Wild, 2002).

Those with renal disease frequently comment on the changes demanded by a diagnosis of renal failure or a dialysis regime. These changes are often expressed through everyday tasks that most people take for granted. Yet for someone who needs dialysis, the world as he or she experienced and understood it has gone. Many comment on the alienation they feel from a world that was once so familiar (Roos, 2002). Other renal patients respond to the major changes dialysis imposes upon them in positive ways. The transition, though not without its share of trauma, goes relatively smoothly. One of the main reasons this is so is that the person's 'perceptions determine not only the impact of the illness but also the patterns of coping with the illness, with treatment and with associated social disruption' (Weinman, 1987).

However, for the majority of patients with renal failure this is not the case. Adapting to a different, unfamiliar way of life is traumatic. Patients feel a sense of loss and they grieve for the life they once knew. Some as a way of coping fall into depression, which Rowe (1996) describes as a place of 'terrible isolation'. In a study conducted in the early 1980s Kaplan-de-Nour concluded that 53% of patients on dialysis experienced moderate or severe depression (Kaplan-de-Nour, 1982). The same could be found today.

When patients begin life on dialysis they enter into a relationship of dependency. Their lifestyle is curtailed and their survival is dependent on a machine and the professionalism of medical and other personnel. This change, particularly of lifestyle, can lead to job loss, job changes and pressure on family, sexual and social relationships (Kidney Alliance, 2001). The paraphernalia of dialysis is familiar to those of us who work in renal medicine, but this familiarity can often blind us to the impact it is having on our patients. We need to frequently remind ourselves, as one nurse puts it, that our patients are 'highly dependent on technology and professional skill for their survival and that this dependence can have a profound psychological impact' (Pritchard, 2000).

# Children

Problems of a particular nature occur when renal failure affects a child. Children have to contend with a chronic illness at an age when they are still developing their sense of who they are. Yet the psychological distress they suffer needs to be addressed as it does if they were adults.

Children are full of hope and dream about what they want to be or do. A diagnosis of renal failure can dent hope and shatter dreams. In the home environment all is familiar. Likes and dislikes, favourite food, books or toys are known. With renal failure, hospitalisation in a paediatric renal unit is a matter of course. There the child finds him- or herself in unfamiliar surroundings, being cared for by people he/she does not know. No matter how good and caring the professionals are, no matter how child-friendly the paediatric renal unit is, the early stages of admission to hospital will leave the child frightened and feeling alone. At the same time the child has to contend with fears about the illness. What children share is the sense that 'an event outside the family's control alters expectations of childhood, of parents' capacity to protect children from trauma' (Altschuler, 1997). The fears the children have need to be addressed by someone professionally trained who can listen to what is being communicated, both verbally and non-verbally. Those working with children need to be acutely aware of their own emotions to seeing children suffering in this way. If they fail to do so it may prevent them hearing what the child is attempting to communicate. Families also need support. The Renal Association (2002) recommends that 'all families should have access to other staff who may be involved in the care of their child with chronic renal failure, including play staff, schoolteachers, psychologists, psychiatrists and youth workers'.

# Psychological support services

Any review of psychological support services in the renal field in the UK shows that the provision of psychological support is patchy. Some units have, as members of the multiprofessional team, people who are professionally trained to respond to the psychological needs of patients. In other units no such person or service exists. The reasons why such a situation exists are many. Yet evidence shows that by failing to address the psychological and emotional wellbeing of patients we run the risk of undermining their physical wellbeing. Nichols (1989) warns against ignoring the psychological as he concludes from his studies that 'preventive psychological care underpins physical treatment such that in its absence the efficiency of physical treatment may be seriously diminished'.

## *Effect on families*

The primary focus is the patient. Yet any chronic illness, like renal failure, affects not only the patient but also his or her family. One mother describes the effect on her as filling her 'with such despair that my immediate reaction was to deny the situation' (Ward, 1986). Often it is the family that assumes the role of primary carer. The role of families in the care of individuals with renal failure is crucial not least because it is estimated that they save the NHS £4 billion pounds a year (Sedgewick, 2002). If families fail to provide the supporting care necessary, the cost would have to be borne by the NHS, with perhaps detrimental consequences to the provision of renal services.

Families also play a crucial role in how the patient perceives and responds to life on dialysis. A report from the Kidney Alliance (2001) emphasises the importance of this role. The report says 'support from families and carers is critical. Families, partners and friends can amplify anxieties of patients or they can absorb stress and provide a positive influence on the perceptions of the patient and become their major support'. There are some studies that question whether families facing a chronic illness are more likely to suffer emotional distress than families where there is no chronic illness (Perrin and McLean, 1988). However, in families where there is psychological distress caused by renal failure, attention must be paid to this, not only in terms of the impact on the levels of support they offer the patient, but also in how they themselves are affected by the illness.

Nichols (1989), in a study that looked at the impact of the illness on partners of those with renal failure, found that '61% of partners felt depressed at how the other had changed, 54% felt exhausted and 27% felt trapped because the other was dependent on them'. Nichols concludes by saying that 'the stressful impact of dialysis on partners must also concern us'.

These papers show the impact renal failure has on partners and families. It is a timely reminder for those of us working in renal medicine that we must also consider the family. A diagnosis of established renal failure (ERF) will involve some reorganisation of the family structure. The family must in psychological terms contend with the 'loss' of a loved one. Just as the life of the patient changes with the diagnosis of renal failure, so also does the life of the family. The loss they feel can be profound and acute. Murray Parkes (1998) reminds us just how devastating this loss can be and how vital it is for us to keep the family in mind. He writes, 'many of the losses that are met with in medicine affect the lives of members of the families of our patients and sometimes their losses are as great as or greater than those experienced by the patient. Whenever a loss extends to affect the family, it is the family, which includes the patient, that should be the unit of care. This conclusion may seem obvious, but members of the medical profession are so used to treating the patient as the unit of care that they regularly neglect the family'.

Everyone needs a certain amount of security in order to be able to live a peaceful life and this sense of security comes from the way we live our lives; it comes from the presence of and the reinforcement from family and friends; it comes from our place of work; and through daily routines. Chronic illness will inevitably provoke a crisis. To move from the known to the unknown provokes feelings of terrible loss and fear, of pain, failure, weakness and anger. Often these feelings search for a scapegoat and the scapegoat is all too often the person or persons who are nearest to the patient – the family members.

It is incumbent upon those of us who work in renal medicine to review our working practices, set ourselves standards and, through our continuous professional development, grow in our knowledge and skill in order to enhance our ability to care for our patients. We do this as part of our working routine, yet it could be questioned how often we review, what could be termed, our 'mindset'. Perhaps the question that needs to be addressed is – in my mind who is the unit of care? Is it the patient, or the family which includes the patient? If the family, as Stein and Wild (2002) describe, is the 'main source of psychological support for the patient', then in order to maintain that level of support we must recognise and respond to the impact renal failure has on the family.

## Multiprofessional approach

As a member of a multiprofessional team, the role of the counsellor involves organising and facilitating a support group for pre-dialysis patients and their families. At each meeting, invited speakers include someone presently on dialysis, someone who has had a transplant and a family member who speak about their experiences. The value of such groups is underlined by the Kidney Alliance (2001) and others, as they see 'support from small groups meetings with patients with a similar condition can also be valuable as a forum for sharing worries and for learning information and new coping strategies'.

It is noticeable that often during the question and answer session that follows, the majority of questions asked are principally directed to the person who has had a transplant. It is as if dialysis, the 'bit in the middle', is excluded from thinking. For many people in the pre-dialysis stage, a transplant is seen as 'the gate' to a return to life as it was before. In this way it reflects their level of psychological distress, as a transplant is viewed as a way out of this distress. For family members, particularly those who fear being trapped or who cannot bear the burden of responsibility of looking after a loved one who is chronically ill, a transplant is viewed with relief, as in their mind it restores their loved one to an independent state, someone who can once again take control of their lives. There are grains of truth in both of these perceptions, but it is sometimes not as hopeful as it is imagined.

The disappointment at the discovery that it is not as it was imagined provokes what Nichols (1989) describes as 'the high incidence of psychological difficulties among people dealing with life after a transplant'. The reason for these difficulties are (1) medication has to be taken for the rest of their lives, (2) there are still limits on what they can and cannot do and (3) it is unknown how long the transplanted kidney will survive. While the percentage figures for successful transplants are very high – 88% are still functioning at the end of the first year (UK Transplant, 2002) – people know their transplant has a limited life span.

## Referral to counselling services

For those involved directly in patient care, the prospect of dealing with the psychological impact of ERF may seem daunting. There is the desire to support and help, but often skills may be limited. Where professionally trained people such as counsellors are available, patients and families may be referred to them. However, before a referral is made the following points are worth considering:

- Staff may be the first point of contact for the patient or family member. This may be the first place and time patients risk mentioning the psychological distress they are in.
- It is important for staff to respond to the patient within the limits of their skills. To refer too quickly could leave the patient feeling unheard, hurt and rejected, thereby increasing the distress felt.
- When contemplating a referral, staff need to consider the attachment the patient has to them. It may be strong and the patient might feel more comfortable talking to already-known staff. Careful handling at this stage may allow for a referral if and when that is appropriate.
- Referring patients runs the risk that patients agree to the referral not because they feel they need psychological help but because someone entrusted with their care has suggested it.

Psychological support services should be integral to the provision of renal care. Multiprofessional teams should count among their number someone professionally trained who can attend to the psychological needs of patients and their families. The Kidney Alliance (2001) speaks of the value of psychological support at all stages of dialysis from pre-dialysis to conservative therapy. For those, for example, whose entry into renal replacement therapy (RRT) is planned, the report states that structured counselling of patients approaching

ERF involving the multidisciplinary team and other patients should aim for the seamless entry onto RRT.

## Review of key issues in psychological care

The importance of professional psychological care for those with ERF has been highlighted. While good listeners among staff are essential, there is a need for a degree of professional training. The origins and the effects of fear around failure and loss are usually to be found in childhood. Parents can make their children feel they have to merit their love, that it is a reward for good behaviour. Under these conditions, children feel that they must be perfect before they deserve to be loved. Worth is something to be proved rather than seeing oneself as having a unique value as a person. When chronic illness strikes, with its ensuing dependence, the patient is forced to look at, often for the first time, unresolved issues from childhood. If life has been constructed on success, social esteem and power, then a chronic illness like renal failure can bring a sense of worthlessness that can have repercussions for the whole family. Counselling provides a space where the patient can allow the needy and vulnerable side to show itself and be accepted. It is a space where issues can be dealt with without the family becoming the place of projection and of seeking approval. It is the place where regression is an acceptable part of the task in hand and not something to be avoided. Psychological care becomes an integral part of the treatment that allows the patient to make full use of the resources and care that is being provided in the renal unit.

The following section demonstrates how renal counsellors can implement evidence-based practice and influence the care and management of living donors.

## Best-practice guidelines for psychological care of living donors

Whilst renal counsellors are well placed to meet the challenges of donor advocacy, they are an under-represented resource within the field of renal medicine. Implicitly this means that many units do not have the appropriate level of psychological support available for potential donors during the transplant work-up period or indeed beyond. With this in mind, evidence-based data from a multicentre study have been disseminated into best-practice guidelines aimed at raising awareness within renal teams of the dynamics of being a donor. The following section will explain how dissemination of data from a four-centre study led to the compilation of best practice guidelines for the psychological care of living donors (see Appendix One).

The well-documented dearth of cadaveric kidneys available for transplantation (Conrad and Murray, 1999) has led to many renal units actively promoting living donation where close family members, spouses or friends are considered as potential donors. Guidelines produced by the Renal Association for living kidney donor transplantation (Renal Association, 2000) promote the concept of *informed consent* and recommend that all living donors should have access to a donor advocate.

A study was carried out to explore the attitudes of transplant surgeons and transplant sisters in relation to (1) living donation and (2) counsellors as donor advocates, whilst also researching potential donors' experiences of (a) 'being worked up' and (b) donors' attitudes towards counsellors on Living Programmes (C. Eggeling, unpublished data, 2002).

Twenty four potential donors attending four renal and transplant units were interviewed. Participants were seen at different stages of their donor work-up, either in hospital or at home. The views of four transplant sisters and three transplant surgeons were also sought.

Data were collected in semi-structured taped interviews lasting between 60 and 90 minutes and were later transcribed and analysed under the tenets of Grounded Theory – a qualitative methodology which aims to produce a detailed and systematic recording of themes and issues addressed in interviews (Strauss and Corbin, 1990).

From this detailed analysis, the following findings emerged.

## Donor search and selection

The system of donor search and selection showed evidence of the competitive struggle that exists in some families (Fellner and Marshall, 1968), together with the effective way in which some members were excluded from the donation process, often by a self-selection process. Other families operated a pecking order culture which seemed to be accepted by potential donors at the point of donor selection, but occasionally led to voluntary withdrawal further along the work-up programme.

## Decision making

In line with other studies (Simmons et al., 1977; Eggeling, 1999), data analysis found a decision-making model of emotional immediacy. As the work-up progressed, several donors spoke of experiencing a sense of surrealism – a sense of feeling 'detached' from the process. This was possibly a defence mechanism – a way of avoiding 'reflection' or thinking too deeply about the implications and consequences of donation – but this, together with the autonomous spontaneity of decision making, surely casts doubt on the donor's ability to give informed consent?

## Significant others

Little has been written about the impact of donation on the partners and families of potential donors in terms of the effect on interpersonal relationships or feelings with regard to the gift that is being offered outside of the nuclear family. (Kemph et al., 1969; Eggeling, 1999). However, the importance and influential abilities of significant others should not be under-estimated, for if they withhold support, donation could be put in jeopardy.

Data analysis found that several donors tended to assume they had the full and unconditional support of their significant others, only to later find that their perceptions were completely inaccurate. One can so easily empathise with significant others who say the needs of the recipient are being put before their own; that loyalty to a sibling, parent or friend is being put before the love and responsibility to a partner.

## Transplant surgeons

There was an awareness that it is not always possible to reconcile the needs of the donor with the needs of the recipient. However, it was acknowledged that psychological screening is an aid to facilitating the surgeon's decision making regarding suitability, which goes some way towards safe-guarding the interests of the donor.

## Transplant nurses

All transplant sisters saw donor advocacy as part of their role and were totally committed nurse practitioners. However, it could be argued that a transplant nurse cannot truly act as a donor advocate when she is also responsible for caring for the recipient. There is the potential for ethical dilemmas and breaches in confidentiality to occur, and the complex psychological issues that may arise during the work-up period may provide great challenges for those without formal counselling training.

## Ethical issues

Pressure and the risk of emotional coercion can be highest in cultures that emphasise family solidarity and build obligations upon it, some with strong religious sanctions. Young eligible donors may have potential responsibilities, such as a spouse or parent, to set against the putative claims of a sibling threatened with renal failure. To decline to donate may provoke family hostility and division and in turn generate feelings of guilt. The main conclusions of the study can be found in Table 13.1.

## Donors' views on counselling

The research concluded that donors felt that the presence of a counsellor facilitated a therapeutic alliance where respectful dialogue and an honest exchange of views, fears and fantasies could take place. It resulted in significant others feeling more included in the process, which enabled all parties concerned to

**Table 13.1** Main findings of study into living donation.

- There is more complexity to living donation than previously acknowledged or recorded in existing literature.
- The desire to restore health rather than the quality of the donor/recipient relationship is the prime motivational influence for donating.
- A decision-making model of autonomy and immediacy casts doubt on the donor's ability to give informed consent.
- Ambivalence and surrealism are not necessarily contra-indications to donation but feelings that need to be acknowledged, worked through and understood.
- Significant others frequently felt the needs of the recipient were being put before their own.
- Transplant teams have much to learn with regard to developing living donor programmes that will meet the complex needs of donors and their families.
- Counselling facilitates donors' understanding and increases levels of awareness and insight in relation to possible or probable implications and consequences arising as a result of donation.
- The role for a counsellor within this framework was clearly identified.

feel more comfortable about re-presenting should a need arise. Perhaps more importantly, it gave donors time to reflect on their decision and to decide whether and when they wished to proceed to the next stage of the work-up.

Unsuitable donors or those who voluntarily withdrew also valued the support that the counsellor was able to offer, seeing it as an ongoing service provision where distress, disappointment, ambivalence or guilt could be verbalised and worked through.

## Summary

Data analysis of this study was shared with multidisciplinary members of renal teams in two renal dialysis and transplant units and it was their feedback that informed the author's decision to produce best practice guidelines, which are shown in Appendix One.

Whilst not set out to teach or enhance existing counselling skills but rather to *raise awareness* of the donor's psychological journey through the work-up programme and beyond, they also demonstrate that psychological management of potential donors cannot be seen separately from their clinical and medical care. Integration offers an holistic framework for potential donors and it is proposed that the renal counsellor is the best health care professional to take this forward.

## Appendix One: best practice guidelines for the emotional care of the living donor

- The object of these guidelines is to raise awareness within multidisciplinary renal teams of the psychosocio-economic experiences of being a living donor and to demonstrate, through evidence-based practice, the need to integrate psychological care into the work-up programme.

- No standards of practice that are truly *evidence-based* are currently available to facilitate better understanding within multidisciplinary renal teams of the donor's emotional journey through the Living Programme.
- Being aware of the complexity of the donor-search, decision-making process and the experiences of being *worked-up* can facilitate a deeper understanding of the donor's world and provide a pathway to a more holistic model of care.
- Best practice guidelines are not intended to be restrictive or prescriptive, but informative – an aid to ensuring *informed decision making* is undertaken. Implicitly this also ensures that professionals are aware of the complexity of living donation and this increased awareness can assist physicians, surgeons and transplant team members in *their* decision making regarding the donor's psychological suitability.
- Best practice guidelines identify possible scenarios and practice suggestions which, in the light of available evidence, appear to offer optimum outcomes for potential donors and significant others who may also be impacted by the decision to donate.
- Best practice guidelines are not static but are continuously evolving as new information or research becomes available.
- Continued assessment of the effect of implementing best practice guidelines on patient care is an integral part of their application.
- Best practice guidelines ensure that bad news (such as donor unsuitability, medical problems being identified during screening which prevent donation) is broken appropriately and with empathic understanding.
- In addition to the potential for improving the holistic care of the patient, best practice guidelines form advice for purchasers of renal services and can be an aid to making purchasing decisions.

## Key sensitive areas of the donor programme and recommended guidelines for best practice

### (A) The donor search

'My sister also wants to do it, but in all respects I think I am the most suited, both psychologically and physically.'

*Guidelines*
- Remain aware of family dynamics within the selection criteria.
- Encourage the donor to explore the donor search pathway and identify areas of pressure that may have been encountered along the way.
- Offer reassurance that this information is the first step to understanding the donor's unique experience and is not intended to undermine or question the donor search process, or the commitment of the donor.
- Elicit the views of significant others who have been impacted by the donor search.

## (B) Decision making

'Watching my sister go through this. . . . I just wanted to help. I just put my hand in the air . . . nobody asked.'

*Guidelines*
- Clarify donors' understanding of their decision making. Is it a commitment to undertake initial tests or proceed to donation?
- Encourage donors to explore their family medical history as this might influence their decision making.
- Explore the donor's understanding of the transplant process within the decision-making framework. Allow time for related fears and fantasies to be explored and seek specialist advice when required.
- Decision making should be a sequence of happenings. Potential donors should be screened for psychosocio-economic risk factors with an evaluation of stability of the individual and the family.
- Potential donors with a psychiatric history should be referred on for psychiatric opinion.
- Interviews with significant others should be written into protocols. They are impacted by their loved one's decision to donate and need an opportunity to talk through any concerns they may have.
- An assessment as to whether financial hardship will be incurred as a result of donation should be undertaken and, if appropriate, approaches made to the recipient's primary care trust (PCT) for reimbursement for loss of earnings and out-of-pocket expenses.
- Offer reassurance regarding the confidentiality of test results in order that the potential donor can withdraw at any stage of the work-up, safe in the knowledge that the decision will be fully respected and supported by the transplant team.
- This may require doctors or transplant sisters to provide donors with a medical excuse not to proceed – a benevolent deception justified by the overall good for both donors and recipients and by the need to protect confidentiality and the integrity of the family system.
- Refer on for counselling to address any ambivalence, guilt, disappointment or distress should donation not be a reality.
- Offer access to specialist counselling if relationship problems arise as a result of living donation.

## (C) Levels of understanding regarding clinical information-giving and organisational liaison

'I watched a fly-on-the-wall documentary so I know quite a lot about it . . . well as much as I want to know. If there's rejection, well I guess the staff will try and compensate.'

*Guidelines*
- Pressure and anxiety increase as the work-up progresses and donors need their own advocate with whom to talk through relevant issues and concerns.
- Some donors experience a diminished sense of personal responsibility in the presence of doctors and may need 'permission' or help to regain control.
- Ensure that the work-up timetable meets the needs of the individual donor and routinely check that he or she is committed to proceeding to the next stage.
- At all stages of the work-up, prepare donors for disappointment. Include this in information packs, together with contact numbers should they wish to access counselling support.

## (D) Medical screening

'I've been told I've got raised blood pressure. I've got to go on medication and I'll be reviewed in 6 months. I feel dreadful. I really feel I have let him down now. He was so looking forward to it.'

*Guidelines*
- Protocols should identify the way in which all test results will be shared with potential donors. This is of great significance in living-related donor situations where genetic linking is inconclusive.
- Sensitively prepare donors for the possibility that they may be excluded from the programme at any time during the medical screening.
- Unsuitable donors should be offered a clinic appointment with a consultant or transplant sister to discuss test results and encouraged to explore what 'being unsuitable' means to them.
- Encourage donors to explore their family medical history, as it might be relevant in their decision-making process.
- Recognise the donor's anxiety during the stressful medical screening period and refer on for counselling if appropriate.
- Having to withdraw from the programme for medical reasons means the donor has to deal with not only concerns about their own health, but also their disappointment at not being able to donate. Offer follow-up psychological care.

## (E) HIV counselling

'I don't remember any specific counselling . . . I was going to have the tests done on my return so as not to blight the holiday but she (recipient) strong armed me into having them done before. It was the first vacation in 3 years and I spent the first week looking over my shoulder wondering what the results of the tests would be.'

*Guidelines*
- Consider offering all donors, and not just those identified as 'high risk', access to specialist counselling.
- Incorporate formal HIV protocols into the living donor programme.
- Preferably share the results during a clinic appointment and have protocols in place for onward referral if necessary.
- Remain mindful of donor anxiety and stress at this time.

## (F) Dissonant emotions

**Fear:** 'I'm just terrified of not waking up . . . what they do when I'm out for the count is fine. You know, I've got this real hang up about dying.'

*Guidelines*
- Ensure patients are fully informed in respect of all aspects of the living donor programme and able to make informed decisions.
- 'Normalise' fear of anaesthesia – recognising it as a commonly expressed concern.
- Acknowledge that concerns for the recipient frequently override concerns for the donor, but remember that donors also need to be 'taken care of'.
- This includes the offer of psychological support should the donor be found to have medical problems that preclude proceeding to donation and which will exacerbate existent feelings of having failed – of having let others down.

**Ambivalence:** 'I feel a little bit worried (laughter) a little bit worried – about myself, that it won't work and you suddenly got something wrong, or I mean infections. Yeah, but if successful, it's OK, but I am a little bit. . . . But I would still like to do it. . . .'

*Guidelines*
- Respect the potential donor's autonomy and right to decide without influence.
- Recognise one's own prejudices.
- Acknowledge that ambivalence is 'healthy', rarely alters the original decision or intention to donate, but needs to be 'given a voice'.
- Refer to the renal counsellor/donor advocate for counselling.

**Pressure:** 'She said she needed it now . . . she wanted to be able to interact with her son . . . all that emotional stuff. I said 'OK, have it now'. Then I lost the plot, I couldn't even go to work. I was like completely. . . .'

*Guidelines*
- Identify areas of pressure and facilitate ways of addressing same.
- Normalise dissonant emotions.
- Recognise when undue pressure is being exerted and help the donor through this process.

- Offer increased support during times of stress.
- Meet with significant others to acknowledge their views and concerns and mediate where necessary.

**Depression:** 'I've had to have more tests done and I'm not sure what's happening next. I really feel I've let him down. It breaks my heart, although he says 'don't worry mum, it will still go ahead but not when we first planned'. It's so hard to see your son going through this . . . it tears you apart.'

*Guidelines*
- Donors with a previous history of depression should be identified and monitored carefully throughout the work-up.
- Anticipate 'at risk' situations.
- Minimise the risk of recurrent episodes of depression by ensuring immediate and ongoing counselling is available when required.
- Ensure donors are fully informed and that support is available in the event of bad news having to be broken.
- Adhere to timetables and keep the donor informed at all times of anticipated planning changes.
- Do not prepare the donor for theatre until all test results are to hand.

**Post-operative depression:** 'I'm usually such a positive person, but I feel I've let the side down. I'm told that all donors are discharged within a few days . . . and I'm still here. I've been made to feel it's my fault. And my wound is really painful . . . I feel so fed up, I could cry.'

*Guidelines*
- Be aware of the psychology of donating and have appropriate support systems in place.
- Advise that post-operative depression is common, watch for signs and refer on for specialist counselling or support if appropriate.
- Offer regular follow-up physical and psychological care.
- Value donors by encouraging them to participate in educational lectures.
- Offer assistance to donors wishing to set up donor support groups.

## (G) Facilitating coping strategies

Emotional distancing: 'I don't want to talk about it. I don't want to be influenced.'
Denial: 'Nothing about this worries me . . . really.'
Compartmentalisation: 'I kind of compartmentalise things – put them to one side.'
Assertiveness: 'I had to say, hang on there, there's only so much I can take in.'
Goal-setting: 'I've given up smoking and lost one stone in weight for this.'
Meditation: 'I took up meditation to regain my focus – to remain strong.'
Blocking: 'I don't think about failure rates – they said it should work.'
Positivism: 'I keep boosting him up – you're alive, that's all that matters.'

Displacement: 'I have faith in the doctors and NHS. If anything goes wrong it's down to them.'

Rescuing: 'My husband's had a horrible year. He can't cope now so I don't tell him.'

Rationalisation: 'My blood pressure has shot up through stress.'

Bargaining: 'If he is half-way back to normal after this, it will be a bonus.'

*Guidelines*
- Recognise and respect the donor's defence mechanisms.
- Encourage and facilitate exploration of these strategies within a safe and non-judgemental environment.

### (H) Significant others

'I've only discussed it with her briefly, but she'll be all right about it. She knows how close (recipient) and me are. So . . . to answer your question . . . I don't talk about it with her.'

*Guidelines*
- Donors often 'assume' they have the unconditional support of their significant others and avoid meaningful discussion around donation.
- Appreciate the importance of significant others and elicit their views.
- Assess for contra-indications, such as risk of family breakdown, financial disadvantage, etc. occurring as a result of donation.
- Liaise with PCTs regarding reimbursement of loss of earnings and out-of-pocket expenses, if appropriate.
- Significant others can influence decision making. Without their support, the donation process could be in jeopardy.
- Encourage open and honest expression of feelings and concerns between all parties impacted by the decision to donate.
- Offer mediation if appropriate.

### (I) Genetically related donors

'I mean I'm 62 – lots of my friends are at this age and having heart attacks and things. Can you just tell my wife I had the tests but wasn't compatible?' (father to son donation)

'There have been lots of times when I have had to help her over a bad patch in the past. In a strange sort of way, it's almost like a marriage really.' (son to mother donation)

'He (the doctor) held his head in his hands and said "I don't know how to tell you this but you are not full brother and sister."' (sister donating to brother)

*Guidelines*
- Do not be judgemental. Respect and work with differences in family values, belief systems and attitudes.

- Be mindful of the impact living related donation can have on family members.
- Emphasise during the work-up that it is possible to find inconclusive genetic links between donors and recipients and ensure protocols are in place for effective management of such outcomes.

### (J) Emotionally related donation – spousal

'I want to do it to get him (husband) back to normal and give the children and him a better life.'

*Guidelines*
- Psychosocio-economic assessment is an essential part of the work-up.
- Clarify motivational influences.
- Be aware of the potential for pressure and emotional blackmail to be exerted on the donor.
- Facilitate consideration and exploration of child care and financial implications that might arise as a result of spousal donation.

### (K) Emotionally related donation – friends

'We're just like sisters, we holiday together and everything. She is so brave and has had so many disappointments (cries), she deserves a break.'

*Guidelines*
- Fully explore motivational influences.
- Ensure potential donors are fully aware of the psychosocial, economic and practical implications that may arise as a result of donation.
- Invite significant others to attend information programmes so that they may fully understand what is involved in the donation programme.
- Significant others can feel the needs of the donor are being put before the needs of the recipient's family and should be made to feel part of the process.
- Be aware of the impact that being found to be 'incompatible' can have on both the donor and the recipient.
- Advise that follow-up counselling for unsuitable or unsuccessful donors is available.

### (L) Ethical responsibilities

'With the shortage of kidneys in general, we can sometimes run the danger of being so focused on the needs and requirements of the recipient, that we forget about the basic needs and rights of the donor.' (transplant surgeon)

*Guidelines*
- Congruence and truthfulness are essential if the donor is to make a fully informed decision to donate.

- Protocols addressing management of ethical issues should be in place.
- At an early stage of the work-up, identify ways for the donor to withdraw from the programme with dignity and with the donor/recipient relationship still intact.
- Provide counselling support, as self-esteem and self-image may have been damaged by the decision to withdraw.
- Appointing an independent advocate for the donor is desirable.

# References

Altschuler, J. (1997) *Working with Chronic Illness*. Macmillan, London.

Ansell, D. and Feest, T. (eds) (2001) *The Fourth Annual Report of the UK Renal Registry*. UK Renal Registry, Bristol.

Buchanan, D.C. and Abram, H.S. (1989) Psychological adaptation to haemodialysis. In: Moos, R.H. (ed.) *Coping with Physical Illness, 2: New Perspectives*, Chapter 8. Plenum Medical Book Co., London.

Conrad, N.E. and Murray, L.R. (1999) The psychological meanings of living related kidney organ donation: recipient and donor perspectives – literature review. *American Nephrology Nurses Association Journal* **26** (1), 485–90.

Eggeling, C. (1999) The psychosocial implications of live related kidney donation. *European Dialysis and Transplantation Nurses Association/European Renal Care Association Journal* **25** (3), 19–22.

Fallowfield, L. (1990) The quality of life in cardiovascular disease. In: Fallowfield, L. *The Quality of Life – The Missing Measurement in Health Care*, Chapter 5. Souvenir Press, London.

Fellner, C.H. and Marshall, J.R. (1968) Twelve kidney donors. *Journal of the American Medical Association* **206** (12), 2703–2707.

Gudex, C.M. (1995) Health related quality of life in end stage renal failure. *Quality of Life Research* **4** (4), 359–66.

Holkamp, S. (2002) *Wrapped in Mourning*. Brunner-Routledge, London.

Kaplan-de-Nour, A. (1982) Psychosocial adjustment to illness scale (PAIS): a study of chronic hemodialysis patients. *Journal of Psychosomatic Research* **26** (1), 11–22.

Kaplan-de-Nour, A. and Czackes, J.W. (1968) Emotional problems and reactions of the medical team in a chronic haemodialysis unit. *Lancet* **988**, 987–91.

Kemph, J.P., Bermann, E.A. and Coppolillo, H.P. (1969) Kidney transplant and shifts in family dynamics. *American Journal of Psychiatry* **125**, 1485–90.

Kidney Alliance (2001) *ESRF – A Framework for Planning and Service Delivery*. www.kidneyalliance.org.uk.

Murray Parkes, C. (1998) The challenge of physical Illness. In: Murray Parkes, C. and Markus, A. (eds) *Coping with Loss*, Chapter 1. BMJ Books, London.

Nichols, K.A. (1984) *Psychological Care in Physical Illness*. Croom Helm, London.

Nichols, K.A. (1989) Renal failure. In: Hubert Lacey, J. and Burns, T. (eds) *Psychological Management of the Physically Ill*, Chapter 16. Churchill Livingstone, London.

Perrin, J.M. and McLean, W.E. (1988) Children with chronic illness: the prevention of dysfunction. *Paediatric Clinics of North America* **35**, 1325–37.

Pritchard, C. (2000) The challenge of care for the long term dialysis patient. *British Journal of Renal Medicine* **5** (3), 6–8.

Radley, A. (1994) Chronic illness. In: Radley, A. *Making Sense of Illness: The Social Psychology of Health and Disease*, Chapter 7. Sage Publications, London.

Renal Association (2002) *United Kingdom Guidelines for Living Donor Kidney Transplantation*. British Transplantation Society Secretariat, London.

Roos, S. (2002) *Chronic Sorrow*. Brunner-Routledge, London.

Rowe, D. (1996) *Depression*, 2nd edn. Routledge, London.

Sedgewick, J. (2002) *The 'Policing' Role of the Carer in the Management of Fluids: A Hidden Dilemma*. Paper presented at the EDTNA/ERCA Conference, 20–22 September 2003, Birmingham.

Simmons, R.G., Klein, S.D. and Simmons, E.L. (1977) *Gift of Life – The Social and Psychological Impact of Organ Transplantation*. Wiley, New York.

Stein, A. and Wild, J. (2002) *Kidney Failure Explained*, 2nd edn. Class, London.

Stevens, P. (2002) Anticipating the impact of the Renal National Service Framework. *British Journal of Renal Medicine* **7** (3), 20–24.

Strauss, A. and Corbin, J. (1990) *Basics of Qualitative Research – Grounded Theory Procedures and Techniques*. Sage, London.

UK Transplant (2002) *United Kingdom Activity Report*. www.uktransplant.org.uk.

Ward, E. (1986) *Timbo, A Struggle for Survival*. Hodder and Stoughton, London.

Weinman, J. (1987) Coping with illness and handicap. In: *An Outline of Psychology Applied to Medicine* (Weinman, J.), 2nd edn, Chapter 12. IOP, Bristol.

# Chapter 14
# Technical Aspects of Dialysis

*André Stragier*

## Introduction

Haemodialysis encompasses many technical aspects, several of which have been addressed in Chapter 4. In this section, the issues of water treatment, water distribution and dialysate quality assurance are reviewed. An evaluation of the technique of on-line dialysis efficacy monitoring concludes this chapter.

## Water treatment

'It is not exaggerated to state that inadequate water treatment is one of the gravest risks posed to the health of the patient on dialysis' (Keshaviah, 1989).

This section will emphasise the large variety of contaminants that tap water may hold and will offer recommendations for a safer water treatment strategy.

### Water origin: underground water

When the stopcock at home or in the renal unit is opened, water may originate from two different sources. The first water type represents underground or well water. In the USA and Europe, nearly half of the tap water is pumped up from underground. This water is generally of excellent quality, though it might be variably charged with minerals that are present in the ground such as calcium, iron or aluminium. Over the last decade, this water has also become periodically contaminated with chemicals from agriculture, fertilisers, such as nitrates, and several phytopharmaceutics. Underground water production stations are numerous and small in size. In such stations, water is pumped up, filtered and added to the distribution network. Though this underground water is usually free of bacterial contamination, chlorine or chloramines are intermittently added as a preservative.

## Water origin: surface water

To cover our ever-growing consumption, over 50% of tap water is produced from surface waters, that is, from rivers or lakes. Here, the scatter of possible contaminants is very large and complex, necessitating a combined filtration, purification and disinfection process. In contrast to underground water retrieval stations, surface-originating drinking water production plants are small in number, but they are larger and more sophisticated. In a surface-originating drinking water production plant, aluminium sulphate is added after pre-filtration and filtration. Aluminium reacts with most contaminants as a coagulation agent that precipitates. In the final stage, water is filtered and disinfected by ozone, but more commonly active chlorine and chloramines are used (less expensive).

Making the difference between underground or well water and surface-treated water makes sense as the latter not only holds extra aluminium, but also may still contain some contaminants drained or dumped in the surface water which were not eliminated by the drinking water production plant. It is also important to realise that tap water originates from different sources and is often mixed, so extra treatment (softening for example) may sometimes also be needed to meet the drinking water standards.

A sophisticated network of pumping stations from large reservoirs, situated at ground level, allows water distribution. Extra water towers serve to maintain a constant hydrostatic pressure, allowing peak flows such as in the morning, when most people take a shower.

## Calcium and magnesium

In the early years of dialysis the 'hard water syndrome' was a well-known problem. This occurred when high levels of calcium and magnesium were not removed from the tap water and created hypercalcaemia and hyper-magnesaemia during dialysis. This was associated with nausea, vomiting, muscle weakness, skin flushing and profound hypo- or hypertension. Today, water softening is necessary to avoid scaling, which subsequently can damage the reverse osmosis (RO) membranes (Lopot, 1988). Scaling is mainly due to calcium carbonate precipitation but also magnesium and iron precipitate in the carbonate form.

Water hardness is most commonly expressed as the amount of calcium carbonate ($CaCO_3$) in milligrams per litre, though different units are utilised in some countries (Lopot, 1988). Water hardness in Belgium varies between 50 and 500 mg/l $CaCO_3$, thus entailing a tenfold variation in the water softener size. In the UK, London tap water is hard, in Manchester it is moderate and in Leeds it is soft. Large water hardness variations are common in most countries and can even vary at any time in the same unit. This can be easily followed up by on-line water hardness monitoring after water softening.

## Iron

Water softeners remove iron, preventing RO membrane scaling by iron carbonate. However, this is not always sufficient. If the RO iron feed water concentration is more than 0.3 mg/l, the use of a special sediment filter as water pre-treatment is recommended. Such filters contain greensand, charged with oxidants, which precipitate iron.

## The aluminium challenge

As water companies deliver a variable proportion of underground- and surface-originating water from different locations, its aluminium concentration (measured in micrograms per litre) varies considerably and may even change over time in the same unit. In the UK only 10 µg/l or less was found in the tap water of Nottingham, up to strikingly high levels of between 1000 and 3550 µg/l occasionally in Glasgow and Leeds (Lopot, 1988). Although it is recognised that aluminium levels may have changed considerably since this investigation in 1998, the challenge of differing aluminium levels remains.

The physical–chemical characteristic of aluminium in tap water is complex and pH dependent. About 60–70% of the aluminium in most water supplies is present as neutral, non-ionised hydrated aluminium hydroxide.

### RO efficiency for aluminium

An RO device is considered the safest and most efficient water purification technique for aluminium. RO membranes very efficiently reject the ionised aluminium fraction, as it is a trivalent positive ion. In addition, the RO membranes will efficiently reject the bulk aluminium, present as a colloid, by size exclusion unless the membranes are fouled. The fouling challenge to RO membranes is obvious as RO membrane pores are 1000 times smaller than those of the pre-filter. The tangential flow succeeds in eliminating most colloids with the reject water. However, a minor part of colloids precipitates progressively at the membrane surface. Under fouling conditions, it has been found that the ability of RO to reject aluminium may be as low as 30–50% (Luehmann et al., 1989).

### The aluminium accident in Portugal

In a south-Portuguese renal unit, in early 1993, 25 patients died of severe encephalopathy linked to aluminium intoxication (Simoes et al., 1994; Stragier, 1994). After a period of very scarce rainfall, high concentrations of suspended particles were found in reservoirs, necessitating the addition of extra aluminium sulphate as coagulation agent. The HD unit was not made aware of this action. This resulted in frequent obstruction of the cartridge filters and RO membrane fouling. During this period, aluminium seeped through the water treatment system, resulting in this tragedy.

*Aluminium accumulation in patients on dialysis*

Acute and chronic aluminium intoxication has been previously reported in Europe (Flendrig et al., 1976) and the USA (Centers of Disease Control, 1982). Eighty to 90% of aluminium binds with patients' proteins (D'Haese and De Broe, 1994). This explains its very fast and efficient accumulation: in practice, diffusion does occur from dialysate to blood, albumin binding increasing the free aluminium concentration gradient. This is the reason why dialysate aluminium should never exceed 10 μg/l.

Simoes and colleagues (1994) reported that several aluminium determinations performed on serum, dialysate and water coming from more than 20 countries pointed to a number of episodes of acute aluminium intoxication, under normal operating conditions. These results demonstrate that, although RO devices are very safe for aluminium removal in good operating conditions, these optimal conditions are not always met and strict monitoring is recommended.

*Prevention of aluminium seepage into dialysate*

Deionisers, with separate cation and anion columns, are the most reliable technique to remove aluminium from tap water. In an acid environment, the neutral aluminium becomes a hydrated cation, and in an alkaline environment it becomes an aluminate anion. As a result, a double bed deioniser efficiently removes all aluminium.

An investigation (Dialysis Technicians Association DTV, Belgium, 1996) performed in 22 units in northern Belgium found that renal units are not very much concerned about the problem associated with RO membrane fouling, as 33% of these units claimed never to perform RO membrane cleaning; 50% of units performed RO membrane cleaning every 6 months to 2 years, whereas 17% cleaned the membranes only after the RO water outlet resistivity had significantly dropped. RO water production technical failure, needing treatment interruption, occurred on average once in 5 years; however, in 50% of cases the dialysis technician could rapidly fix the problem.

## From free chlorine to chloramines

Free chlorine has been the standard disinfectant used in municipal water distribution networks to avoid bacterial and algae growth. However, since the mid 1970s, the potential of free chlorine to react with organic substances, such as humic acids, present in surface water became a cause for concern. Indeed, this reaction results in the genesis of potentially carcinogenic compounds, called trihalomethanes (e.g. chloroform). The detection of trihalomethanes in tap water in Belgium (Van Roosbroeck and Quaghebeur, 1982) and Germany (Bommer and Ritz, 1987) and its uptake by patients on dialysis from dialysate in France (Cailleux et al., 1989) were subsequently reported.

Carbon filters are the only available efficient technique to eliminate trihalomethanes and other low molecular weight organics from water.

Thus, free chlorine has been replaced in most countries by chloramines, a less effective but more stable disinfectant, avoiding the generation of trihalomethanes, but also making its removal in dialysis water purification techniques more difficult.

## The chloramine accident in Spain

A dialysis unit in Madrid suffered a chloramine accident due to a water treatment sub-unit failure in the 1990s (Lorenzo et al., 1996). This resulted in severe haemolysis in 66 patients, 15 of whom required transfusions, and the remaining patients needed extra erythropoietin. Several chloramine accidents have also been previously reported in the USA (Tripple et al., 1988; Food and Drug Administration, 1998).

## Water purification for chloramines

Active chlorine and chloramines permeate through ion exchangers and are only removed to a minor extent by RO. Activated charcoal is the most suitable purification technique. One third of units in the USA and Europe deal with chloramines in tap water. However, the concentrations of active chlorine and chloramines in tap water vary considerably in Europe and thus its purification requirement. For example, in Belgium and the Netherlands, chloramine concentrations in tap water are generally low, but in France and Spain they are often high (1.5–5 mg/l).

In the latter case, a carbon filter exposure time of 6 and 10 minutes respectively is required to reduce active chlorine and chloramines to the AAMI (Association for the Advancement of Medical Instrumentation) norms (0.5 mg/l for active chlorine and 0.1 mg/l for chloramines). The reason for this long adsorption contact time is that although chloramine adsorption performs fast at a low water pH, its adsorption progressively slows down when the water pH increases. Water pH is not always stable and there is a tendency to increase it in order to reduce piping corrosion. Daily monitoring is necessary.

What sort of protection is recommended for countries with low chlorine and chloramine levels in tap water? An investigation by the Dialysis Technicians Association DTV, Belgium (1996) clearly illustrates that no consensus exists. However, it is observed that water companies operate in these locations with chloramine boluses rather than with a continuous infusion. The chloramine concentration close to the injection point is high and progressively attenuates over the distribution network. The users are unaware of the point or of the time of injection.

Chloramine-induced erythropoietin resistance has been demonstrated in two UK studies in Leeds (Richardson et al., 1999) and London (Fluck et al., 1999). It is agreed that carbon adsorption is much cheaper than extra erythropoietin and also much safer for patients. Thus, carbon adsorption is always required.

## Other water contaminants

Four hundred herbicides, fungicides and insecticides are registered in Belgium and even more in Europe (Lamotte, 1994). After pulverisation, they can seep into the drinking water. This is illustrated by the fact that a water company in the region of Antwerp had permission to temporarily exceed tenfold the European drinking water norms of 0.1 µg/l for each and 0.5 µg/l for total phytopharmaceutics of four compounds: atrazine, simazine, diuron and isoproturon (herbicides).

Furthermore, many thousands of chemical compounds do exist and 2000 new ones are created yearly and can seep into water supplies, with potential toxicity (Keshaviah, 1989). Contamination of surface water is much more problematic than underground or well water. Throughout Europe, water companies reserve the right to transfer at any time and without warning from one type of water to another as water distribution networks are inter-connected. Our water purification equipment has thus to be as complete and efficient as possible to deal with all possible known and unknown contaminants.

## Review of water treatment

Two recent severe European accidents illustrate that water treatment for haemodialysis is not as safe and easy as anticipated. Technical development of on-line water contaminant monitoring, such as the use of chloramines, active chlorine and total organics, seems within our reach and should be encouraged. Water treatment for haemodialysis still often remains a neglected problem. This is disappointing as the investment for water treatment represents only a very small fraction of the total haemodialysis cost. The following recommendations should be considered:

(1) Generalised use of carbon adsorption with a minimum of 10 minutes' contact time.
(2) Generalised use of RO for any haemodialysis, with a proper membrane cleaning frequency.
(3) Promotion of a better communication between water distribution companies and renal units: confidential warning by water companies of exceptional water contaminant challenges should be advocated.

# Water distribution

Dialysate endotoxin interferes with patients' blood cells, creating chronic inflammatory reactions that should be prevented (Canaud et al., 2000). Tap water contains high amounts of endotoxin and low levels of bacteria. RO should be used in water purification for any haemodialysis as it produces endotoxin- and bacteria-free water. As endotoxin is a by-product of gram-negative bacteria, bacterial quality of the water distribution after the RO should also be monitored and strictly controlled.

## Prevention of stagnation

Bacterial growth is not a major problem in water distribution during operation, but it is during standstill. Bacteria have the affinity to depose and attach to the walls of dialysis systems and colonise. This is the onset of biofilm formation, a situation that should be avoided. Keeping a turbulent flow (more than 1.5 m/s speed) in a water distribution loop significantly reduces bacterial sedimentation (Andrysiak and Varughese, 2002). RO water loop stagnation can be limited by automatic, intermittent rinsing of the loop, during the time of no operation, the return being switched to the RO inlet. Also, dead-spaces and tanks should be avoided in a water distribution system, as they represent zones of stagnation. If an RO water tank is necessary, measures should be taken to minimise bacterial growth and carry out easy disinfection. Such preventive measures may include the use of UV filters, ultrafilters, RO product water recirculation over the RO and more frequent disinfection of the water distribution system.

## Water standards and guidelines

The European Pharmacopoeia (EP) has put forward maximum norms for RO water of less than 100 colony forming units (cfu)/ml and less than 0.25 endotoxin units (EU), which are supported by the European Renal Association/ European Dialysis and Transplant Association (ERA/EDTA) Best Practice Guidelines (ERA-EDTA, 2002).

The European Dialysis and Transplant Nurses Association/European Renal Care Association (EDTNA/ERCA) endorses these norms and is also offering guidelines (EDTNA/ERCA. 2002) on how to manage this by advising on the frequency of testing and sampling conditions. The frequency of microbiological/endotoxin testing should be deduced from the historical data and the disinfection frequency of the water system. If frequent disinfection is performed and the results are good, monthly testing is sufficient. However, if the disinfection interval is long and/or the bacterial results are elevated or no historical data are available, then weekly testing should be performed.

## Disinfection principles

To meet the EP water standards at any time, action levels are proposed at 25 cfu/ml and 0.125 EU (Lindley and Canaud, 2002). Samples for culture/ endotoxin testing should be taken just before disinfection is planned (the worst case).

Disinfection should be performed at least monthly, covering the RO, the water distribution loop and the machine connections to the water loop, by putting the machines in rinsing phase. This is important to avoid biofilm formation in all parts of the water distribution system. The latest progress in this field represents automatic overnight hot water disinfection of the complete water distribution system, including the connections to the machines (Nystrand, 2001). The investment in overnight heat disinfection is higher, but it saves staff work, representing an excellent strategy for maintaining very high standards.

## *Ultrapure RO water*

Ultrapure RO water for haemodialysis relates to a much higher bacterial/endotoxin quality norm of 0.1 cfu/ml and 0.03 EU, respectively (ERA/EDTA, 2002). Its rationale is to prevent inflammatory patient reactions to endotoxins, entailing long-term patient morbidity (Canaud et al., 2000). To keep RO water distribution in compliance with this higher quality standard, extra measures are necessary, such as optimal dead-space free water loop configuration, continuous recirculation of the water loop over the RO and very frequent disinfection. Automatic, very frequent heat disinfection of the water loop and dialysis machines is an excellent option for this purpose (Nystrand, 2001). Ultrapure RO water may be recommended as a better quality standard for any dialysis but especially for dialysis techniques with a high convection rate such as haemodiafiltration and haemofiltration (see Chapter 4).

# Dialysate quality

Dialysate is an important fluid as it comes into direct contact with the dialysis membranes. When dialysate bacterial/endotoxin results do not meet the quality standards, all sources should be more closely investigated: the RO water, the liquid bicarbonate if used and machine disinfection.

Endotoxin is a by-product of gram-negative bacteria; of which *Pseudomonas aeruginosa* (PA) is a typical example. It was demonstrated (Favero et al., 1975) that the PA replication time is 40 minutes in dialysate (rich milieu), nearly the same as in an ideal broth; by contrast, in purified (distilled) water it was nine times slower (poor milieu). This slow replication time explains why bacteria are unable to increase in number during machine operation; therefore it is not important at which time during dialysis samples for bacterial/endotoxin assessment are withdrawn. However, this should be performed on Monday morning and just before the water distribution disinfection is planned (the worst case).

Machine standstill is the biggest problem regarding bacterial growth; during this period of time, machines should always be filled with RO water. Also, spare machines and machines in repair should be disinfected at a minimum of once a week. Completely emptying a system during prolonged stagnation is of course the best solution; however, this might not be possible with most dialysis machines.

## *European dialysate quality norms*

Lindley et al. (2000) surveyed 69 haemodialysis facilities in 62 centres. They found that while European dialysis facilities normally aim to produce water for dialysis that meets the requirements of the EP, many do not check the quality of the water routinely. This situation arose because there were no mandatory requirements for testing in most European countries.

Since that survey, the EDTNA/ERCA has established a working group to draft guidelines for the monitoring of water quality and these were published in 2002. ERA/EDTA also published guidelines in 2002.

The EP specifies an endotoxin norm of 0.5 EU for dialysis concentrate after proper dilution into dialysate with pyrogen-free water. A bacterial dialysate norm of 100 cfu/ml with 0.25 EU is recommended (EDTNA/ERCA, 2002; ERA-EDTA, 2002); the norms for ultrapure dialysate are 0.1 cfu/ml and 0.03 EU respectively. Dedicated sampling ports and proper hygienic procedures are important to withdraw representative samples for bacterial/endotoxin assessment, avoiding false positive results.

## *Disinfection principles*

A recommended principle is 'Clean first and only disinfect thereafter!' (Stragier, 1995). To succeed well, bacteria (job 1), organic (job 2) and inorganic (job 3) deposits such as calcium and magnesium carbonate, and iron carbonate deposits (job 4) must be regularly eliminated (Stragier, 1995). Dialysis machine manuals fail to offer clear instructions on this issue and this can lead to confusion. For example, a small survey in 30 renal units in Spain revealed that seven different chemicals were used for this purpose in 16 different combinations (Mayado, 1996).

If any of the deposits are not regularly removed from the interior dialysis machine fluid pathway, bacteria will nestle down, developing a biofilm. In this situation endotoxin dialysate results may be beyond the EP norm. Upon inspection, technicians should identify the non-removed deposits and correction should immediately be performed for the missing 'job'.

## *Dialysate endotoxin filters*

Dialysate endotoxin filters have the ability to efficiently 'catch up' bacteria and endotoxin from the dialysate, meeting the ultrapure dialysate norms. However, this should not be the compromise solution dealing with RO water or liquid bicarbonate of insufficient bacterial quality nor with inadequate machine disinfection procedures.

It is good to note that water and dialysate standards and guidelines are voluntary (non-mandatory) and have the purpose of stimulating renal units to achieve high-quality care. Each renal unit should keep its own dialysis fluids bacterial-/endotoxin-related protocols and results in a dedicated file; results should be shown and discussed on a regular basis during staff meetings.

# On-line dialysis efficacy monitoring

Traditionally, dialysis efficacy is assessed monthly by withdrawing pre- and post-dialysis blood samples. The urea reduction ratio (URR) or Kt/V and sometimes the protein catabolic rate (PCR) are deduced from these blood urea results. In contrast, on-line dialysis efficacy monitoring offers monitoring of specific dialysis efficacy and the expected Kt/V at the start of each dialysis and blood sampling is not required. If dialysis efficacy is hampered for any reason (access recirculation, inadequate blood flow, coagulation, etc.), a pre-set alarm system will alert the renal team, who can then make any adjustments and corrections.

## The urease principle

The ™UM 1000 is a typical example of an on-line dialysis efficacy monitoring method, using the urease principle. This is an independent monitor, which can be added to any dialysis machine. Other companies (such as Gambro and Bellco) have integrated this principle into their machines. After daily calibration, the patient's data are introduced (or selected from the previously stored database). The patient is connected and intermittently a dialysate outlet sample is passed over a small urease cartridge, converting urea into ammonium. Urea is non-conductive whereas ammonium is. So by measuring the conductivity difference after this reaction, the actual dialysate urea removal is monitored, from which the patient's Kt/V and PCR are calculated. Results are printed out and can also be electronically transferred.

## The ionic dialysance principle

Typical examples of the ionic dialysance principle are Diascan™ (Hospal) and OCM™ (Fresenius). Ionic dialysance assessment is integrated into the machine and consists of a conductivity measurement situated at the dialyser inlets and outlets. The patient's data are introduced (or selected). Every 30 minutes, inlet conductivity is changed by 10% for 2 minutes and the outlet difference measured. Dialysate electrolytes diffuse through dialysis membranes at the same speed as urea, and indirectly reveal the actual urea clearance. This clearance is displayed together with the Kt/V and data can be electronically transferred.

## Evaluation

The urease principle quantifies the urea amount removed during dialysis, and also the patient's PCR, whereas the ionic dialysance principle assesses the actual urea clearance. Both methods offer Kt/V calculation. Ionic dialysance does not measure PCR but has the advantage of not needing any disposables.

On-line efficacy assessment is more reliable, but the results are lower compared to those obtained with conventional methods (Depner et al., 1996). The reason is that blood urea is not equilibrated just after dialysis due to the diffusion delay between intra- and extracellular compartments; hence efficacy is overestimated by the conventional method.

Ionic dialysance correlates with effective urea clearance, corrected for recirculation and ultrafiltration (Petitclerc et al., 1995) and ensures that a more constant dialysis dose is delivered (Katopodis and Hoenich, 2002).

## Summary

This section has discussed four important technical aspects of dialysis: water treatment and distribution, dialysate quality and on-line dialysis efficacy monitoring. There is growing evidence of the negative impact of dialysate endotoxin on the immunity system of patients; hence an evolution towards ultra-pure water and dialysate is likely to occur in the near future. Also, patient on-line efficacy monitoring will most likely become easier and more available, leading to improved health outcomes for patients.

## References

Andrysiak, P. and Varughese, P.M. (2002) Design requirements for a water distribution system in a hemodialysis center. *Dialysis and Transplantation* **31**, 683–90.

Bommer, J. and Ritz, E. (1987) Water quality – a neglected problem in haemodialysis. *Nephron* **46**, 1–6.

Cailleux, A., Subra, J.F., Riberi, P. and Allain, P. (1989) Uptake of trihalomethanes by patients during hemodialysis. *Clinica Chimica Acta* **181**, 75–80.

Canaud, B., Bosc, J.Y., Leray, H., Morena, M. and Stec, F. (2000) Microbiologic purity of dialysate: rationale and technical aspects. *Blood Purification* **18**, 200–213.

Centers of Disease Control (1982) *Dialysis Dementia from Aluminium. Epidemic Investigation Report EPI 81–39.* Centers of Disease Control, Atlanta.

Depner, T.A., Keshaviah, P.R., Ebben, J.P., Emerson, P.F., Collins, A.J., Jindal, K.K., Nissenson, A.R., Lazarus, J.M. and Pu, K. (1996) Multicenter clinical validation of an on-line monitor of dialysis adequacy. *Journal of American Society of Nephrology* **7**, 464–71.

D'Haese, P.C. and De Broe, M.E. (1994) Aluminium toxicity. In: Daugirdas, T. and Ing, T.S. (1994) *Handbook of Dialysis*, 2nd edn. Little Brown, Boston/Toronto, pp. 523–36.

Dialysis Technicians Association DTV, Belgium (1996) *Water Treatment Enquiry.* Dialysis Technicians Association DTV, Aalst. Belgium.

EDTNA/ERCA (2002) EDTNA/ERCA guidelines for the control and monitoring of microbiological contamination in water for dialysis. *EDTNA/ERCA Journal* **28** (3), 107–115. www.edtna-erca.org.

ERA-EDTA (2002) ERA-EDTA European Best Practice Guidelines for haemodialysis IV – dialysis fluid purity. *Nephrology Dialysis Transplantation* **17** (Suppl 7), 45–62.

Favero, M.S., Peterson, N.J., Carson, L.A., Bond, W.W. and Hindman, S.H. (1975) Gram negative water bacteria in hemodialysis systems. *Health Laboratory Science* **12**, 321–34.

Flendrig, J.A., Kruis, H. and Das, H.A. (1976) Aluminium intoxication: the cause of dialysis dementia? *Proceedings of EDTA* **13**, 355.

Fluck, S., McKane, W., Cairns, T., Fairchild, V., Lawrence, A., Lee, J., Murrey, D., Polpitiya, M. and Taube, D. (1999) Chloramine-induced haemolysis presenting as erythropoietin resistance. *Nephrology Dialysis Transplantation* **14**, 1687–91.

Food and Drug Administration (1998) *FDA Safety Alert: Chloramine Contamination of Hemodialysis Water Supplies*. FDA, Rockville, Maryland.

Katopodis, K.P. and Hoenich, N.A. (2002) Accuracy and clinical utility of dialysis dose measurement using online ionic dialysance. *Clinical Nephrology* **57**, 215–20.

Keshaviah, P.R. (1989) Pretreatment and preparation of city water for hemodialysis. In: Maher, J.F. (ed.) *Replacement of Renal Function by Dialysis*, 3rd edn. Kluwer, Dordrecht, pp. 189–98.

Lamotte, P. (1994) Feu orange sur les nappes. *Le Vif Express* **12**, 21–2.

Lindley, E. and Canaud, B. (2002) New European guidelines for microbiological quality of dialysis fluid: a review. *Nephrology News and Issues* **16**, 46–9.

Lindley, E.J., Lopot, F., Harrington, M. and Elseviers, M.M. (2000) Treatment of water for dialysis – a European survey. *EDTNA-ERCA Journal* **26** (4), 34–40.

Lopot, F. (ed.) (1988) *EDTNA/ERCA Water Treatment Monograph*. EDTNA/ERCA, Lucerne.

Lorenzo, I., Medina, N., Calderon, P., Castro, S. and Lazaro, R. (1996) Use of erythropoietin in emergencies: massive intoxication by chloramines. *EDTNA/ERCA Journal* **22** (1), 31–3.

Luehmann, D.A., Keshaviah, P.R., Ward, R.A. and Thomas, A. (1989) *A Manual on Water Treatment for Hemodialysis*. Food and Drug Administration, Rockville, Maryland.

Mayado, D.E.M. (1996) Estudio Multicétrico sobre riesgos y precauciones en Unidades de Dialysis. In: *Proc 6th Spanish EDTNA/ERCA Seminar*, 21–22 March, Murcia, pp. 104–121.

Nystrand, R. (2001) Dialysis fluid contamination. *EDTNA/ERCA Journal* **27** (3), 135–9.

Petitclerc, T., Bene, B., Goux, N., Saudon, M.C. and Jacobs, C. (1995) Non invasive monitoring of effective dialysis dose delivered to the hemodialysis patient. *Nephrology Dialysis Transplantation* **10**, 212–16.

Richardson, D., Barlett, C., Goutcher, E., Jones, H.J., Davidson, A.M. and Will, E.J. (1999) Erythropoietin resistance due to dialysate chloramine: the two-way traffic of solutes in haemodialysis. *Nephrology Dialysis Transplantation* **14**, 2625–7.

Simoes, J., Barata, J.D., D'Haese, P.C. and De Broe, M.E. (1994) Cela n'arrive qu'aux autres. *Nephrology Dialysis Transplantation* **9**, 67–8.

Stragier, A. (1994) Aluminium intoxication: are we protected at our unit? *Nephrology News and Issues* **2**, 5–6, 14.

Stragier, A. (1995) Disinfection of dialysis machines: why and how? *EDTNA/ERCA Journal* **21** (4), 11–14.

Tripple, M.A., Bland, I.A., Favero, M.S. and Jarvis, W.R. (1988) Investigation of hemolytic anemia after chloramine exposure in a dialysis center. *American Society for Artificial Internal Organs Transplantation* **34**, 1060.

Van Roosbroeck, G. and Quaghebeur, D. (1982) De problematiek van trihalomethanen in drinkwater. *Water* **4**, 111–16.

# Chapter 15
# Clinical Governance

*Anne M. Keogh*

## Introduction

Clinical governance is at the heart of the Government's commitment to improving health and health services. The term 'clinical governance' has been widely used, but is less commonly fully understood, and is often defined as 'a framework through which National Health Service (NHS) organisations are accountable for continuously improving the quality of their services and safeguarding high standards of care, by creating an environment of excellence in which clinical care will flourish' (Department of Health, 1998).

The introduction of clinical governance was designed to bring a systematic approach to the delivery of high-quality health care. The relationship between quality improvement and organisational culture has been successfully understood and used in business and industry for many years. Achieving meaningful and sustainable quality improvements in the NHS requires a fundamental shift in culture, to focus effort and enable and empower NHS workers to improve quality locally. At its simplest, clinical governance has two dimensions: firstly, to drive upwards overall standards of care delivery at institutional level by tackling poor performers and encourage others to aspire to clinical excellence; and secondly, satisfying public demand to regulate the quality of an individual professional's work.

In this chapter, the implications of clinical governance will be considered for a wide range of nephrology health care professionals focusing on established renal failure (ERF) as this constitutes the largest workload in renal services and is also perhaps the area most at risk to variations in quality. Much has been written on this subject, but there is still a bias towards theory and a relative shortage of straightforward and practical guidance on how practitioners can make effective progress at a clinical level, especially within nephrology. For effective clinical governance to be successfully introduced, all clinical staff require access to clearly written, reliable information on clinical governance and to be equipped to deliver these complex and challenging roles within an ever-changing nephrology health care environment. The implementation of clinical governance is crucial if quality of health care is to become the driving force for the development of renal services.

## Clinical governance and high-quality care

A review of the literature related to clinical governance highlights the common themes of quality improvement and maintenance, professional and organisational accountability, safety and culture as being the key components of clinical governance (Secretary of State for Health, 1998; Wallace et al., 2001; Currie and Loftus-Hills, 2002; McSherry and Pearce, 2002).

Since April 1999, all NHS bodies in England have had a statutory duty of clinical governance placed upon them (Swage, 2000). This introduced corporate accountability for clinical quality and performance, with NHS Trust Chief Executives holding ultimate responsibility for delivery of care of appropriate quality. The underlying strategy for quality care, of which clinical governance forms a critical part, has a number of features, paramount of which is a focus on patient-centred care, which should be at the heart of every NHS organisation to ensure that patients are kept well informed and are given the opportunity to participate in their care (Donaldson and Muir Grey, 1998).

All health professionals need to work in teams to a consistently high standard, identify ways to provide safer and even better care for their patients and develop an environment where good evidence-based practice and research evidence are systematically adopted. Accurate and relevant information has been identified as being essential to the monitoring of clinical practice (Roderick and Roderick, 2001).

Quality care also means ensuring that risks and hazards to patients are reduced to the lowest possible level, creating a safety culture throughout the NHS. Risk management has become an important area of corporate responsibility, with a central initiative for an 'organisation with a memory' intended to share experience of identifying and reducing risk across the NHS (Department of Health, 2000).

Over a similar time scale, introduction of appraisal, professional portfolios of clinical activity and professional development, and periodic registration/ revalidation have led to closer regulation of individual professional quality for both nursing and medical staff.

## The challenge of clinical governance implementation

Successful implementation of clinical governance will require changes by individual health care professionals, teams and organisations (Miller, 2002). It is about changing the way people work and demonstrating that communication, teamwork and leadership are equally important contributors to high-quality care as risk management and clinical effectiveness. One of the reasons for clinical governance not working is that people look at isolated problems and not at the whole system.

Many staff will already have implemented aspects of clinical governance, and it may only need them to review these practices and put them into a more structured framework. However, for successful implementation across an organisation or even across a department, managers and professional leaders need to ensure an appropriate cultural and organisational infrastructure (Wallace et al., 2001).

## Ownership and communication

Unless individual professionals feel a personal commitment to high-quality clinical care, and the organisation's strategy to achieve it, then they are unlikely to collaborate with initiatives and unlikely to perform at optimal level. To achieve a sense of ownership an organisation must show that it values its staff, their opinions and abilities. This can be demonstrated by having a strategic human resource management plan of collaborative management, empowerment and development of individuals (Swage, 2000).

Staff in turn will give commitment which will result in employees who are more satisfied, productive and adaptable, thereby allowing managers to maximise these attributes within teams. Ownership can be encouraged by involving staff at all levels in planning changes and initiatives designed to improve the quality of care, and having representatives of all staff groups on any executive committees or working parties that implement clinical governance (Haslock, 1999).

## Teamwork

Employing a multidisciplinary team approach to health care is beneficial not only for the individual and the patient, but also for the employer, who gains from a highly motivated and clinically skilled professional workforce (Styles, 1994). Working together involves acknowledging that all participants bring equally valid knowledge and expertise from their professional and personal experience. Making collaboration work is not about what people have in common, but about their differences, as it is those differences that make collaborative work much more powerful. The challenge for health care organisations is to understand how systems work at optimum capacity without exploiting staff in the process whilst maintaining a flexible approach to task allocation. Do not assume that people know the goals and values just because there is a published document.

Renal teams need to become true multidisciplinary groups, where understanding members' respective roles, sharing information and knowledge and support for each other become part of everyday practice (Bolton, 1998; Campbell, 1999; Keogh, 1999). Reflective practice and clinical supervision are two key activities inextricably linked and hold much promise in the support of quality care.

## Individual professional responsibility

Individual health care professionals need to embrace change by adopting reflective practice, which places patients at the centre of their thinking. As well as thinking about best practice in the context of the individual patient, it is a personal and professional responsibility to maintain professional development and participate in audit of care outcomes. Committed individuals will also wish to participate in other aspects of clinical governance including research, quality control, risk management and peer review.

## Leadership

Successes should flow from interventions that are supported by active leadership. Leadership is described by Wickens (1995) as 'getting people to do what you want them to do because they want to do it'. Managers are members of the team as well as leaders of it. The team needs to address specific issues and projects, rather than broad generalisations. Managers should be visionary, strategic and provide inspiration and opportunities to fully engage all team members, setting realistic yet stretching standards and leading by example. Managers who seek scapegoats when things go wrong create an environment in which people avoid experimenting and taking risks.

Realistic leaders foster a climate in which it is acceptable to make mistakes, as long as they are not caused by carelessness, stupidity or negligence. Whether you are the chief executive, the ward manager or the nurse in charge of a particular shift, the way you lead is the single biggest success factor for everyone you work with. Leaders change the organisations around them. Leadership is about what you do. It involves learnable skills that can be applied to the tasks that occur in every health care environment.

## Risk

One of the key responsibilities of clinical governance is the management of risk. Getting things right and delivering a safe and reliable service to patients can reduce litigation costs which can be reinvested in the service to create a better environment for patient care. *An Organisation with a Memory* (Department of Health, 2000) and *Building a Safer NHS for Patients* (Department of Health, 2001b) identify the significant opportunities that exist to reduce unintended harm to patients arising during NHS care.

Around 10 000 new claims were received in 1999–2000 (Comptroller and Auditor General, 2001) and currently outstanding claims for clinical negligence total £2.4 billion (Crouch, 2003). Claimants often want a wider range of remedies such as an apology, an explanation or reassurance that it would not happen again.

The Clinical Negligence Scheme for Trusts (CNST) is a payment made by trusts to insure against litigation. In a service as large and complex as the

NHS, hazard is unavoidable, but the risk can be minimised by a culture of openness, robust working systems and effective staff education. When things do go wrong, the response should not be one of blame and retribution, but of learning, concern for staff who may suffer as a consequence and a determination to reduce risk for future patients (Department of Health, 2001a).

The National Patient Safety Agency (NPSA) has developed a causal analysis checklist (National Patient Safety Agency, 2001) designed to analyse near-misses, to change ineffective systems and to prevent incidents from happening. All NHS Trusts and many Primary Care Trusts are expected to provide data to the national adverse event reporting system.

# Professional audit

Involvement in clinical audit is a professional responsibility for all medical and nursing staff, and monitoring and improving the quality of clinical care via the 'audit cycle' should now be familiar to all staff.

Professional audit can take many forms, but given the range of professions involved in renal care these peer reviews should be multiprofessional.

## Commission for Health Audit and Inspection

The Commission for Health Audit and Inspection (CHAI) brought together the work of the Audit Commission, Commission of Health Improvement (CHI) and the private health care role of the National Care Standards Commission. The CHAI uses a systematic framework to carry out reviews in every NHS organisation in England and Wales to provide independent and systematic scrutiny of the clinical governance arrangements within each Trust. The CHAI model illustrates its belief that effective clinical governance depends upon a culture of continuous learning, innovation and development, which improves the patient's experience of care and treatment in hospital (Bevan and Bowden, 2001) and complements the Department of Health's definition.

Prior to a review, the Trust provides data and documents demonstrating how clinical governance is working within its services, allowing CHAI to identify areas for detailed review during the site visit and briefing of the review team.

The CHAI review team is made up of a nurse, a doctor, an NHS manager, a lay member and another clinical professional, who visit the trust to interview trust staff, observe practice, verify information already obtained and gather further information. The aim of the visit is to collect information about how clinical governance is working throughout the organisation and to examine the experience of patients first hand. The review team compile an assessment of the clinical governance arrangements which are presented to the Trust verbally as well as in a written report. After the site visit, the CHAI and the Trust jointly hold a workshop to consider areas for action, identify future priorities and interpret them into achievable and measurable objectives. The resulting action plan is approved and monitored by the Strategic Health Authority. Clinical governance reviews by the CHAI do not attempt to comment on or measure actions that a Trust is taking to improve performance or comment on how well an organisation is doing against national performance indicators. This can sometimes result in irritation and resentment being directed at the CHAI that work to improve performance is not acknowledged (Fradd, 2002).

# Applying clinical governance in nephrology practice

The implementation of clinical governance within a nephrology department will involve two main areas: the training and development of clinical and non-clinical staff to ensure the effective delivery of health care, and timely and accurate information on which to base clinical decisions and monitor performance and outcomes. Quality improvements may be achieved through greater emphasis on evidence-based practice, the setting and monitoring of standards and clinical audit. Making the necessary changes to achieve quality may involve relatively minor changes to routine working practice or may merit redesign of a whole process of care.

To make clinical governance a reality, the concept of multidisciplinary clinical improvement groups needs to be developed (Hewer and Lugon, 2001). As there is always a world of difference between having a good idea and it being implemented successfully in practice, their establishment will not happen overnight. Good practice in one service, department or organisation should be recognised and shared with others. Nephrology care already has many of these structures in place to achieve this.

## Setting standards of care

Nephrology staff may not always appreciate how much of their day-to-day practice already depends on internally or externally defined standards: routines, treatment regimens, criteria for performing certain procedures, protocols and guidelines. Such standards are real even when unwritten. Standards can be either personal or service-related. Personal standards relate to the individual's professional practice and personal professionalism – derived from employment experience, knowledge, skills and practice.

For these to contribute to clinical governance they need to be formalised throughout the organisation and not just happening on an ad hoc basis. Service standards can be further subdivided into clinical and non-clinical standards. Non-clinical standards are already accepted as part of the normal practice. Risk management would be a good example of this.

Clinical standards would include standards derived from the results of clinical research and trials, an evidence-based approach, and increasingly standards from the specialist nephrology societies (Renal Association, EDTNA/ERCA,

RCN Nephrology Forum), the recently published Part One of the Renal National Service Framework (NSF) (Department of Health, 2004) and the National Institute for Clinical Excellence (NICE).

So what externally defined standards are available for nephrology staff to use? Most nephrology staff are aware that in 1995 the Renal Association, together with the Royal College of Physicians of London, produced a consensus statement of recommended standards and good practice for treatment of renal failure. These were updated in 1997 and the third edition was published in August 2002 (Renal Association, 2002). This document provides a framework for delivery of standards of renal care which have been widely accepted by purchasers and providers of renal services in the UK.

In January 2001, the Kidney Alliance launched a framework for planning and service delivery for established renal failure (ERF). This proposed seven national service standards which constituted the core objectives of a strategic plan for renal services for the next decade to ensure adequate and equitable nephrology care across the patient care continuum. This document identified that whilst much of the infrastructure that has been developed in the UK for established renal disease was sound, too few patients were receiving treatment, some of the treatment was insufficient and, perhaps most importantly from a clinical governance viewpoint, there were glaring inequalities in access to service and in the quality of services across the country (Kidney Alliance, 2001).

One example of this inequality are regional variations in the frequency of haemodialysis sessions. When this service inequality is viewed within a clinical governance framework, there are implications for many different areas, including the Regional Specialised Commissioning Groups (RSCGs) who need to have robust baseline assessment of need, appropriate service level agreements between the commissioners and the Trust, vigorous methods of data collection that can provide services and commissioners with measures of progress and performance, and finally human resources to deliver the care to patients and their families. Delivery of some of these service standards will represent a considerable challenge in many areas, particularly in view of the shortage of human resources.

The Renal National Service Framework (NSF) (Department of Health, 2004) aims to raise standards, reduce variations in services and improve the health care of patients with renal disease. The development process started in 2002 and two modules will be produced and published at intervals, comprising standards in: (1) dialysis and transplantation, and (2) prevention, primary care, acute renal failure and end of life care.

The UK Renal Registry was established by the Renal Association, with support from other renal organisations in the UK; participation is voluntary, but the expectation is that all UK renal and transplant units will ultimately take advantage of the opportunities offered by the Renal Registry database (see www.renalreg.com). The Renal Registry enables benchmarking by individual units, although currently the registry does not cover the entire country and boundaries between individual units are ill-defined.

During 2002 the need for increased home dialysis provision was appraised by NICE who recommend that all suitable patients should be offered the choice between home haemodialysis or haemodialysis in a hospital/satellite. Many units do not currently support home haemodialysis. Their recommendations could mean a fivefold increase in the number of patients conducting their own haemodialysis in the community and has implications for how patients are prepared for dialysis and how units achieve comprehensive choice for patients (National Institute for Clinical Excellence, 2002a).

The professional nursing literature offers limited explanation of the meaning of clinical nursing excellence, and thus few strategies to facilitate and maintain excellence in practice. However, most nurses will have examples of nursing excellence from their clinical experience. EDTNA/ERCA have published standards, which remain relevant to clinical practice today (Van Waeleghem and Edwards 1994).

## Audit changing practice

Clinical audit, and critically implementing changes in practice to 'close the audit cycle', is central to achieving optimal quality care. Most experienced clinicians are able to give examples from their own work where clinical audit has changed practice for the better, as in the example below.

Increasingly, central venous catheters (CVCs) are the only available option for vascular access due to the loss of viable peripheral access sites or urgency in the timing of dialysis requirement. Many practitioners will associate with the example of a renal unit who noted that there seemed to be an increase in the number of infections in their haemodialysis patients with CVCs. Following a detailed audit, results identified a lack of clear and consistent documentation of all aspects of CVC management, which made it impossible to know if the infection rate was higher than expected. The unit implemented changes in its information system to record these aspects for future audits. To look at only the infection rate in isolation would have been inadequate and would only result in a knee-jerk response to one aspect of CVCs in haemodialysis patients. Using a structured framework, nephrology staff would start by exploring the incidence and use of CVCs in haemodialysis patients within the unit.

Whilst the preferred access in any haemodialysis patients is a native arteriovenous fistula (AVF), most renal units are unable to achieve this. The UK Renal Association suggests that 67% of patients presenting within 3 months of dialysis should start haemodialysis with a usable native AVF (Renal Association, 2002). After 2 years of data, the Dialysis Outcomes and Practice Patterns Study (DOPPS) showed that only 47% of UK patients in the study started haemodialysis with a functioning AVF, whereas the European average is 66% (Young et al., 2000). The European average is still less than in the USA, suggesting that a facility's preferences and approaches to vascular access practice are major determinants of vascular access use (Pisoni et al., 2002).

The prevalence of AVFs and the number of planned patients who start dialysis with permanent access should be audited as this may well be a reflection of the efficiency and effectiveness of the service. Infection does represent a major complication associated with CVC use. Appropriate procedures, protocols, staff training and governance are therefore essential to maintain optimum outcomes in CVC management.

For those patients in whom CVCs are unavoidable, recent direction from NICE on the use of ultrasound-locating devices for placing CVCs (National Institute for Clinical Excellence, 2002b) advises that two-dimensional (2-D) imaging ultrasound guidance is recommended as the preferred method for insertion of CVCs into the internal jugular vein (IJV) in adults and children in elective situations and should be considered in most clinical circumstances.

Not only does this have implication for the delivery of care, but also units will have to ensure that those involved in placing CVCs using 2-D imaging ultrasound guidance have undertaken appropriate training to achieve competence. Units will have to demonstrate how they have implemented this guidance into practice. So, already, what started as an audit to look at infection has widened to a much larger issue.

## Process redesign

A particular example of how change can shape teams and result in much improved care for patients was evident when a review of a renal home care programme took place at a large NHS Trust (Wilde and Macefield, 2001). Staff in the home care teams were responsible for over 250 patients dialysing in the community on both peritoneal and haemodialysis. With over 150 new patients per year, they identified that the care was fragmented from initial referral through to ongoing care once dialysis was established. A cohort of professionals was involved in the delivery of care, resulting at times in duplication and inconsistency in information given to patients and their relatives.

After the process redesign (Figure 15.1), four home care teams comprising qualified staff and support workers were established, with each team having responsibility for a caseload of patients within a specified geographic location. Patients are seen in the community pre-dialysis, where an holistic assessment to identify the life goals of the patient can be done, and only after that was appropriate dialysis information given. The advantage for patients is that they are then in a continuous supportive cycle for all their non-inpatient care, throughout their replacement therapy.

Clinical governance recommends greater collaboration, consultation and involvement with the public and patients to ensure they have confidence in the service. Questionnaires were sent to patients who had been part of the change process 12 months after the change was introduced, to evaluate their satisfaction with the redesigned service; 76% of those who replied were very satisfied with the care they received during the pre-dialysis stage of their treatment and 80% were very satisfied with the care they had received once on dialysis. This is

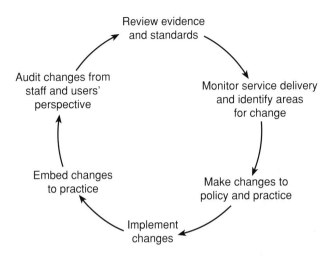

**Figure 15.1**  Process redesign home teams.

an example of how several staff members had a vision of how care could be delivered and inspired the teams to change practice for the benefit of patients.

## *Assessment and appraisal*

People generally do not perceive their capabilities in the same way as others. As a result, they may not fully understand or anticipate the impact of their actions and decisions on others. At best, this means that unintended consequences may result from their decisions. At worst, their individual effectiveness as well as their team's effectiveness may be compromised. In order to maximise their strengths and improve performance, individuals need clear and unambiguous feedback.

A technique that is gaining increasing popularity is the '360° Assessment' which provides structured multisource feedback on an individual staff member's competence (France, 1997). Feedback is sought from managers, professional supervisors and peers, other members of the multidisciplinary team, patients and other stakeholders on the individual's performance. A standard set of questions based on their experience with the individual is completed by all those giving feedback. At the very simplest level this could be a single question such as 'Do you have any concerns about this individual's professional practice? Yes/No. If so, please give details below'.

Data from assessors are aggregated and feedback is based on these aggregated data. Information provided by all sources is both confidential and anonymous. A 360° Assessment provides an opportunity for individuals to compare how they see themselves with how others view their performance. Both strengths and gaps become apparent and attention can be given to development in the right areas. A 360° Assessment is a complement to other systems of feedback and enhances other sources of feedback (France, 1997).

Formal annual appraisal has now been introduced throughout the NHS for both nursing and medical staff, giving the opportunity for each professional to meet with their manager/supervisor in a formalised setting. This will form a critical part of the implementation of clinical governance in an organisation, but to be successful it will need to be fully informed by structured data on personal performance, including data on actual work performed, results of clinical audit and data on attendance of audit, governance and continuing educational meetings within and outside the department.

## Data from clinical information systems

In order that collection and analysis of data for clinical governance and audit do not become hugely time-consuming and costly, as much as possible of the data collection process should be electronic.

Health care professionals should be able to rely on information systems and technology to support them in undertaking specific care activities with individual patients and in the operational management of those care services. Effective information technology will be vital to ensuring that there is easy access to relevant timely sources with excellent intercommunications. Hospitals usually have more than one system to capture data, for example, complaints, clinical risk management and library databases, as well as the relevant administrative support information and these do not interface with each other.

The current NHS information strategy provides a clear pathway to the development, over the next decade, of a fully integrated care record spanning all clinical and administrative aspects of a patient's care within the NHS (Department of Health, 2001c). Such an information system will become an essential audit tool to examine individual and departmental performance.

A review of 22 randomly selected CHI inspections reports examined the use of clinical information (Lugon, 2002) and concluded that attention needed to be given to using what is available now, and making it available to clinical teams. Also relevant information is not always either accessible or understandable to patients, and few organisations have yet managed to establish an information network across the primary/secondary care interface.

There is still a great deal to be done using currently available systems. In one NHS Trust, members of a multiprofessional team identified that nursing documentation of clinical assessments, interventions and outcomes was not being recorded on all of the patient caseload and that most of the nursing documentation was not accessible by other members of the multiprofessional team (Gorrod et al., 2003). The authors initiated a project to review the existing recording system, identify changes and training required for the nursing staff, deliver training and ensure that changes were in keeping with initiatives for improving quality as part of clinical governance. This reconfiguration project facilitated audit, captured nurse specialist activity in terms of clinical/educational assessment, intervention and outcomes and was able to identify best practice and care deficits.

## Inspiring excellence

How do staff ensure that rhetoric gets turned into reality and that staff are inspired and achieve excellence for all their patients? This requires effective and dynamic leadership. Health care traditions have emphasised hierarchy and bureaucratic rule-following. One of the mistakes made has been the assumption that leadership is about the post rather than personal qualities and ways of behaving. Leadership can happen at any level in an organisation or profession and relates to an individual shift or how staff lead themselves with integrity through day-to-day activities.

Effective leaders in nephrology care will ensure that they set parameters of safe legal and ethical frameworks within which excellence can develop and prosper. They will have a sense of personal integrity, a vision for the delivery of the service, a sense of reality, political awareness and a competency in the professional field.

## Research changing practice

It is known that, on its own, the dissemination of research evidence is insufficient to alter clinical practice (Grimshaw et al., 1995). No single intervention alone will be optimal in stimulating such change and a combination of approaches is generally recommended. Effective strategies therefore tend to be resource intensive and there continues to be a need for new, simple approaches that might produce benefit for relatively modest input (Ewings et al., 2000). A supportive environment is crucial to the nurture of a climate of innovation, and consideration of the environment and those who will be affected by the practice change provides a good starting point.

## Patients

Although both clinical governance and involving service users in the NHS are current priorities, they are all too often seen as being in separate boxes. Listening to the experiences of patients is a process, not an event, and it is most important to ensure that it is at the centre of clinical governance, and not at the periphery.

Patients themselves can also play a key role in optimising the quality of the care they receive, by making sure that they understand as much as possible about their condition, the care they receive and about how this might differ from any standard recommendations (Chamber, 2000). As renal replacement therapy is intensive and time-consuming, a well-informed patient will be able to detect areas where care is less than optimal, but it also makes it easier to achieve optimal outcomes in areas where the process of care is already well designed and implemented.

Patients' experiences should be integral to clinical governance in all nephrology departments. There is a wealth of readily available material to support clinicians and managers in obtaining and valuing patients' experiences (Kelson, 2000).

Clinical governance systems and processes cannot be assumed to be robust unless the views of actual and potential patients are sought and taken into account (Levenson, 2000). Equally, the experiences of service users must be integrated into all aspects of quality improvement, including clinical matters, in order to justify the efforts made by service users and voluntary organisations in giving their views, as well as the efforts made by NHS staff in seeking them.

The National Kidney Federation (NKF) has always advocated patients knowing, understanding and participating in all aspects of their nephrology care, including their investigation results. During 2000 the NKF surveyed its members to find out what they knew about their haemoglobin results (National Kidney Federation, 2000). Of the 400 patients who replied, 84% had heard of haemoglobin, 67% knew their own level, 47% had never heard of national standards, 20% said they had never discussed haemoglobin, anaemia or any other result numbers with a doctor and 87% would like to have a printed leaflet giving such information. Such a leaflet was subsequently produced and distributed in 'Z-card' format – hopefully empowering patients to ensure that management of their own anaemia in ERF is optimal (see www.kidney.org.uk).

## Summary

Clinical governance is becoming embedded in daily nephrology practice and many nephrology staff express positive feelings about the concept and associated tasks. For the individual nephrology practitioner in clinical practice, this will mean that you will:

(1)  Be aware of best practice guidelines and ensure they are adopted as part of clinical audit within your clinical area and your individual practice development.
(2)  Contribute to your department and organisation's assessment of its present ability for quality improvement.
(3)  Lead and participate in quality improvements within clinical areas.
(4)  Work within multiprofessional teams to identify ways to improve.
(5)  Assume a full part in continuing professional and personal development programmes.
(6)  Ensure users and carers are involved in the planning of service improvements.

Most units welcome the publication of Part One of the Renal NSF and the influences that it will have on nephrology care delivery, such as auditing, significant-event auditing, dealing with complaints, collecting data, establishing comparable databases, but most importantly the delivery of patient care.

Professional learning plans, staff appraisals, departmental away days, continuing professional development and using evidence-based practice are all integral to full implementation of clinical governance. Difficulties at a clinical level will relate to pressure of time, lack of resources, lack of support and to some emotional and conceptual concerns around the implementation of a clinical governance framework. Clinical governance leaders within nephrology departments and Trusts need to continue to invest time and resources so that early progress can be maintained. Its implementation is crucial for the quality of health care to become the driving force in the development of renal services.

# References

Bevan, G. and Bowden, D. (2001) Clinical data and information, and clinical governance. *Clinical Governance Bulletin* **2** (2), 2–3.

Bolton, W.K. (1998) The role of the nephrologist in ESRD/Pre-ESRD care: a collaborative approach. *Journal of the American Society of Nephrology* **9** (Suppl 12), S90–95.

Campbell, A. (1999) Improvement of patient care through a collaborative approach to patient education and triage. *Advances in Renal Replacement Therapy* **6** (4), 347–50.

Chamber, R. (2000) *Involving Patients and the Public.* Radcliffe Medical Press, Oxford.

Comptroller and Auditor General (2001) *Handling Clinical Negligence Claims in England.* Stationery Office, London.

Crouch, D. (2003) Breaking the error chain. *Nursing Times* **99** (3), 22–5.

Currie, L. and Loftus-Hills, A. (2002) The nursing view of clinical governance. *Nursing Standard* **16** (27), 40–44.

Department of Health (1998) *A First Class Service, Quality in the New NHS.* NHS Executive, London.

Department of Health (2000) *An Organisation with a Memory.* Department of Health, London.

Department of Health (2001a) *A Commitment to Quality, A Quest for Excellence.* Department of Health, London.

Department of Health (2001b) *Building a Safer NHS for Patients.* Department of Health, London.

Department of Health (2001c) *Building the Information core – Implementing the NHS Plan.* Department of Health, London.

Department of Health (2004) *The National Service Framework for Renal Services. Part One: Dialysis and Transplantation.* www.doh.gov.uk/nsf/renal.

Donaldson, L.J. and Muir Grey, J.A. (1998) Clinical governance; a quality duty for health care organisations. *Quality in Healthcare* **7** (Suppl), S37–44.

Ewings, P., Pearson, N., Myers, P. and Speakman, M. (2000) A strategy for supporting the implementation of evidence-based practice. *Clinical Governance Bulletin* 1 (3), 7–8.

Fradd, L. (2002) The ultimate wake-up call. *Nursing Times* **98** (45), 17.

France, S. (1997) *360 Degree Appraisal.* Spiro Press, Newbury.

Gorrod, R., Keogh, A.M., Stribling, B. and Howlett, T.A. (2003) Reconfiguration of diabetes nurses' record keeping within a clinical workstation. *Journal of Diabetic Nursing* **7** (1), 28–32.

Grimshaw, J., Freemantle, N. and Wallace, S. (1995) Developing and implementing clinical practice guidelines. *Quality in Health Care* **4**, 55–64.

Haslock, I. (1999) Introducing clinical governance in an acute trust. *Hospital Medicine (London)* **60**, 744–7.

Hewer, P. and Lugon, M. (2001) Clinical governance – putting it into practice in a trust. *Clinical Governance Bulletin* **2** (1), 8–9.

Kelson, M. (2000) User involvement in clinical governance: good practice guidance and examples. *Clinical Governance Bulletin* **1** (1), 2–3.

Keogh, A.M. (1999) Teamwork and the renal nurse. *Nursing Times* **95** (25), 52–4.

Kidney Alliance (2001) *End Stage Renal Failure – A Framework for Planning and Service Delivery.* Kidney Alliance, London.

Levenson, R. (2000) Involving patients – an opportunity for the whole organisation. *Clinical Governance Bulletin* **1** (1), 11–12.

Lugon, M. (2002) Clinical governance – rhetoric or reality? *Clinical Governance Bulletin* **3** (3), 1–2.

McSherry, R. and Pearce, P. (2002) *Clinical Governance. A Guide to Implementation for Healthcare Professionals.* Blackwell Science, Oxford.

Miller, J. (2002) *Nursing Times Monographs: Clinical Governance.* Emap Healthcare, London.

National Institute for Clinical Excellence (2002a) *Guidance on Home Compared with Hospital Haemodialysis for Patients with End-Stage Renal Failure.* Technology Guidance 48. NHS Executive, London.

National Institute for Clinical Excellence (2002b) *Guidance on the Use of Ultrasound Locating Devices for Placing Central Venous Catheters.* Technology Guidance. NHS Executive, London.

National Kidney Federation (2000) Knowing your numbers. *Kidney Life* **1** (Autumn).

National Patient Safety Agency (2001) *Doing Less Harm.* National Patient Safety Agency, London.

Pisoni, R.L., Young, E.W., Dykstra, D.M., Greenwood, R.N., Hecking, E., Gillespie, B., Wolfe, R.A., Goodkin, D.A. and Held, P.J. (2002) Vascular access use in Europe and the United States: results from the DOPPS. *Kidney International* **61** (1), 305–316.

Renal Association (2002) *Treatment of Adult Patients with Renal Failure*, 3rd edn. Royal College of Physicians, London.

Roderick, N. and Roderick, A. (2001) The myth of accurate clinical information. In: *Advancing Clinical Governance* (Lugon, M. Secker-Walker, J., eds), pp. 111–24. RSM Press, London.

Secretary of State for Health (1998) *A First Class Service, Quality in the New NHS.* NHS Executive, London.

Styles, B. (1994) Viol bodies. *Health Service Journal* **104** (5388), 30–32.

Swage, T. (2000) *Clinical Governance in Health Care Practice.* Butterworth Heinemann, Oxford.

Van Waeleghem, J.P. and Edwards, P. (1994) *EDTNA/ERCA European Standards for Nephrology Nursing Practice.* EDTNA/ERCA, Ghent.

Wallace, L.M., Freeman, T., Latham, L., Walshe, K. and Spurgeon, P. (2001) Organisational strategies for changing clinical practice: how trusts are meeting the challenges of clinical governance. *Quality in Health Care* **10** (2), 76–82.

Wickens, P. (1995) Why 'how' is as crucial as 'what'. *People Management* **1** (6), 38–9.

Wilde, C. and Macefield, J. (2001) Improvement in care: a collaborative approach to rehabilitation. *EDTNA/ERCA Journal* **27** (2), 69–71.

Young, E.W., Goodkin, D.A., Mapes, D.L., Port, F.K., Keen, M.L., Chen, K., Maroni, B.L., Wolfe, R.A. and Held, P.J. (2000) The Dialysis and Outcomes and Practice Study (DOPPS): an international haemodialysis study. *Kidney International* **57** (Suppl 74), S74–82.

# Chapter 16
# Caring for Staff in Renal Care

*Cordelia Ashwanden*

## Introduction

One of the nephrology challenges of the 21st century is how to care for the ever-growing numbers of people with renal failure. The number of people requiring renal replacement therapy (RRT) continues to grow and the number of specialist health care providers needed to care for this section of the population is not increasing commensurately (Winearls, 1999; Charter, 2002; Hawkes and Norfolk, 2002). Renal care is total care of the patient, involving all members of the health care team, and shortage of any of its members affects the whole team and the provision of care, which in turn can affect the treatment outcome.

Nurses have been shown to be the pivotal force in the care of those with renal failure (Bevan, 1998; Kidney Alliance, 2001). Their expertise is highly regarded within renal units and their knowledge sought by renal physicians and the manufacturers of dialysers (Bevan, 1998). Because of their pivotal nature to the provision of RRT, this chapter will concentrate to a greater extent on the care of nurses, but this care should be extended to all the health care team. The chapter will discuss the methods of recruiting nurses into renal care and how it is possible to promote retention of this specialised health care force. The benefits of specialised further education will be evaluated.

This chapter will discuss the aggression and violence that are becoming increasingly common in dialysis units and which for some is a deterrent to staying in this speciality. Finally, the specialist role of the renal nurse is evaluated in terms of how far this role can be expanded and what implications there are for the nurses and renal units of the future.

## Method

The information in this chapter has been gathered by observations that have involved the author in participating in the life of dialysis units, both as a member of the team and as a researcher. Data were gathered from informal interviews with hermeneutical interpretations, which as Taylor (1993) suggests is a special kind of interpretation that facilitates the discovery of the hidden meanings within the interpretation of phenomena. A questionnaire was used to find information about the perceived benefits of specialist education. The electronic databases of CINAHL, Web of Science, MEDLINE and the RCN database (1997–2002) were some of the information services used to guide and substantiate the discussion in this chapter.

## Staffing challenges

This chapter cannot do more than briefly explore some of the reasons for the lack of recruits for general nursing, but this shortage is significant since it underlies the shortage of nurses working in renal care. The various surveys that have been conducted to discover the number of people entering nursing offer diverse results as to the state of nursing recruitment and it can depend on the evidence read as to the conclusions drawn.

A review prepared by Buchan and Seccombe (2002) considered that the Department of Health statistics were over optimistic and that a further 20 000 nurses are still needed to fulfil the Government's promise of the numbers of trained nurses working in the NHS (RCN, 2002). This difference in numbers was in part due to the different interpretations of data. However, it is a fact that the population of the UK is an ageing one, affecting the numbers of young people applying to train as nurses as well as increasing those who will be retiring, and affecting the number of potential patients (Buchan and Seccombe, 2002).

It is important to consider why the young people of today do not wish to enter the profession of nursing. The answers are complex and not fully under-stood, although there is much literature written exploring the reasons for the staffing crisis [see Cunningham and Kitson (2000) and Jackson et al. (2002) amongst others]. Peach (1999) attempts to rationalise the reluctance of people to enter the profession, but he also admits that no one can give the definitive reason. Financial rewards although important are not the only consideration. Nursing is considered to be an unattractive career choice and is seen by young people to be a 'low status job' (United Kingdom Central Council for Nursing, Midwifery and Health Visiting, 1999b) where the nurse is not valued enough for her/his knowledge and expertise (Jowett et al., 1999).

Nursing is without the social status that is awarded to many post-university careers. Moreover, nursing is still a predominately female profession which leads to other conflicts caused by the accepted women's social role. Managing home, social and work life becomes ever more complicated, and even the introduction of flexible working hours can only be of significant value to a small percentage of nurses (Brooks and Swailes, 2002). Combining the nursing work schedules on a busy ward with caring for the home and children is extremely difficult (Brooks and Swailes, 2002). Also Jowett et al. (1999) did find that the work of the nurse is grossly underestimated and the expectations of what should be accom-plished in the daily routine have increased significantly over the last decade.

For many outside the NHS the nurse is still 'the hand maiden of the doctor' acting solely under orders (Nightingale, 1859). This is changing, and, as Peach (1999) explains, nurses' expertise is continuing to increase, but for the general public it is often only after a stay in hospital that nurses are recognised for their skills and knowledge. The NHS advocates partnership in care between all members of the multiprofessional team, but for this to happen in the true sense when all the partners are valued equally, there has to be a change in the culture in health care (Bristol Royal Infirmary Report, 2001).

The career structure for nurses is not well defined, in fact there is little advertised about what employment opportunities there are for the trained staff nurse (Brooks and Swailes, 2002; Major, 2002). Work in the renal unit reflects this apparent lack of structured opportunities; but as knowledge and expertise increase so there are many paths of further specialisation that are possible for the renal nurse. Some units today have too many nurses who cannot achieve promotion as the budget does not allow for this, despite increased experience; conversely, in some units there are no suitable people capable or willing to accept the responsibilities of the higher grades, which is symptomatic of the difficulties encountered by the woman/nurse when juggling her two lives. Why should people come into nursing where the pay is not equal to that in business, hours are difficult and the rewards or job satisfaction are no longer great? The frustrations of not having time to care or to care in the way that had been expected are voiced as one of the primary reasons for people to leave the profession (Peach, 1999; Finlayson, 2002).

## What is renal nursing and why is it different?

### *Medical complexity*

Renal nursing is nursing people with renal disease, a disease that is often superimposed on other medical problems and may lead to a variety of other complications. Nursing the person with renal failure is complex. Co-morbidities such as diabetes, cardiac problems and psychological illnesses are exacerbated or caused by the renal disease and its treatment. Munshi et al. (2001) in their study of older people (more than 75 years of age) found that 93% of those starting haemodialysis had co-morbidities. The renal nurse requires knowledge and understanding of the changing technical and pharmaceutical treatments available, and this is constantly being updated as medical knowledge increases, which means that renal nurses have to be prepared to continue their education throughout a career in the renal speciality.

### *Stress*

Treatment of those with renal disease is a highly specialised field of nursing with special stresses. It is often a unique involvement of staff with a patient over a long period of time, either as a haemodialysis nurse providing intensive technical care over long periods, or as a peritoneal nurse in repetitive procedures and intensive learning and teaching. Whichever therapy is being used, renal nursing means nursing the chronically sick with its attendant problems, but also every dialysis treatment is a major unique critical intervention without which the patient will eventually die (Bevan, 1998). With any chronic illness there is no cure; it is adaptation to the illness and its demands that make life hard for those on dialysis (Auer, 2002).

The satisfactions for the nurse cannot come from cure but rather from the care involved with dialysis and transplantation, and the interactions between the carer and recipient of that care. It is the commitment of patients to their survival that will help them to optimise the treatment outcomes, but the provision of good treatment by the whole health care team can influence the treatment outcome (Kidney Alliance, 2001).

## Long-term care

Nursing in the renal unit offers the chance of commitment over long periods of time, and caring for people over many years may mean that special relationships can develop (Tschudin, 1997). One aspect that sets the renal unit apart from other units in hospital is the partnership between the multidisciplinary team and the patient and the patients' commitment to survival. It is through this partnership that the team of patient and carer works towards the common goal of better treatment outcomes. While completing her research the author was continually being told how important the concept of one's 'own nurse' was. Too often because of pressure of work and non-appreciation of this important concept, the named nurse was unable to be with 'her' patient in the planning of the daily work schedule.

## Frustrations

Caring for the chronically ill has frustrations for the carers as well as the sick. There is no cure and for those with renal failure there are the stresses and uncertainties of the ever-present treatment to be coped with. Patients feel that someone has to be blamed for their condition and accepting not only the limitations of renal disease but also the frustrations of the omnipotent treatment is one of the hardest parts of the adjustment process. Renal disease takes over the body and the health carers take over the person. There is inevitability about the treatment that makes it difficult to adapt to the limited life style. There are nurses who become so overtaken with technology that they forget the human care the patient requires to mitigate the technological aspects of the treatment (Bevan, 1998).

Nursing in the renal speciality is both frustrating and rewarding. Renal nurses have time to develop relationships that enable them to empathise with the patients and understand the daily stresses of life with renal failure. The small victories are of great importance for the patient. A dialysis session that goes well after a period of problems can enable the patient to do something he or she has not done for a long time, such as walking, cooking or even gardening. This may provide a feeling of satisfaction for nurse and patient: 'Life has to be more than dialysis' as was voiced by one young man.

However, renal nurses need special skills to help develop partnerships with patients and families, and they have to appreciate the latter's frustrations as well as understanding their own emotions. The nurse has specialised knowledge to share and through sharing can inspire patients to take more control and care about their blood results and the progression of treatments. The longevity of those receiving dialysis means that there is time for these relationships to develop. Good partnerships are therapeutic for both nurses and patients.

## Caring

Tschudin (1997) offers the idea that people enter nursing because they are in some way needing to be cared for. This is hard to prove, but it does provide a challenging idea about why people enter nursing. If a nurse is searching for someone to care for her/him, perhaps that is why people do not remain in nursing, when they realise that nursing cannot fulfil their personal needs. Society has changed from when the ward sister was a figure of awe but also benevolence, who could be turned to for help in most situations.

The modern matron does not necessarily have time to spend physically and emotionally caring for her/his nurses. Generally, the modern matron or ward sister is trying to cope with family and social life as well as the increasing demands of the hospital and the ward. However, if this idea is turned around, it is possible that the best ward sisters or unit managers are those who are no longer looking for someone to care for them, but who have the time and maturity to care for those under them. Beech (2002) and Welford (2002) both discuss how good leadership can motivate and care for those within the team. Staff will remain where they are motivated in their work and where they know they are valued. Renal units need good leaders.

## Skills

In the renal unit some practices (such as insertion of central lines) are now performed by renal nurses rather than medical staff. These opportunities mean that the professional boundaries are changing and the Department of Health (2000) has registered the need to document these changes. However, a dialogue is needed about how far these roles should be further expanded; as discussed by Scholes and Vaugham (2002), there can be problems in the nurses taking on the traditional doctors' roles.

The Kidney Alliance (2001) describes the role of the renal nurse and the report accepts the expanded practice for those working in renal units. Part One of the Renal National Service Framework (Department of Health, 2004) will help to clarify the special needs of the renal nurse and will evaluate how much further these roles need to be expanded to provide the right care in the right place for the good of the patient.

## *Continuity of care*

Freeman et al. (2000) evaluate the importance of continuity of care for the wellbeing of the patient; they consider that in most cases patients benefit from having as few people as possible involved in an individual's care. In the dialysis units, nurses are the constant factor and it is they who can provide the constant care. Scholes and Vaugham (2002) discuss the benefits and problems of training the nurse to undertake some of the doctors' roles. Certainly when trained these nurses can provide the expertise that the continually changing junior doctors are unable to give. However, the caring role, which is the essence of nursing (Kitson, 1993), has to be acknowledged and should not be superseded by medical and technical wizardry.

It is the skills and expanded knowledge that should be used by the renal nurse to consolidate continuity of care, providing expert knowledge for the benefit of the patient and the multidisciplinary team. Specialist nurses are settled in their post and not only can they undertake extended practices as a regular part of their role, but also because they understand the principles and practices of dialysis they can give the person receiving and giving RRT understanding and support. They also can be present in the unit to give advice and help to all the team. There are, as yet, no long-term studies to show whether, by removing the opportunity to learn from junior doctors, the care that future consultants can offer will be compromised.

## Recruitment of nurses

The section looks at the different strategies that can be used to attract nurses into the renal speciality. The review 'Fitness to Practice' (United Kingdom Central Council for Nursing, Midwifery and Health Visiting, 1999a) sets out the problems facing the delivery of health care within the NHS, which has significance for the provision of care in renal units. The Department of Health (DoH) has recently claimed that the shortage of nurses has been addressed and there are increasing numbers of nurses in the profession, but Buchan and Seccombe (2002) challenge the DoH's statistics.

In practice, renal units do have a continuing shortage of nurses (Kidney Alliance, 2001) and other members of the health care team, which influences the provision of treatments in units. Those working in the NHS do know there has to be rationing of health care because of the shortage of staff. In a specialised field such as renal nursing this problem is exacerbated (Winearls, 1999). The methods used at present to recruit nurses into the renal field need to be evaluated and innovative ways to attract more recruits need to be explored.

## *Methods of recruitment*

The 1990s were times when 'Open Days' and 'Road Shows' were commonly used (apart from the usual advertising) to attract staff. However, neither of these innovative methods proved particularly successful. As one manager reported, 'they only came for a look', and another reported that out of the 32 people who attended an open day she had four enquiries and only two were finally recruited. Therefore, in renal care, these methods have largely been rejected. Advertising in glossy magazines and journals has only a limited use and again should be carefully looked at as it is expensive and too often it does not bring forth the necessary applicants.

Because the majority of the nursing workforce are women with families, family considerations influence the choice of where one works. The concentration on getting nurses 'back to work' has helped to fill some of the staffing gaps. Peach (1999) discusses how flexibility in work patterns may attract some people back to nursing, but nursing remains a 24-hour occupation. If those with family commitments are rostered into the most attractive working patterns, such as school hours and no night working, this can cause resentment between team members.

Renal units have to find some unique way to encourage nurses into the units. The unit has to become well known as a progressive and supporting environment to work, and this is possible through staff attendance at conferences and publications. It is surprising how people, when asked why they came to a unit, said they had heard about it from colleagues, or read articles written by staff in a particular unit. The renal community is small enough for people to know about other units and how they function. The reputation of good management is appreciated and if people have a choice of where they will work this is one of the prime attractions. The unit should have a good reputation for caring for staff through good leadership.

## *Renal care*

The person wanting to specialise has already spent time as a registered nurse with the responsibilities and rewards that are involved, but now has to make the decision to 'start again'. Previous general nursing experience is essential to be a successful renal nurse, but often that experience is unrecognised. Units have different policies about the grading of a nurse coming into a new speciality, and certainly it is not helpful for recruitment if the novice renal nurse is downgraded. However, the question has to be acknowledged: where does a novice nurse fit within the structure of the renal health care team?

Acquired skills, experience and pre-knowledge have to be recognised, but this does create challenges when there is a wealth of new knowledge and practice to be learnt. Some recruits are not willing to face the perceived ignominy of working with more junior nurses as their mentors (Major, 2002). Some admit to being scared about the technology of haemodialysis or peritoneal dialysis and the new practices that have to be understood. Machinery can make some people feel helpless and it does take time to appreciate the finer workings of the machines that offer life to people with renal failure.

The rewards of renal nursing have been cited as the special opportunities to form long-term partnerships, and the expansion and use of specialised knowledge. The author, during her research, was provided with various reasons for entering renal nursing such as 'I want new knowledge', 'because I want to be able to expand my practice and use new techniques'. This is supported by Cunningham and Kitson (2000) who claim that new knowledge motivates people. However, there were many to whom the practicalities of working on a renal unit were the important factors such as: 'no working on Sundays', 'no night duty' or 'because I will have time for my patients'.

## Overseas nurses

The employment of nurses from overseas has helped the recruitment challenge in the immediate present, but this staff drain from other countries has posed ethical problems. The government has had to provide guidelines to designate those countries from which it is acceptable to employ nurses in order to mitigate the effects of the drain on the foreign home health services (RCN, 2002). However, it could be argued that taking overseas nurses affects the health care of the home country, as the countries themselves lose some of their highly trained work force and the country of employment is only gaining a temporary reprieve. Although some of the most pressing crises have been assisted by employment of overseas nurses, they are not the answer to the long-term problem (Witchell and Osuch, 2002). The long-term effects of employing overseas nurses in the NHS need further investigation.

Once here the nurse often has to have extra training or 'adaptation' to reach the required competency levels, but it could be argued that the pre-knowledge and experience gained in their home country has not been fully recognised or respected. Assessment can be a poor guide as there are too many dependencies, and it must be extremely frustrating as well as demoralising for an experienced renal nurse to be assessed badly and to then spend time re-learning what she/he already knows (Daniel et al., 2001).

It takes time and understanding to help these nurses from different cultures adapt to the UK's way of working and there are reported instances of bullying and discrimination (Witchell and Osuch, 2002). There has been some perceived 'unfairness' about the packages offered to the overseas nurse, as was expressed to the author: 'Why could not the money which is being spent attracting these nurses be spent on better remuneration for nurses already in the system?' Some believe that the expense involved in interviewing nurses from the other side of the world with offers of attractive packages to encourage them to abandon home and family for short periods of time seem to be short-sighted.

However, a wider view is needed to objectively evaluate the situation, and although the overseas nurses are a most valued immediate answer to the staffing crisis, they do not solve the long-term problem. If more effort was put into supporting nurses already within the UK system, perhaps this would lessen the need to take nurses from countries who can ill afford to lose the best of their workforce.

## Nursing schools

Nursing schools in the UK now offer a predominately university-style training, where nurses are taught theory and practical skills, and have supernumerary status on practice placements.

Despite the fact that renal failure and its treatment is now recognised as one of the fastest growing challenges in health care (Casey, 2002), there is too little taught in nursing schools about renal practice. The European Dialysis and Transplant Nurses Association/European Renal Care Association (EDTNA/ ERCA) has identified that few nursing schools have a planned renal programme for students. EDTNA/ERCA (Fuchs et al., 2002) recently published guidelines on the number of hours that should be devoted to renal nursing in a basic core curriculum. This curriculum should be well prepared to give the student nurse an overall insight into the general care of renal patients (Fuchs et al., 2002), and 16 hours of learning and teaching is recommended.

# Retention of staff

Education, specialisation, job satisfaction, support and good management are all factors in the retention of staff. Once having attracted the qualified staff into the renal units, we need to discuss how this workforce can be maintained and how specialisation can promote better care. To provide the best renal care, nurses should have the specialist training that enables them to understand renal disease.

## Education

Post-registration renal courses which prepare nurses for the daily phenomena in the units offer a wide knowledge base from which nurses are able to practise as renal practitioners. However, there is nothing that can give the nurse experience better than the daily work. Nurses in this specialist field have to become confident practitioners responsible for their actions and able to qualify those actions through their theoretical and practical knowledge. Experience and intuition are vital and these can only be gained through practice based on knowledge, and the nurse develops from the 'novice' through to the 'expert practitioner' (Benner, 1984). Increased knowledge and experience can affect the outcomes of treatments for both the giver and receiver of the care.

EDTNA/ERCA (Kuntzle and Thomas, 1995) has developed a post-basic core curriculum in nephrology nursing, which may, in the future, be recognised by all the authorities in Europe. This Association has encouraged nursing schools and hospitals to use this curriculum upon which to base their post-registration nephrology courses. To take this a stage further, EDTNA/ERCA in 2001 began a system of accreditation of post-basic renal courses which will in the future improve standardisation of renal nursing education in Europe.

## *Practical education*

The renal unit is a frightening environment for the novice practitioner. The first few days in this new environment are most important. First impressions make a difference to future happiness and job satisfaction and can influence the nurse's desire to remain in the unit (Obrey, 2002). To belong to a well-functioning team mitigates the fear of the unknown and promotes good working practices and the motivation to remain in the renal field (Welford, 2002). As has been stated, to have renal failure does not exclude being affected with other diseases, and knowledge of renal failure has to be used in the context of other illnesses. Too often when discussing renal care, it is the dialysis unit where the main focus lies.

However, a renal unit comprises the haemodialysis and peritoneal dialysis units as well as renal clinics and a renal ward. A renal ward should be staffed with specialist renal staff, who understand the complexities of renal disease in conjunction with other illnesses, amongst other general trained staff. Transplant facilities are not available in every renal unit, but the specialist renal nurse needs to have first-hand experience of working therein.

The continuing discussions about the rotation of staff within the various areas of the renal units show that there are divergent opinions. Managers consider that staff remain more interested in their work when there is variety, but some nurses when questioned stated they did not like rotation. Others were in favour as, like the managers, they saw it as having the benefit of diversity. However, there are practical problems to be overcome when working in the wards rather than on a unit, where night duty is an essential requirement. One of the main senior nurses' concerns about having rotation of staff was that expertise such as the skilful placing of needles would be lost to the detriment of both the patient and the practitioner. The National Service Framework (Department of Health, 2004) gives more concrete proposals for the motivation of the workforce, recognising the expertise within the health care team.

## *Teachers*

Education is the way forward for the renal nurse, but specialised renal education necessitates a highly trained teacher. It is essential that the educationalist is also a skilled practitioner who understands the needs of the care providers and receivers and can work in the renal units as well as teach. Too many nurses in education have forgotten the reality of the dialysis units or the work on a stressful ward full of acutely sick people. The clinical trainer is present on the wards to ensure that practice is following research findings and best clinical practice, but the teachers who run the courses also need to have current experience in renal care. There are other roles that need specialist renal knowledge such as the renal social worker, the renal nutritionist and podiatrist, to name but a few. The list appears endless, but it has to be appreciated that all in the multidisciplinary team require specialist education in order to be able to provide good renal care.

## Violence and aggression as a factor in retaining staff

Having examined some of the reasons why nurses enter renal nursing, this section looks at why some nurses leave this specialist field. Jackson et al. (2002) and Wells and Bowers (2002) discuss aggression towards the nursing staff, but also the aggression of the nursing staff towards the patients and to each other. Aggression is not necessarily physical and the psychological aggression and verbal abuse that humans can display towards each other have to be considered. The literature shows that overseas nurses particularly have to cope with discrimination and bullying amongst all the other problems they face when away from the familiar (Witchell and Osuch, 2002).

Nursing the chronically ill is frustrating and can be responsible for feelings of aggression (although the rewards of renal nursing are great) and this does need to be considered when discussing violence and aggression. Jackson et al. (2002) discuss the probability of violence being a factor in recruitment and retention of staff. From experience this author would agree with Farrell (1999) that it is the covert harassment or intimidation of staff towards each other that makes staff wish to leave the work place, rather than the threat of actual violence.

### Incidence of violence

Violence in health care has been defined as any aggressive behaviour aimed at inflicting harm or discomfort on its victims (Felton, 1997). Violence and aggression are now a fact of general working conditions in the NHS (Wells and Bowers, 2002). They argue that it is not a new phenomenon, but the reporting of it and interest in it have grown. The real prevalence of violence against nurses is unknown because the literature demonstrates that there is under-reporting, despite hearsay evidence that the episodes of violence are increasing according to Adib et al. (2002), Jackson et al. (2002) and Wells and Bowers (2002).

### Causes of violence

Renal patients can suffer from mental illness along with any other illnesses and some mental illnesses increase the instances of violence. Renal disease carries with it the problems of reduced brain function caused through dialysis and renal impairment (Levy and Cohen, 2000). Some of the medication prescribed for these patients has an adverse effect on personality (Levy and Cohen, 2000). The frustrations and loss of control that are inherent in the treatment of kidney disease are also factors that can predetermine acts of violence. Aggression can be exacerbated by anxiety and pressures within the work place (Paterson et al., 1997). It could be asserted that the renal unit with its usual overcrowding of long-term chronically ill patients is a situation ready for aggression.

It has to be assumed that violence and aggression are increasing in renal units as everywhere in the NHS. There are reported instances of violence and aggression, most of which take the form of verbal abuse, but there are growing instances of actual violence against the staff from patients (O'Connell et al., 2000). In the environment of the unit with its ever-increasing population and workload, the likelihood of violence and aggression is increased (Jackson et al., 2002).

O'Connell et al. (2000) suggest that the more common form of aggression which causes 'harm and discomfort' to the individual is sexual harassment or verbal abuse. Nurses working outside the hospital, such as the community peritoneal nurse, are also exposed to a high risk of violence and there has to be some form of security for these nurses when doing home visits (O'Connell et al., 2000; Jackson et al., 2002). However, all health care staff need protection from the increasing violence both in and out of hospitals. Some units have the system of giving 'cards' for unacceptable behaviour. A dialysis patient may receive a yellow card as a warning, but once a red card is issued he or she will be refused treatment in that particular unit and be transferred elsewhere. This cannot in many cases help the situation, but the dialysis nurse has few options. The patient has to receive treatment or will die, but moving him or her from one unit to another may only serve to increase that patient's isolation and feelings of frustration, which could increase his or her violent behaviour.

Loss of control is a cause of anxiety, which is a common feature in renal disease. Unfortunately kidney failure means patients lose control over their life, over the treatment and over their body. In ERF the prognosis is uncertain, and the regular dialysis treatments have uncertain outcomes. Even daily living is uncertain when the body is an unreliable refuge. Changing lifestyles and adaptation to chronic illness all contribute to anxiety. Abusive language and threatening behaviour are an outward sign of anxiety.

The dialysis units are places where both staff and patients suffer from stresses leading to anxiety which frustrates the development of partnerships, so the causes of stress need to be addressed where possible. Good communications are the first way to mitigate stress (Bristol Royal Infirmary Report, 2001). Information about the disease and foreseen problems are an immediate help, but care is required to ensure that the information is not only given but understood. Anxiety about the unknown is sometimes difficult to allay because there are so many unsolved questions associated with kidney disease. However, there are ways of alleviating some of the daily worries that accompany RRT and these should be utilised where possible.

Knowledge of what is happening as the patient waits for treatment is a prime way to relieve daily anxiety. Nurses are desensitised by repetitive practice so that they do not always appreciate some of the anxieties of the patients. Acknowledgement and sympathetic handling of these anxieties will help relieve situations that can cause aggression.

### Peer violence

Violence does not occur without provocation. It is recognised in the literature that nursing itself conspires to promote an environment where all sorts of violence, including bullying and sexual harassment, can develop (O'Connell et al., 2000; Major, 2002). O'Connell et al. (2000) found that 32.7% of nurses identified the source of bullying or intimidation as coming from their peers and senior nurses. Major (2002) and Scholes and Vaugham (2002) both discuss the problems engendered through poorly functioning teams.

The continuing staff shortages mean that nurses are vulnerable to intimidation from their senior staff about working hours and off-duty. The working lives of the nurses have to fit into their home social lives and too often an unsympathetic manager can make life even more difficult. Part-time workers can ease the staff crises, but the needs of the full-time worker have to be included in the overall time schedules in the units (Brooks and Swailes, 2002). Team working and good relations which can develop into working partnerships will ease the stressful environment which may promote aggression of both the staff and patients.

## Specialisation

### The benefits of specialisation

The United Kingdom Central Council for Nursing, Midwifery and Health Visiting (1999b) has recognised the need to set out guidelines for the development of a higher level of practice which will protect the practitioner and also the patient. There are university courses that offer academic knowledge together with practical skills, ending in a degree of advanced practice, which prepare the nurse for expanding practice (Casey, 2002). The concentration of knowledge into one field is certainly for the benefit of the patient, but in specialisation it could be argued that other skills are potentially lost.

Because renal failure does not exclude other illnesses it can mean that general nursing knowledge has to be at the base of most decisions; therefore previous knowledge and experience will add to the sum of the renal nurses' knowledge. Nurses appreciate the renal training and the exclusivity it brings. A large survey carried out in Australia on specialist paediatric nurses (Johnson and Copnell, 2002) found that the most highly rated benefit of specialist training was the ability to link theory to practice. This was reinforced by the results of a small questionnaire ($n = 15$) conducted by the author where this ability to relate theory to practice came second to increased self-confidence which was voted by 50% of those replying as the most important benefit.

The importance of the increased self-confidence that was gained from the course poses the question 'do we not value our nurses enough?' Is it the lack of self-esteem that nurses feel about the profession that is responsible for the shortage of nurses? As Jackson et al. (2002) suggest, is it the lack of confidence that creates vulnerability to intimidation and bullying, which again influences the retention of nurses? Knowledge gives confidence, confidence to be oneself and be an autonomous practitioner, which again brings job satisfaction.

## *The specialist nurse*

Specialist renal nurses not only have to know the aetiology of renal disease, but also understand the effects of renal disease on all the systems in the body. Renal nursing is complex with a wide variety of treatment modalities. The specialist role of the renal nurse calls for many skills which in other parts of the hospital would be considered as 'expanded practice'. There are many opportunities for the renal nurse to specialise further within that role, such as the renal-diabetes nurse, the pre-dialysis nurse or the anaemia co-ordinator. However, it needs to be considered whether further specialisation will fragment the total care of the patient, as if there is a specialist pre-dialysis nurse, for example, it may mean that she/he is excluded from practice within the units.

Scholes and Vaugham (2002) discuss the need to create a workforce that has the skills and flexibility to deliver the right care to those who need it. This is so apposite for the renal unit where nurses already accept that their skills will provide the right care in the right place – the unit – for the patient receiving RRT. Therefore it would appear that renal units are the ideal environment for the development of expanded roles. At this time there is much literature about expanding practice for nurses in general practice, but little is documented about renal care, where expanded practices are accepted as normal.

## The expanding role of the renal nurse

The role of renal nurse consultants who provide care that is different but complementary to the care that doctors can provide is now being developed. The absence of literature would suggest that the job descriptions are deline-ated by the Health Authorities by whom these nurses are employed. The provision of nurses specialised in renal nursing but also specialists in some of the effects of renal disease can provide good continuity of care for the renal patient. There are problems of role delineation as discussed by Scholes and Vaugham (2002), but when these are addressed the well-functioning multidisciplinary team can benefit the patient and the members of the team. The nurse is not taking over the doctor's role but adding to the team's knowledge through her/his unique knowledge and expertise. Kennedy (2001) in the Bristol Inquiry stresses the importance of good communications to prevent some of the problems that occur in cross-boundary working. Nurse specialists are of great importance to the efficiency of the team functioning and their different knowledge adds to the provision of better care (Spilsbury and Meyer, 2001).

## Recommendations

### Care of staff

There appears to be no distinct pattern to define why nurses stay in renal care, some for many years and some only for a few months. Some units request information about reasons for leaving on the exit form, which bears the leaver's name; therefore the reliability of the answers is questionable, despite the promises of confidentiality. Having asked leavers face to face, the author can offer some of the replies, but reiterating that there is no guarantee of truth. The most common answer from those leaving within a year of coming to a unit was: 'I couldn't stand the stress', or words to that effect.

Other statements include: 'I hate seeing these patients and not be able to do anything for them, I know they will all die. It's horrible', 'I feel it's like a factory, no time to stop and care' and 'there must be a better way to help these people'. These examples show that frustration for the nurse was one of the prime reasons for leaving. The lack of being able to care or do something positive is shown to be an important factor in reasons for leaving the renal field. It should be noted that many of these replies were from those who left the renal units without much renal experience. This emphasises the need for good teaching which will demonstrate how renal nursing is multifaceted, and as one nurse who had been the manager for over 10 years said, 'the more you learn the more you know you don't know'.

Then some long-term renal nurses were asked why they had stayed and here are some examples of their answers: 'I couldn't leave my patients, they are used to me'; 'I am always hoping to see L get a transplant'; 'I enjoy doing the things you can't do elsewhere in the hospital'; 'I think seeing the same people and having a really good relationship with the patients is super'; 'I like being specialised'; 'I think autonomy is a good thing for a nurse and here we have to be autonomous'; 'I like using my own initiative'. Motivation to stay comes from someone or something. People enjoy the long-term relationships with their patients which is unique to caring for those with renal failure.

The shortage of specialist trained nurses means that those who stay must have their expertise recognised. The renal unit is a place where the doctors do recognise that nurses have many and diverse skills, but is this knowledge shared amongst the whole team? From experience it would seem that in many units the nurses are not valued in an overt fashion, although their expanded practices are accepted. The consultants may not acknowledge the nurses' expertise and the lack of team working means that others in the health care team are not aware of the specialist knowledge of the renal nurses (Scholes and Vaugham, 2002).

One of the ways to promote self-esteem is to praise the jobs well done and to thank the team after the day is over (Finlayson, 2002). Too often the nurses will leave the unit knowing they have done their best but without recognition. RRT is an acute treatment without which the patient will die; thus lives are saved on a daily basis, but this goes unacknowledged (Bevan, 1998). The patients accept the treatments as routine and complain when there are problems; this is how it should be as this regular treatment can only be acceptable if it is considered a routine event.

However, treatment does have uncertain outcomes which may lead to death, and the stress of providing this treatment takes its toll on the nurses. They complain of a lack of job satisfaction and no appreciation. They complain about the production-style processing of patients which leaves no time to care in the traditional fashion. In the general wards there is satisfaction to be gained from the appreciation of patients and relatives when the illness episode is over and the person recovers. However, renal failure is a chronic illness without a cure, and therefore thanks and appreciation are often not forthcoming. The members of a well-functioning team acknowledge hard work with a quick word or gesture, which enables people to go home feeling satisfied and appreciated.

## Recognition

To keep specialist nurses in renal units they need recognition and to be valued for their contribution to the therapeutic treatment of the patients. A good manager who cares for her/his team and recognises and values individual contributions will motivate staff to remain in their posts. The health care team should be encouraged to function as a real team, as team-working is a vital part of ensuring quality of care and job satisfaction (Major, 2002; Scholes and Vaugham, 2002). There is infinite scope for renal nursing to expand its practice further. New knowledge and skills will improve patient care and the stimulation of acquiring new knowledge is a prime motivation for retention of staff (Jowett et al., 2001).

## Autonomy

The idea of autonomy although it did not feature frequently in the reasons given for remaining in nursing is backed up by Peach (1999) in his review of health care practice. Pearson and Peels (2002) also feel that autonomy must allow for the expertise and accountability of the practitioner. Autonomy gives satisfaction and increased self-esteem which can be seen through increased confidence and expert practice. Smith and Gray (2000) continue the idea that caring still matters for job satisfaction and suggest that caring is a prime reason given by young people for going into nursing.

Caring is the essence of nursing (Kitson, 1993) and in renal units there is hopefully time and the opportunity to care. There are also the opportunities to practice with autonomy and accomplishing one's own set standards, thereby achieving job satisfaction and the motivation to remain in the renal field.

## Summary

This chapter has discussed the various methods of recruiting and retaining renal staff. Renal nursing is a specialist branch of nursing which encompasses other nursing knowledge, and more information about renal nursing should be encouraged in the nursing schools. The expanded practices that are involved in routine renal nursing should be acknowledged and the specialist renal practitioners valued and recognised.

Because renal nursing is nursing the chronic sick with all the accompanying problems, the daily acute nature of the work has to be recognised and valued. It is only through work satisfaction that nurses will remain in a highly stressful area such as a renal unit.

There are some simple ways with no financial implications that help renal care practitioners feel more satisfied and appreciated. The importance of good team working cannot be emphasised too much, and at the end of the day the small words of thanks help the practitioner feel valued.

## References

Adib, S., Al-Shatti, A., Kamal, S., El-Gerges, N. and Al-Raqem, M. (2002) Violence against nurses in healthcare facilities in Kuwait. *International Journal of Nursing Studies* **39**, 469–78.

Auer, J. (2002) Dialysis – a family matter. A personal tribute to the relatives of kidney patients. *EDTNA/ERCA Journal* **28** (3), 141–4.

Beech, M. (2002) Leaders or managers: the drive for effective leadership. *Nursing Standard* **16** (30), 35–6.

Benner, P. (1984) *From Novice to Expert*. Addison-Wesley, California.

Bevan, M. (1998) Nursing in the dialysis unit: technical enframing and declining art, or an imperative for caring. *Journal of Advanced Nursing* **27**, 730–736.

Bristol Royal Infirmary Report (2001) *Learning from Bristol: The Report of the Public Inquiry into Children's Heart Surgery at the BRI. 1984–1995*. Command Paper CM 5207. HMSO, London.

Brooks, I. and Swailes, S. (2002) Analysis of the relationship between nurse influences over flexible working and commitment to nursing. *Journal of Advanced Nursing* **38** (2), 117–26.

Buchan, J. and Seccombe, I. (2002) *Behind the Headlines – A Review of the UK Nursing Labour Market in 2001*. RCN Press Archive. RCN, London.

Casey, J. (2002) The advent of advanced nursing in renal medicine. *British Journal of Renal Medicine* Spring, 25–7.

Charter, D. (2002) Organ shortage puts transplant service at risk. *The Times* August, 17.

Cunningham, G. and Kitson, A. (2000) An evaluation of the RCN Clinical Leadership Development Programme: part 2. *Nursing Standard* **15** (13–15), 33–40.

Daniel, P., Chamberlain, A. and Gordon, F. (2001) Expectations and experiences of newly recruited Filipino nurses. *British Journal of Nursing* **10** (4), 254–65.

Department of Health (2000) *A Health Service for All Talents*. Department of Health, London.

Department of Health (2004) *The National Service Framework for Renal Services. Part One: Dialysis and Transplantation*. www.doh.gov.uk/nsf/renal.

Farrell, G. (1999) Aggression in clinical settings: nurses' views – a follow-up study. *Journal of Advanced Nursing* **29** (3), 532–41.

Felton, J. (1997) Violence prevention at the health care site. *Occupational Medicine* **12**, 701–715.

Finlayson, B. (2002) *Counting the Smiles: Morale and Motivation in the NHS*. King's Fund Research, www.kingsfund.org.uk.

Freeman, G., Shepperd, S., Robinson, I., Ehrich, K. and Richards, S. (2000) *DSO Scoping Exercise. Continuity of Care*. National Coordinating Centre for NHS Service Delivery Organisation, London.

Fuchs, S., Kuntzle, W. and Thomas, N. (eds) (2002) *European Core Curriculum for a Basic Course in Nephrology Nursing*. EDTNA/ERCA, www.edtna-erca.org/education.

Hawkes, N. and Norfolk, A. (2002) Transplant service fails to learn from Spain. *The Times* August, 2.

Jackson, D., Clarke, J. and Mannix, J. (2002) Who would want to be a nurse? Violence in the workplace – a factor in recruitment and retention. *Journal of Nursing Management* **10**, 13–20.

Johnson, A. and Copnell, B. (2002) Benefits and barriers for registered nurses undertaking post-graduate diplomas in paediatric nursing. *Nurse Education Today* **22**, 118–27.

Jowett, S., Peters, M., Reynolds, H. and Wilson-Barnet, J. (1999) The impact of Scope – practitioners' views on its relevance and potential for service development. *Nursing Times Research* **4**, 422–31.

Jowett, S., Peters, M., Reynolds, H. and Wilson-Barnet, J. (2001) The UKCC's Scope of Professional Practice – some implications for health care delivery. *Journal of Nursing Management* **9** (2), 93–100.

Kennedy, I. (2001) Forward. In: *Bristol Royal Infirmary Inquiry. Command Paper CM 5207. Learning From Bristol. The Report of the Public Inquiry into Children's Heart Surgery at the BRI. 1984–1995*. HMSO, London.

Kidney Alliance (2001) *End Stage Renal Failure – A Framework for Planning and Service Delivery*. Kidney Alliance, London.

Kitson, A. (1993) Formalising concepts related to nursing and caring. In: *Nursing: Art and Science* (Kitson, A., ed.). Chapman and Hall, London.

Kuntzle, W. and Thomas, N. (eds) (1995) *European Core Curriculum for a Post-Basic Course in Nephrology Nursing*. EDTNA/ERCA, Gent.

Levy, N. and Cohen, L. (2000) End-stage renal disease and its treatment: dialysis and transplantation. In: *Psychiatric Care of the Medical Patient*, 2nd edn (Stoudemire, A., Fogel, B. and Greenberg, D., eds). Oxford University Press, London.

Major, S. (2002) Dysfunctional teams: a health and resource warning. *Nursing Management* **9** (2), 25–8.

Munshi, A., Vijiyakumar, N., Taub, N., Bhullar, H., Lo, T. and Warwick, G. (2001) Outcome of renal replacement therapy in the very elderly. *Nephrology Dialysis Transplantation* **16**, 128–33.

Nightingale, F. (1859) *Notes on Nursing*. Republished 1980. Churchill Livingstone, Edinburgh.

Obrey, A. (2002) Securing the future of the NHS: developing and supporting staff nurses. *Nursing Management* **9** (2), 15–17.

O'Connell, B., Brooks, J., Hutchinson, J. and Lofthouse, J. (2000) Nurses' perceptions of the nature and frequency of aggression in general ward settings and high dependency areas. *Journal of Clinical Nursing* **9**, 602–610.

Paterson, B., McCornsih, A. and Aitken, I. (1997) Abuse and bullying. *Nursing Management* **3** (10), 8–9.

Peach, L. (1999) *Fitness to Practice: The UKCC. Commission for Nursing and Midwifery Education*. UKCC, London.

Pearson, A. and Peels, S. (2002) The nurse practitioner. Special supplement. *International Journal of Nursing Practice* **8** (4), s5–10.

RCN (2002) Government called on to ensure nurses are not recruited from developing countries. *RCN News and Campaigns* 17 July, www.rcn.org.uk/news/.

Scholes, J. and Vaughan, B. (2002) Cross-boundary working: implications for the multiprofessional team. *Journal of Clinical Nursing* **11** (3), 399–408.

Smith, P. and Gray, B. (2000) *The Emotional Labour of Nursing: How Student and Qualified Nurses Learn to Care*. www.health-fc.sbu.ac.uk/emlab/.

Spilsbury, K. and Meyer, J. (2001) Defining the nursing contribution to patient outcome: lessons from a review of the literature examining nursing outcome, skill mix and changing roles. *Journal of Clinical Nursing* **10** (1), 3–14.

Taylor, B. (1993) Phenomenology: one way to understand nursing practice. *International Journal of Nursing Studies* **30**, 1243–51.

Tschudin, V. (1997) The emotional care of care. In: *Caring: The Compassion and Wisdom of Nursing* (Brykczynska, G., ed.). Hodder Headline, London.

United Kingdom Central Council for Nursing, Midwifery and Health Visiting (1999a) *Fitness for Practice: The Report of the UKCC Commission for Nursing and Midwifery Education*. UKCC, London.

United Kingdom Central Council for Nursing, Midwifery and Health Visiting (1999b) *A Higher Level of Practice*. UKCC, London.

Welford, C. (2002) Matching theory to practice. *Nursing Management* **9** (4), 7–11.

Wells, J. and Bowers, L. (2002) How prevalent is violence towards nurses working in general hospitals in the UK? *Journal of Advanced Nursing* **39** (3), 230–40.

Winearls, C. (1999) Crisis in renal replacement service provision. *British Journal of Renal Medicine* Spring (4).

Witchell, L. and Osuch, A. (2002) Managing international recruits. *Nursing Management* **9** (3), 10–14.

# Index

*Note:* ERF in subentries refers to 'established renal failure', PD to 'peritoneal dialysis' and PKD to 'polycystic kidney disease'.